MEDICAL MASTERCLASS

Infectious Diseases and Dermatology

Disclaimer

Medical Masterclass

EDITOR-IN-CHIEF

John D. Firth DM FRCP
Consultant Physician and Nephrologist
Addenbrooke's Hospital
Cambridge

Infectious Diseases and Dermatology

EDITORS

William Lynn MB BS MD FRCP
Consultant
Ealing Hospital
London

Karen Harman MA MB BChir MRCP
Specialist Registrar
King's College Hospital
London

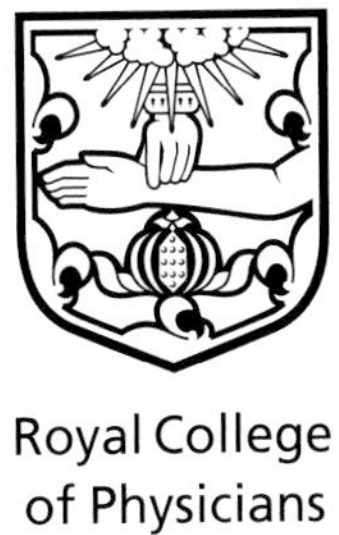

Royal College
of Physicians

First published 2001 Blackwell Science Ltd
Reprinted 2004 Royal College of Physicians of London

Published by:
Royal College of Physicians of London
11 St. Andrews Place
Regent's Park
London NW1 4LE
United Kingdom

Set and printed by Graphicraft Limited, Hong Kong

ISBN: 1-86016-219-3 (this book)
ISBN: 1-86016-210-X (set)

Distribution Information:
Jerwood Medical Education Resource Centre
Royal College of Physicians of London
11 St. Andrews Place
Regent's Park
London NW1 4LE
United Kingdom
Tel: 0044 (0)207 935 1174 ext 422/490
Fax: 0044 (0)207 486 6653
Email: merc@rcplondon.ac.uk
Web: http://www.rcplondon.ac.uk/

Contents

Dermatology

List of contributors

Alec Bonington BSC MBCHB MRCP DTMH MD
Specialist Registrar
North Manchester General Hospital
Manchester

Karen Harman MA MB BCHIR MRCP
Specialist Registrar
King's College Hospital
London

Carolyn Hemsley MRCP BM BCH MA
Specialist Regsitrar
John Radcliffe Hospital
Oxford

Michael Jacobs MA PHD MRCP DTMH
Specialist Registrar
Northwick Park Hospital
Harrow

Paul Klenerman MRCP DPHIL
Wellcome Trust Research Fellow
University of Oxford
Nuffield Department of Medicine
John Radcliffe Hospital
Oxford

William Lynn MB BS MD FRCP
Consultant
Ealing Hospital
London

Graham Ogg BM BCH MRCP DPHIL
MRC Fellow
John Radcliffe Hospital
Oxford

Natalie M. Stone BA HONS MRCP
Specialist Registrar
Churchill Hospital
Oxford

Foreword

Since its foundation in 1518, the Royal College of Physicians has engaged in a wide range of activities dedicated to its overall aim of upholding and improving standards of medical practice. *Medical Masterclass* is one of the most innovative and ambitious educational resources the College has developed, and while it continues the tradition of pioneering and supporting high quality medicine, it also makes use of modern day technology by offering computer-assisted learning.

The MRCP(UK) examination is crucial to the progress of physicians through their training. Preparation is not only essential for success in the examination, but it is also important for the acquisition of requisite knowledge, skills and attitudes appropriate for further training. With a pass rate of about 40% at each sitting of the written papers, the exam is a challenge. The College wishes to encourage excellence, and with this in mind has produced *Medical Masterclass*, a comprehensive distance-learning package designed to help candidates with the preparation that is key to making the grade.

Medical Masterclass has been produced by the RCP's Education Department. It represents a formidable amount of work by Dr John Firth and his team of authors and editors. I congratulate our colleagues for this superb educational product and wholeheartedly recommend it as an invaluable MRCP(UK) study aid.

Professor Carol M. Black CBE
President of the Royal College of Physicians

Preface

Medical Masterclass comprises twelve paper-based modules, two CD-ROMs and a companion website. Its aim is to help doctors in their first few years of training to improve their medical skills and knowledge.

The twelve paper-based modules are divided as follows: two cover the scientific background to medicine, one is devoted to general clinical issues, one to emergency medicine and practical procedures, and eight cover the range of medical specialities. Medicine is often fairly straightforward when the diagnosis is clear, but patients rarely come to their doctor and say 'I've got Hodgkin's disease': they have lumps. The core material of each of the clinical specialities is defined by case presentations in the first part of each module: how do you approach the man who has lumps? Structured concise notes on specific diseases follow later. All practising doctors know that medicine is much more than knowing lots of facts about diseases: how do you tell someone they've got cancer? How do you decide when to stop treatment? Most medical texts say little about these issues: *Medical Masterclass* does not avoid them, nor does it talk in vague and abstract terms.

The two CD-ROMs each contain 30 interactive cases requiring diagnosis and treatment. The format is remarkably close to real life: you see the patient and are told the story; you have to decide how to investigate and treat; but you can't see all the results before you start to make decisions!

The companion website, which will be regularly updated, includes self-assessment questions and mock MRCP(UK) exam papers. How much do you know, and are you improving? You will see how your score compares with your previous attempts, and also how your performance compares with others who have logged on to the site.

The *Medical Masterclass* is produced by the Education Department of the Royal College of Physicians. It has been specifically designed to support candidates studying for the MRCP(UK) Examination (All Parts). I have no doubt that someone putting effort into learning through the *Medical Masterclass* would be in a strong position to impress the examiners.

John Firth
Editor-in-Chief

Acknowledgements

Medical Masterclass has been produced by a team. The names of those who have written and edited material are clearly indicated elsewhere, but without the efforts of many other people *Medical Masterclass* would not exist at all. These include Professor Lesley Rees and Mrs Winnie Wade from the Education Department of the Royal College of Physicians of London, who initiated the project; Dr Mike Stein and Dr Andy Robinson from Medschool.com and Blackwell Science respectively, who have enthusiastically supported it from the beginning; and Ms Filipa Maia and Ms Katherine Bowker, who have run the office with splendid efficiency and induced authors and editors to perform to a schedule rarely achieved. I and the whole of the team of editors and authors are immensely grateful to all of these people for the energy that they have poured into *Medical Masterclass* in various ways.

John Firth
Editor-in-Chief

Key features

We have created a range of icon boxes to help you identify key information and to make learning easier and more enjoyable. Here is a brief explanation:

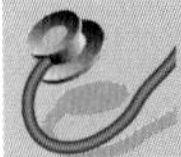

Clinical pointer

This icon highlights important information to be noted.

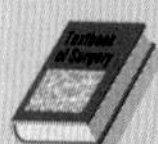

Further information

This icon indicates the source of further information and reference.

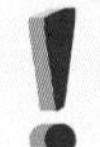

Hints

This icon highlights useful hints, tips and mnemonics.

Key points

This icon is used to highlight points of particular importance.

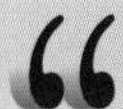

Quote

This icon indicates useful or interesting citations from notable individuals, including well-known physicians.

Think about

This icon indicates what the reader should reflect on after having read a passage from the text.

Warning/Hazard

This icon is used to indicate common or important drug interactions, pitfalls of practical procedures, or when to take symptoms or signs particularly seriously.

Infectious Diseases

AUTHORS:
A. Bonington, C. Hemsley, M. Jacobs, P. Klenerman, W. Lynn

EDITOR:
W. Lynn

EDITOR-IN-CHIEF:
J.D. Firth

1 Clinical presentations

1.1 Fever

Case history

A 43-year-old man who is feeling feverish and unwell comes to the accident and emergency (A&E) department. The casualty officer asks you to review him.

Clinical approach

Fever has a complex pathogenesis and is a frequent presenting feature of illness [1,2]. Infections are by far the most common cause of fever, and much the most likely cause of the problem in this case, but it shouldn't be forgotten that non-infectious causes are possible (see Section 1.10, p. 27). In view of the wide range of possible diagnoses, there is no substitute for a detailed history and complete physical examination. It is a useful exercise to formulate two differential diagnoses, first infectious and then non-infectious. If you know or suspect that the patient is immunocompromised, generate separate differential diagnoses—first for an immunocompetent and then for an immunocompromised individual.

During your assessment, keep in mind the key questions that will direct initial management of a patient with suspected infection:

- What is the site of infection?
- What is (are) the likely infecting organism(s)?
- What has the patient been exposed to?
- Is empirical therapy appropriate?

History of the presenting problem

Documentation of fever

In many illnesses, fever is not continuous. In keeping with the normal circadian temperature rhythm, fever usually peaks in the evening. At the time you see the patient, fever may be absent, especially if he has taken antipyretic medication. Ask the following detailed questions:

- Have you been feeling hot and cold? These subjective sensations are commonly reported by patients who are well and subsequently found not to have fever. Exactly what does the patient mean by 'fever'?
- Have you measured/how did you measure your temperature? Digital thermometers are the most reliable, mercury easily misread and thermal paper strips hopeless.
- Have you been having sweats? Drenching sweats, commonly at night, are an objective symptom and indicate significant pathology. Ask about having to change the sheets as a result of sweats.
- Have you been having shivers/chills? Ask specifically about rigors, i.e. uncontrollable shaking of the whole body, often with teeth chattering, lasting for minutes. Rigors are particularly, but not exclusively, associated with bacterial sepsis or malaria.
- How long have you noticed the fever? In general, as the duration of fever increases, the likelihood of an infectious cause decreases. You will gain little by trying to analyse the fever pattern.

Site of infection

What else have you noticed? The key aim is to gain a clue to target appropriate examination and investigations. A detailed history of symptoms associated with fever is required. Give particular weight to volunteered symptoms and perform a detailed systematic enquiry in relation to all organ systems. Common things are most common, hence ask about the following:

- Urinary symptoms: dysuria, frequency, smelly urine, suprapubic pain, loin pain
- Chest symptoms: breathlessness, pleuritic pain, sputum production
- Spots/boils/abscesses
- Diarrhoea/vomiting
- Meningitic symptoms: severe headache, photophobia, neck stiffness, rash.

Remember that fever of any cause may be accompanied by a constellation of symptoms, including anorexia, myalgia and mild headache.

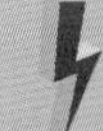

Serious infection (such as bacterial sepsis or malaria) may present with 'false localizing' symptoms and signs such as headache, breathlessness, vomiting or diarrhoea.

Therapeutic drug history

Pay special attention to the following:

- Immunosuppressive drugs, e.g. steroids
- Recent antibiotics
- Adverse reactions to antibiotics.

Exposure history

Asking carefully about what the patient has been doing may suggest certain infections:

- Has anyone whom you know had a similar illness?
- Have you travelled abroad? (See Section 1.20, p. 53.)
- What do you do in your job?
- Do you have any particular hobbies?
- Do you have any pets or other animal exposure?
- Recreational drug use?

A sexual history is an important aspect of the assessment of suspected infection and, if the cause of the problem is not immediately apparent, you should not avoid the subject out of a misplaced sense of politeness (see Section 1.31, p. 76). Tact and care are required (see *General clinical issues*, Section 2).

Relevant past history

Very many conditions—not only obvious immunosuppression—are associated with a particular risk of infection, and so a detailed past history is required. A history of previous infections may suggest immunocompromise.

When the cause of fever is not obvious, consider the following:

- Primary and secondary immunodeficiencies
- Structural abnormalities—such as an abnormal heart valve, indwelling prosthetic material or a chronic urinary catheter
- Non-infectious causes.

Examination

Is the patient pyrexial (Fig. 1)? A full examination is required. Your primary survey should ensure that breathing and circulation are adequate, followed by a detailed examination of each system. Is the patient well, ill, very ill or nearly dead? Your general impression is critically important in deciding whether to give 'best guess' empirical antimicrobial treatment or to wait for the results of tests.

Approach to investigation and management

Investigations

Blood tests

- Blood count, electrolytes, renal and liver function tests, C-reactive protein (CRP) [3], erythrocyte sedimentation rate (ESR), ask microbiology or virology to save serum.

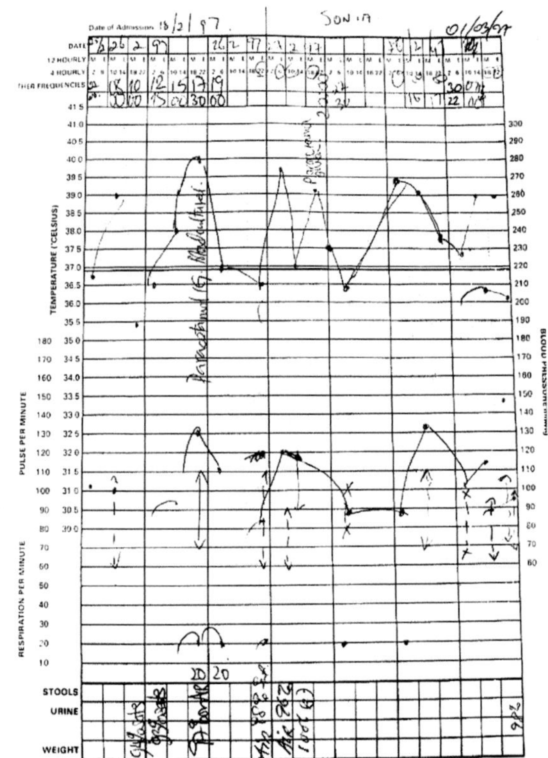

Fig. 1 Temperature chart from a patient with tuberculosis. Temperature recording is essential to establish the presence or absence of a fever, but the pattern of fever cannot reliably distinguish bacterial, viral, parasitic, fungal and non-infectious causes of fever.

Cultures

Blood and urine cultures should be performed in all cases. Other specimens should be sent according to the clinical picture. (See Section 3.2, p. 151.)

Imaging

A chest radiograph is needed in all cases with no obvious cause of fever, to look for areas of consolidation and mediastinal lymphadenopathy.

Management

In general, it is not necessary to abolish fever except for giving symptomatic relief [4]. You may be clear about the likely site of infection from your initial assessment of the patient. You can then initiate specific management, including antimicrobial therapy if appropriate.

Fever of unknown cause

If a positive diagnosis cannot be made, your management depends on your judgement of the most likely diagnoses and how severely ill the patient is. Those whom you judge to be (or at risk of becoming) seriously unwell should be given 'best guess' empirical antimicrobial therapy once specimens for culture have been obtained. In other cases, it will almost certainly be more appropriate to wait for the results of further investigations.

Admission

Admission for observation is the right course if you are worried about the patient's current or future condition. In time, the diagnosis may become apparent (re-evaluate the history and examination regularly), or the illness may persist or deteriorate, necessitating empirical antimicrobial therapy.

Empirical antibiotic therapy

Because right is right, to follow right were wisdom in the scorn of consequence. (Alfred, Lord Tennyson)

Most hospitals have guidelines for initial antibiotic treatment of infections. You will probably find these helpful in guiding your selection of antibiotics, but remember that you must apply these guidelines thoughtfully to ensure that you choose appropriate treatment for individual cases. Usually, the choice of empirical antibiotic therapy is a matter of probability (Fig. 2). For patients who are reasonably well, you should choose antibiotics that treat the most likely organisms. However, if you judge that a patient is seriously ill, you should seek expert advice and use an antimicrobial regimen that also treats less likely, but possible, pathogens.

Further management

As results become available, especially from the microbiology laboratory, you may be able to target antimicrobial treatment more precisely. You will also need to consider modifying antimicrobial treatment if the illness fails to respond to the initial therapy.

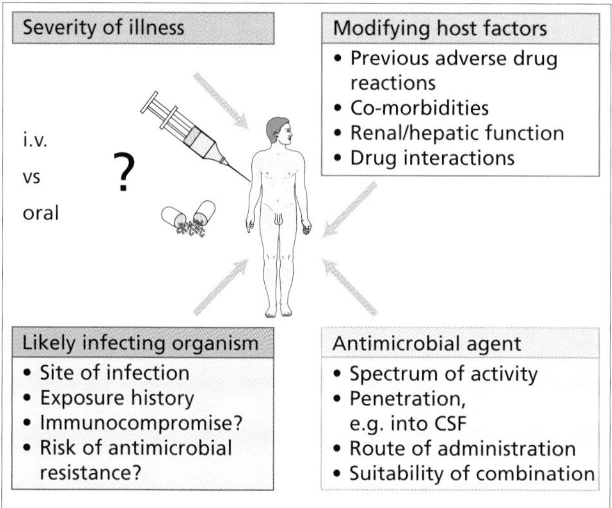

Fig. 2 Factors influencing choice of empirical antimicrobial therapy.

Persistent fever despite antimicrobial therapy

- Antimicrobial spectrum does not include the infecting organism
- Infecting organism has developed antimicrobial resistance
- Failure to achieve adequate drug concentrations at site of infection (compliance, dose, absorption, penetration into a sequestered site)
- Non-infectious cause of fever (see Section 1.10, p. 27)
- Antibiotic-induced (drug) fever.

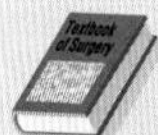

1 Mackowiak PA. Concepts of fever. *Arch Intern Med* 1998; 158: 1870–1881.
2 Dinarello CA. Thermoregulation and the pathogenesis of fever. *Infect Dis Clin North Am* 1996; 10: 433–439.
3 Povoa P, Almeida E, Moreira P *et al.* C-reactive protein as an indicator of sepsis. *Intensive Care Med* 1998; 24: 1052–1056.
4 Plaisanse KI, Mackowiak PA. Antipyretic therapy: physiologic rationale, diagnostic implications and clinical consequences. *Arch Intern Med* 2000; 160: 449–456.

1.2 Fever, hypotension and confusion

Case history

A 20-year-old female university student presents with a 12-h history of fever, chills, and generalized aches and pains. On arrival she is confused, breathless and hypotensive, with a sinus tachycardia.

Clinical approach

You must act quickly. The immediate priority has to be resuscitation. With this presentation, the diagnosis is septic shock until proved otherwise. Once resuscitation is under way (intravenous colloid and oxygen therapy; see *Emergency medicine*, Section 1.2), you need to identify the source. If none is obvious, consider meningococcal septicaemia or toxic shock, and look thoroughly for the purpuric/petechial rash of meningococcal disease (Fig. 3) or the more diffuse erythema associated with toxic shock syndrome.

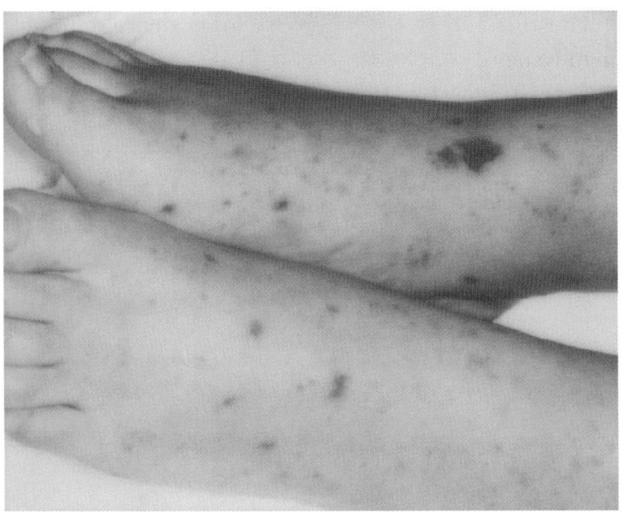

Fig. 3 Petechial/purpuric rash associated with meningococcal bacteraemia. A similar rash can occur with disseminated intravascular coagulation resulting from other infectious agents, although in the UK it is most commonly seen in meningocccal disease.

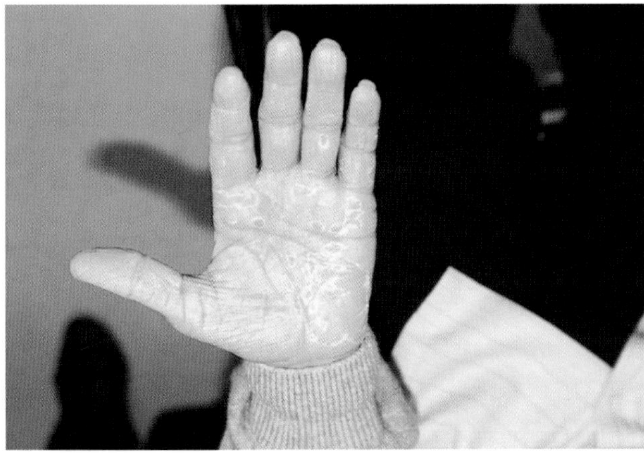

Fig. 4 Palmar desquamation after staphylococcal toxic shock. This may also occur with scarlet fever, Kawasaki's disease or drug reactions.

Differential diagnosis

- Toxic shock syndrome: a severe illness caused by toxin-producing staphylococci. It occurs particularly in women in association with tampon use. Onset is acute with high fever, myalgia and shock. An erythematous sunburn-like rash and renal impairment are both common. Palmar desquamation is common after toxic shock (Fig. 4).
- Meningococcal septicaemia: occurs mainly in children and young adults, and may occur in the absence of meningitis. You must look for the characteristic petechial/purpuric rash (see Section 1.14, p. 37) although this is not always present.
- Non-meningococcal septic shock: look for focus of infection, e.g. cutaneous, pulmonary, urinary tract or intra-abdominal, such as cholangitis.

History of the presenting problem

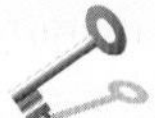

In any who are severely ill—resuscitate first, ask questions afterwards.

It may be difficult to obtain any history from this woman, but while beginning to resuscitate get as much information as possible from her and from any friends or family who are available.

When, where and how

Try to assess the severity/rate of progression of the illness along with the likely focus and aetiological agent. (See Section 1.1, p. 3.)

- When did the symptoms start?
- How did the illness start and how have the symptoms changed? In bacterial sepsis, rapid progression of symptoms indicates severe disease.
- Any rashes? If so where did the rash start and how has it progressed?

Associated symptoms

These symptoms may help to localize the site of infection but can also be misleading, e.g. diarrhoea is frequently seen in bacterial sepsis and does not necessarily indicate an intra-abdominal focus of infection:

- Cough, chest pain, sputum production?
- Nausea and/or vomiting? Common but non-specific, e.g. occurring with meningitis, intracerebral events and migraine.
- Associated earache, sinusitis or cough? Pneumococci are more likely as the aetiological agent.
- Any focal neurological signs or diplopia? If so, need to exclude brain abscess. (See Section 1.14, p. 36.)
- Don't forget to ask about any genitourinary symptoms such as vaginal discharge.

Additional clues

Look for any unusual features that might suggest a particular underlying infection:

- When was her last menstrual period? If currently menstruating, could she have left a tampon *in situ*—think of toxic shock syndrome.
- Contact with anyone with meningococcal infection?
- Travel abroad? Think of malaria. Viral haemorrhagic fever if returned within 3 weeks from West Africa. (See Section 1.20, p. 52.)

Relevant past history

The following could be relevant:
- Immunocompromised, e.g. immunosuppressive therapy, risk factors for HIV infection, immunosuppressive diseases, history of recurrent infection
- Intravenous recreational drug use makes endocarditis and infection with *Staphylococcus aureus* more likely
- Recent hospitalization: this raises the possibility of antibiotic-resistant infection
- Previous surgery and indwelling prosthetic material.

Examination

A full general examination should be performed, taking particular note of the following:
- Pulse, blood pressure, respiratory rate and temperature.
- Rash: in the setting of shock, a petechial/purpuric rash is highly suggestive of meningococcal septicaemia. An erythematous rash suggests toxic shock in this setting.
- Evidence of meningism, i.e. neck stiffness and Kernig's sign.
- Ears and throat for evidence of source of infection.
- Fundoscopy for signs of elevated intracranial pressure or focal signs of infection, i.e. endophthalmitis or Roth's spots.
- Chest for evidence of pneumonia.
- Cardiac murmurs and signs of bacterial endocarditis.
- Needle marks suggesting intravenous drug use makes *Staph. aureus* infection more likely.

Approach to investigation and management

Investigations

Investigations are performed to identify the site and nature of the infection and to monitor disease severity/complications.

Blood tests

Check the following:
- Full blood count (FBC) and differential: neutrophilia is common in bacterial sepsis but in severe cases the white cell count (WCC) may be normal or low; thrombocytopenia may occur as part of disseminated intravascular coagulation (DIC) in septicaemia.
- Electrolytes and renal function tests: renal failure may occur in septicaemia and is common in toxic shock syndrome.
- Liver function tests: can be non-specifically raised in bacterial sepsis, but may also indicate a hepatic source, particularly cholangitis.
- Blood glucose: to exclude hyper-/hypoglycaemia, as hypoglycaemia can complicate severe sepsis and is a poor prognostic sign.
- Clotting and fibrin degradation products (DIC in meningococcal septicaemia).
- Creatine phosphokinae (CPK): for evidence of muscle involvement.
- Arterial blood gases: to assess level of hypoxia and acidosis.

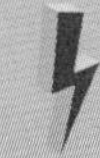

Febrile, breathless patients need arterial blood gas measurement. In bacterial sepsis, breathlessness is often the result of lactic acidosis and may be the only sign of severe disease early in meningococcal septicaemia. Breathlessness is not a feature of uncomplicated influenza.

Cultures

- Blood cultures are essential in all cases before giving antibiotics. (See Section 3.2, p. 151.)
- Urine culture
- Culture other body sites as clinically indicated, e.g. high vaginal swab in this case
- Save serum.

Imaging

- Chest radiograph: exclude pneumonia and look for evidence of adult respiratory distress syndrome (ARDS).
- Liver ultrasonography: if cholangitis suspected as source of sepsis.
- Ultrasonography/computed tomography (CT): as indicated for focal infection. Cranial CT scan in suspected intracranial infection. (See Section 1.14, p. 38; see also *Emergency medicine*, Section 1.22.)

Other tests

If meningitis or encephalitis is suspected, a lumbar puncture will need to be performed. (See Section 1.14, p. 38; see also *Emergency medicine*, Sections 1.22 and 3.5.)

Management

The management of severe bacterial sepsis is based on the identification and treatment of the likely causative organism and intensive support of organ function [1]. For details of how to resuscitate the patient with profound hypotension, see *Emergency medicine*, Section 1.2.

Resuscitation of the patient with profound hypotension

- Check airway, breathing, circulation
- Call for assistance
- Give high-flow oxygen
- Establish intravenous access: place large-bore drips in both antecubital fossae, or insert a femoral venous line
- Give colloid or saline as fast as possible until the blood pressure (BP) restored or jugular venous pressure (JVP) clearly visible
- Establish diagnosis and treat if possible.

In this case the two most likely diagnoses are meningococcal septicaemia and toxic shock syndrome.

Toxic shock syndrome

- Resuscitation and supportive treatment [2]
- Removal of tampon or drainage of pus
- Intravenous flucloxacillin 1–2 g four times daily.

Meningococcal septicaemia

- Resuscitation and supportive treatment [3]
- Antibiotics as for meningococcal meningitis (see Section 2.5.2, p. 107)
- Notification to Consultant in Communicable Diseases Control (CCDC) and prophylaxis for contacts (see Section 1.38, p. 91).

Sepsis with unknown source

- Resuscitation and supportive treatment
- High-dose intravenous antibiotics based on the clinical setting (Section 1.1, p. 3).

See *Emergency medicine*, Sections 1.2 and 1.28.

1 Lynn WA, Cohen J. Management of septic shock. *J Infect* 1995; 30: 207–212.

2 Waldvogel FA. *Staphylococcus aureus* (including staphylococcal toxic shock). In: Mandell GL, Bennett JE, Dolin R (eds) *Principles and Practice of Infectious Diseases* (5th edn). Philadelphia: Churchill Livingstone, 2000: 2069–2092.

3 Pollard AJ, Faust SN, Levin M. Meningitis and meningococcal septicaemia. *J R Coll Physicians Lond* 1998; 32: 319–328.

1.3 A swollen red foot

Case history

A 32-year-old man accidentally cut his left foot with a fork while gardening. Three days later he is admitted with redness and swelling surrounding the injury and a high fever.

Clinical approach

The likely diagnosis is a cellulitis affecting the left leg (Table 1). However, when there is a recent history of a wound contaminated with soil, it is important to consider gas gangrene. Also check that the patient has been immunized with tetanus toxoid within the last 10 years. In any patient presenting with a cellulitis, particularly if severe systemic symptoms are present, the diagnosis of necrotizing fasciitis should always be considered.

Table 1 Aetiological agents of cellulitis.

Scenario	Likely pathogens
Most common	*Streptococcus pyogenes*
Common	*Staphylococcus aureus*
Uncommon	*Clostridium perfringens*—cellulitis or gas gangrene Other *Streptococcus* spp. such as group C or G
Saltwater injury	*Vibrio* spp., particularly *vulnificus*
Freshwater injury	*Aeromonas hydrophila*
Hospital-acquired infection	Staphylococci: consider antibiotic resistance, i.e. methicillin-resistant *Staphylococcus aureus* (MRSA), Gram-negative bacilli
Patient with diabetes	Streptococci and staphylococci plus Gram-negative bacilli and anaerobes

History of the presenting problem

The injury

Confirm the following:
- Site of and how the injury occurred?
- Duration of symptoms?
- Pain, redness and swelling?
- Is it spreading?
- Associated systemic upset? If this is out of proportion to the cellulitis, necrotizing fasciitis must be considered.

Specific risk factors

- Injury in saltwater: consider *Vibrio vulnificus* as a possible causative agent, particularly in patients with underlying liver disease
- Injury while swimming in fresh water: consider *Aeromonas hydrophila*
- Soil contamination of wound (as in this case): consider *Clostridium perfringens*
- Animal or human bite: may inoculate pathogens; bites are associated with a high incidence of infection
- Could there be a foreign body within the wound?

Relevant past history

Look for factors that may impair systemic or local immune responses:
- Previous cellulitis of the same limb: may have caused mild lymphoedema, thereby predisposing to a further attack of cellulitis
- Previous deep venous thrombosis or lymphoedema
- Immunocompromise: must consider a broader range of aetiological agents including Gram-negative bacteria
- Diabetes mellitus: necrotizing fasciitis more common.

Examination

Look for the site of entry of the causative organism. In cellulitis, the affected limb is usually hot, red, tender and

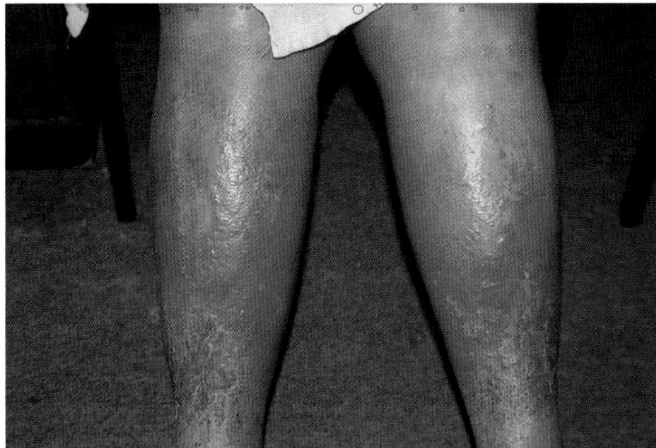

Fig. 5 Bilateral lower leg cellulitis caused by *Streptococcus pyogenes* in a patient with chronic lymphoedema.

swollen (Fig. 5). Fever is usual. If the patient is more unwell than the degree of skin involvement would suggest, don't forget necrotizing fasciitis. Pay particular attention to the following:

- Vital signs: pulse, BP and temperature.
- Note area of redness and draw a line around the edge with a pen—progression will be easy to monitor.
- Evidence of lymphangitis? A red line tracking up the limb along the line of the lymphatic drainage confirms the presence of distal infection.
- Tender lymphadenopathy at the proximal end of the affected limb?
- Any areas of necrosis? If present you must immediately suspect necrotizing fasciitis.
- Any evidence of crepitus within the affected area suggests gas within the tissues—indicating gas gangrene/necrotizing fasciitis.
- Athlete's foot in lower limb cellulitis: often a portal of entry for organisms and recurrent infection will result unless treated appropriately.

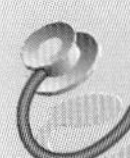

Deep venous thrombosis

Deep venous thrombosis (DVT) is a common differential diagnosis of cellulitis. Both are associated with fever, leg swelling, redness and pain. However, DVT is associated with a woody texture and tenderness to the posterior calf. In cellulitis, the fever and redness are typically more pronounced, the tenderness is circumferential, and lymphangitis and lymphadenopathy are commonly present.

Necrotizing fasciitis/gas gangrene

- Cellulitis with evidence of skin necrosis (but note that necrosis may be deep to the skin and not visible)
- Severe pain
- Rapid progression
- Gas detectable in tissues on examination and/or radiologically
- Typically the patient is more systemically unwell than the degree of skin involvement would suggest.

Approach to investigation and management

This will be dictated by the severity of the illness. If the patient is very unwell, proceed as indicated in Section 1.2 (p. 5), but if not (as in this case) then the following are appropriate.

Investigations

Blood tests

- FBC: neutrophilia usually present; CRP to assess inflammatory response
- Electrolytes and renal function tests: to establish baseline renal function.

Cultures

- Blood cultures: may yield the organism responsible
- Swab for bacterial culture of any open wound around or within the cellulitis.

Imaging

Take a radiograph of the affected limb, to look for gas in the subcutaneous tissues, if gas gangrene or necrotizing fasciitis is suspected. A radiograph may reveal osteomyelitis in chronic infection.

Management

The aims of management are to control the infection, reduce swelling and monitor for evidence of tissue necrosis [1–3]. Surgical intervention may be required. Check that the patient has been immunized with tetanus toxoid in the last 10 years.

Cellulitis

SIMPLE MEASURES

- Keep the affected limb elevated while resting—this reduces oedema and speeds healing
- Analgesia as required.

SPECIFIC TREATMENT

Appropriate antibiotics are given orally if mild or intravenously if severe.

- Streptococcal/staphylococcal: intravenous benzylpenicillin 1.2–2.4 g four times daily will cover a streptococcal cellulitis, but flucloxacillin 0.5–1.0 g four times daily may be added if a staphylococcal aetiology is suspected. Oral co-amoxiclav is a good alternative for mild cases. If the patient is allergic to penicillin, use a macrolide (such as erythromycin) or clindamycin.

- *Aeromonas hydrophila*: use ciprofloxacin or gentamicin.
- *Vibrio vulnificus*: use tetracycline or doxycycline.

Necrotizing fasciitis

Treatment of this condition is an emergency. Don't waste any time.

- Surgical exploration and debridement of all dead tissue are mandatory [1–3].
- High-dose intravenous antibiotics to cover *Streptococcus pyogenes* and other possible aerobic and anaerobic bacteria.

Gas gangrene

This is caused by *Clostridium perfringens* and other *Clostridium* spp. (See Section 2.5.1, p. 103.)

- Aggressive surgical debridement
- High-dose intravenous benzylpenicillin and clindamycin
- Hyperbaric oxygen therapy if available.

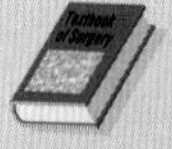

1 Swartz MN. Cellulitis and subcutaneous tissue infections. In: Mandell GL, Bennett JE, Dolin R (eds) *Principles and Practice of Infectious Diseases* (5th edn). Philadelphia: Churchill Livingstone, 2000: 1037–1057.
2 Cox NH, Colver GB, Paterson WD. Management and morbidity of cellulitis of the leg. *J R Soc Med* 1998; 91: 634–637.
3 Urschel JD. Necrotizing soft tissue infections. *Postgrad Med J* 1999; 75: 645–649.

1.4 Fever and cough

Case history

A 44-year-old smoker presents to A&E with a 4-day history of fever and cough.

Clinical approach

The important things to establish initially are whether this is likely to be an upper (URTI) or a lower (LRTI) respiratory tract infection, and whether it is likely to be bacterial or viral. An URTI does not usually require antibiotic treatment. The term 'chest infection' should be avoided because it is too non-specific.

History of the presenting problem

Upper or lower respiratory tract infection

URTIs are not an immediate danger but predispose to subsequent LRTIs, and can also precipitate severe bronchospasm. An URTI is suggested when the patient:

- Appears clinically well
- Has a sore throat and/or rhinorrhoea
- Has an unproductive cough, or cough productive of clear or white sputum
- Has no chest signs.

A LRTI is clearly of more concern than an URTI because pneumonia can be life threatening. A LRTI is suggested by the following:

- Dyspnoea (in the absence of wheeze)
- Going blue (cyanosis)
- Pleuritic chest pain—must be LRTI
- Haemoptysis—and consider also the possibility of underlying carcinoma
- Focal chest signs.

Aetiological agent

Many organisms can cause a LRTI (Table 2) and a careful history is required to spot risk factors predisposing to the more unusual causes [1].

- Onset sudden or gradual over a few days? Sudden onset with high fever, purulent sputum, pleuritic chest pain and/or dyspnoea is suggestive of pneumococcal pneumonia. Gradual onset with prodrome of fever and malaise lasting a few days followed by dry cough suggests an atypical organism.
- Colour of sputum? Green suggests bacterial infection; a dry cough or white or clear sputum suggests viral infection. However, remember that cough is usually dry for the first few days in atypical pneumonia.
- Travel abroad? An air-conditioned hotel room suggests Legionnaire's disease. Caving in North America may lead to acute histoplasmosis. (See Section 2.9.4, p. 123.)
- Any pet birds at home and, if so, are they ill? Consider psittacosis.
- Recent stay on a farm where there were goats? Consider Q fever.
- Preceding 'flu-like illness? Consider secondary bacterial pneumonia, particularly *Staph. aureus.*
- Systemic symptoms? Diarrhoea, jaundice and confusion are more common in Legionnaire's disease. Severe ear ache suggests *Mycoplasma* spp.

Table 2 Aetiology of community-acquired pneumonia.

Frequency	Pathogen
Most common	*Streptococcus pneumoniae*
Common	*Haemophilus influenzae*
	Mycoplasma pneumoniae
	Chlamydia pneumoniae
Less common	*Legionella pneumophila*
	Chlamydia psittaci
	Coxiella burnetii
	Moraxella catarrhalis
	Staphylococcus aureus
	Influenza virus

Relevant past history

Ask about the following:
• Respiratory symptoms that may suggest a diagnosis of chronic obstructive airway disease (COAD). Although *Strep. pneumoniae* is still the most common cause of a LRTI in this setting, organisms such as *Haemophilus influenzae* and *Moraxella catarrhalis* are more common than in the general population. (See *Respiratory medicine*, Sections 1.3 and 2.3.)
• Bronchiectasis or cystic fibrosis: consider organisms such as *Staph. aureus*, *Pseudomonas aeruginosa* and *Burkholderia cepacia* (see *Respiratory medicine*, Section 2.4).
• Immunocompromise such as HIV. Bacterial pneumonia is significantly more common in HIV-infected patients, but don't forget tuberculosis, *Pneumocystis carinii* and fungal infection. (See Section 1.26, p. 65.)
• Past history of tuberculosis. (See Section 1.5, p. 13.)
• Smoking history: even in the absence of chronic lung disease, smoking increases the risk of pneumococcal disease [2] and increases the severity of many pulmonary infections.

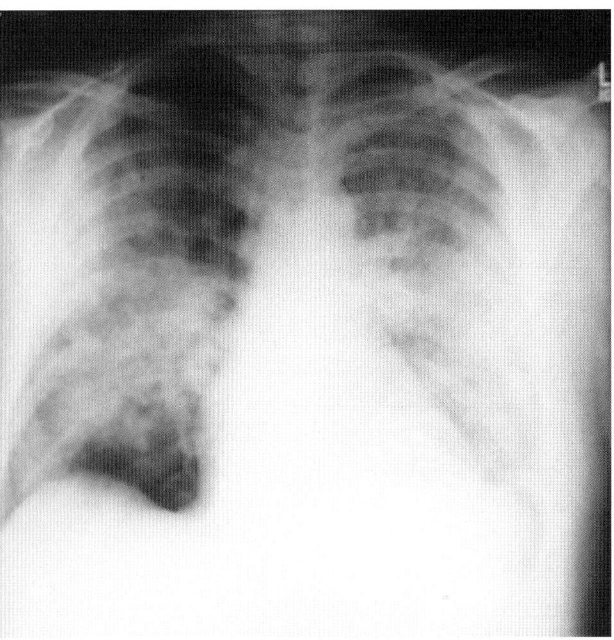

Fig. 6 Chest radiograph from a patient with severe Legionnaire's disease. The patient was a smoker who had recently returned from a package holiday in Europe. The chest was clear on examination, but he was markedly hypoxic and the radiograph revealed extensive consolidation.

Examination

General

Is the patient well, ill, very ill or nearly dead? For details of the clinical approach to the patient who is very breathless, see *Emergency medicine*, Section 1.5.

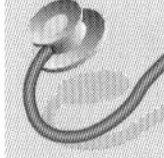

Don't forget that atypical pneumonias commonly present with a gradual onset, dry cough and absence of focal chest signs. It is therefore important to perform a chest radiograph if you suspect atypical pneumonia (Fig. 6).

Respiratory

Look for evidence of respiratory failure and signs of acute or chronic lung disease. Pay particular attention to the following:
• Vital signs: pulse rate, BP, respiratory rate, temperature
• Central cyanosis
• Exclusion of pneumothorax
• Focal lung signs: consolidation, pleural rub or pleural effusion/empyema
• Check peak flow rate and monitor arterial oxygen saturation (pulse oximetry)
• Look at the sputum (and make sure that it is sent for culture).

Note that wheeze signifies bronchospasm, probably as a result of exacerbation of COAD or asthma in this context, but it can also be generated by pulmonary oedema. Is there finger clubbing, suggesting chronic suppurative lung disease or an underlying bronchial carcinoma?

A normal respiratory rate (10–16 breaths/min) is consistent with the following:
• Normality
• Near death: respiratory rate falls as the patient gets exhausted, reaching zero when he or she dies.
Always think 'Is this person getting tired?' If he or she is, call the intensive care unit (ICU) for help.

Approach to investigation and management

Patients may die from respiratory failure or failure to control infection: investigations and management must be aimed at both aspects.

Investigations

Blood tests

Check the following:
• FBC: a marked neutrophilia suggests bacterial pneumonia. In pneumococcal pneumonia, a low WCC is a poor prognostic sign. The WCC is often normal in atypical pneumonia with the exception of Legionnaire's disease where a neutrophil leucocytosis is seen. Low haemoglobin (Hb) may be the result of haemolysis, e.g. *Mycoplasma pneumoniae*.
• Electrolytes and renal function: renal impairment and hyponatraemia are markers of severe disease, the latter being particularly likely in Legionnaire's disease.
• Liver function tests: mild hepatitis may occur in infection as a result of *Mycoplasma pneumoniae*, *Legionella pneumophila*, *Coxiella burnettii* and *Chlamydia psittaci*.
• Arterial blood gases in any patient with O_2 saturation <95% on pulse oximetry, or who is very unwell, or who looks

as though he or she might retain CO_2. (See *Emergency medicine*, Section 1.10.)

Cultures and serology

• Respiratory tract: sputum for bacterial culture (see Section 3.1, p. 150). Always aspirate any pleural effusion to exclude an empyema. Use bronchial lavage in selected cases.
• Blood cultures: may yield the responsible organism.
• Serology: acute and convalescent for atypical organisms if suspected. Rapid diagnostic tests for *Legionella* spp. can be performed on urine and blood. (See Section 3.1, p. 150.)

Imaging

Chest radiograph: look for evidence of consolidation, cavitation and lymphadenopathy. However, do not forget that changes on a chest radiograph may suggest certain diagnoses but are not diagnostic of specific pathogens (Fig. 7).

Management

You need to act quickly if the patient looks very unwell, is centrally cyanosed, very tachypnoeic (≥30 breaths/min), or looks as though he or she is becoming exhausted. For discussion of the management of the patient who is very breathless and has respiratory failure, see *Emergency medicine*, Section 1.5 and *Respiratory medicine*, Section 2.12.

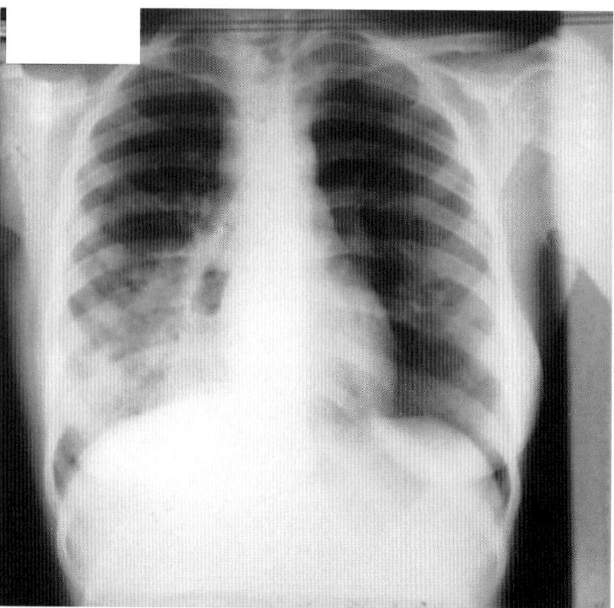

Fig. 7 Chest radiograph from a patient admitted with right lower lobe consolidation and treated for bacterial pneumonia. When the patient failed to respond to antibiotics, an acid-fast sputum smear was positive, indicating tuberculosis.

Immediate management of the very breathless patient

- Check airway, breathing, circulation
- Exclude tension pneumothorax
- Sit patient up and give high-flow oxygen
- Give nebulized bronchodilator
- Monitor with pulse oximetry
- Check blood gases
- Establish diagnosis and treat if possible
- Call for help from the ICU sooner rather than later.

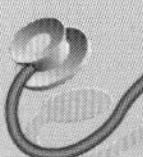

Definition of severe pneumonia

The British Thoracic Society definition of severe pneumonia [3] states that one or more of the following must exist in a patient with clinical and/or radiological signs of pneumonia:

- Respiratory rate >30 breaths/min
- Signs of systemic sepsis: hypotension BP <90 mmHg systolic
- Hypoxia: $Pa\text{O}_2$ <8.0 kPa breathing room air
- Multilobar involvement on chest radiograph
- Elevated urea >7.0 mmol/L

Supportive care

The following are important aspects:
• Give high-flow oxygen, monitoring oxygen saturation with pulse oximetry and repeating blood gases if there is deterioration or any chance of CO_2 retention. (See *Emergency medicine*, Section 1.10.)
• Give intravenous fluids.
• Give adequate analgesia if coughing is painful.

Empirical therapy

Antimicrobial therapy is based on the assessment of the probable aetiological agent and the severity of illness [2]. The British Thoracic Society guidelines recommend an extended spectrum penicillin or macrolide alone for uncomplicated LRTI, with a second- or third-generation cephalosporin plus a macrolide for more severe disease. When a patient fails to respond to first-line therapy, consider the possibility of underlying immunocompromise, tuberculosis (TB), lung cancer, bronchial obstruction, lung abscess or empyema formation.

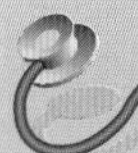

Treatment of community-acquired pneumonia

The British Thoracic Society Guidelines for the treatment of community-acquired pneumonia [3,4]:

- Mild-to-moderate infection: extended-spectrum penicillin (amoxicillin) alone or plus a macrolide (erythromycin). In mild cases and penicillin allergy, a macrolide alone may be sufficient. Oral therapy unless unable to use the oral route.
- Severe pneumonia: parenteral therapy with a second- or third-generation cephalosporin plus a macrolide (oral or intravenous).
- Suspected Legionnaire's disease: high-dose parenteral erythromycin, 1 g 6-hourly, plus consider adding oral rifampicin.

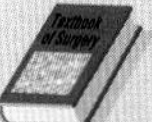

See *Emergency medicine*, Section 1.9.

1 Finch R. Community acquired pneumonia. *J R Coll Physicians Lond* 1998; 32: 328–332.
2 Nuorti JP, Butler JC, Farley MM *et al.* Cigarette smoking and invasive pneumococcal disease. *N Engl J Med* 2000; 342: 681–689.
3 British Thoracic Society. Guidelines for the management of community-acquired pneumonia in adults admitted to hospital. *Br J Hosp Med* 1993; 49: 347–350.
4 British Thoracic Society: www.brit-thoracic.org.uk (the BTS will post updates of the guidelines for the management of community-acquired pneumonia on this site).

1.5 A cavitating lung lesion

Case history

A 48-year-old woman presents with two episodes of haemoptysis. A chest radiograph reveals a cavitating lesion in the left upper lobe. She has had a cough and fever for 5 weeks.

Clinical approach

The key to this case is the cavitation on the chest radiograph. The differential diagnosis will include both infectious and non-infectious conditions. It is essential to consider pulmonary TB in all cases of pulmonary cavities because of the potential infectious risk that TB poses. Patients should therefore be considered as potentially infectious and isolated until TB has been excluded.

History of the presenting problem

Length of illness

The duration of the history is critical in establishing a differential diagnosis. Common possibilities with a short duration (<1 week) include lung abscess resulting from *Staph. aureus* or *Klebsiella pneumoniae*, or cavitation after pulmonary infarction. If the duration is longer, think of pulmonary TB, invasive fungal infection or non-infectious causes, such as primary or secondary carcinoma of the lung or Wegener's granulomatosis.

Infective cause

Ask about features suggesting an infective cause:

- Aspiration: epilepsy, blackouts, alcohol abuse and recent dental work can all lead to aspiration.
- Travel abroad: increased risk of pulmonary TB if the patient has travelled to developing countries; invasive fungi with travel to North or South America (see Section 2.9, p. 123).
- Drug use: active intravenous drug use is a risk factor for right-sided endocarditis, with resultant infected pulmonary emboli and abscess formation.

Note that general symptoms, e.g. fever or night sweats, suggest an infectious aetiology but are non-specific, as is a history of weight loss.

Non-infective cause

The following features suggest a non-infective cause:

- Dyspnoea or pleurisy is suggestive of pulmonary embolism, as would be a history of a recent deep venous thrombosis.
- A history of ear (discharge, bleeding, deafness), nose (discharge, bleeding), eye (scleritis), skin (vasculitic rash) or neurological (particularly mononeuritis) problems would support the diagnosis of Wegener's granulomatosis. (See *Nephrology*, Section 1.12 and *Rheumatology and clinical immunology*, Section 2.5.2.)

Relevant past history

- Is there a previous history of TB? If yes, which antituberculous drugs were given and for what duration of treatment? Consider relapse of TB or invasive fungal infection.
- Is there chronic lung disease? Aspergilloma (fungus ball, see Section 2.9.2, p. 122) occurs in pre-existing lung cavities.

Risk factors for tuberculosis

- Contact with a person with TB, particularly a family member
- Ethnic origin, foreign residence or recent immigration, particularly from a developing country
- Heavy alcohol intake or intravenous drug use
- Immunocompromise as a result of HIV, immunosuppressive drugs, renal failure, etc.
- Homelessness, poverty and overcrowding.

Differential diagnosis

- Bacterial lung abscess: usually a short history but not always, copious sputum, high fever, neutrophil leucocytosis. The common organisms include *Staph. aureus*, particularly postinfluenza, and *K. pneumoniae*.
- Pulmonary embolus: pulmonary infarction may occasionally cavitate. There is usually associated dyspnoea and pleuritic chest pain and there may be specific thrombophilic risk factors present. (See *Haematology*, Section 1.20.)
- Lung neoplasm: particularly in older patients with a history of smoking, the possibility of primary (particularly squamous cell carcinoma) or secondary lung cancer needs to be considered (see *Respiratory medicine*, Section 1.2). However, always send three sputum samples for smear and TB culture if there is any doubt.

Examination

A full physical examination is required. The patient with pulmonary TB may appear rather wasted but look reasonably well otherwise—with advanced disease they are likely to look very ill. Always weigh the patient: increasing weight is a good indicator of response to antituberculous therapy.

Look for evidence of HIV infection if this is suspected—oral hairy leucoplakia (see Section 1.28, p. 71), oral thrush, Kaposi's sarcoma or evidence of old shingles scarring.

In addition, take specific note of the following:

- Finger clubbing is rare in TB and likely to result from bronchial carcinoma.
- Are there any signs to support the diagnosis of Wegener's granulomatosis? (See *Nephrology*, Section 1.12 and *Rheumatology and clinical immunology*, Section 2.5.2.)
- Cervical or supraclavicular lymphadenopathy.
- There are no specific features on respiratory examination in pulmonary TB, and there may or may not be any localized signs at the site of disease.
- Hepatomegaly.
- Signs suggesting DVT.
- Fundoscopy for choroidal tubercles.

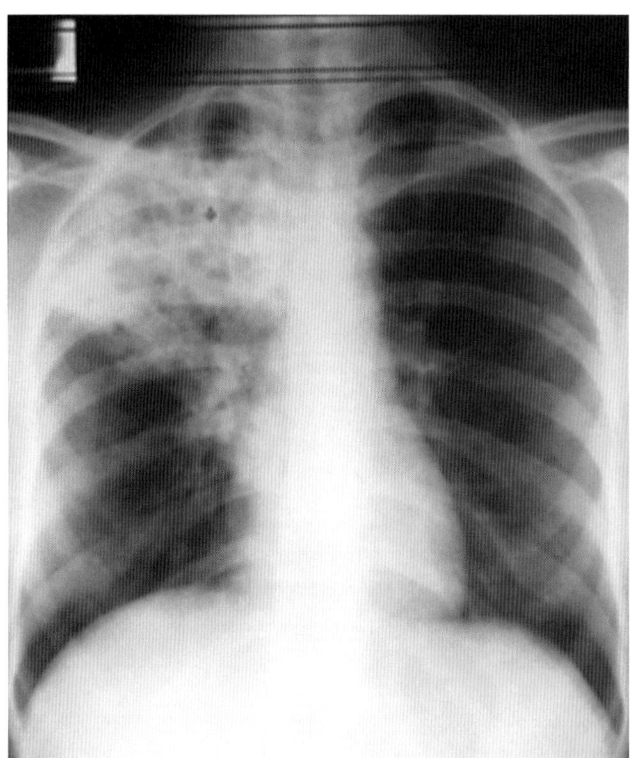

Fig. 8 Right upper lobe cavitating pneumonia caused by *Mycobacterium tuberculosis*.

Approach to investigation and management

Investigations

Urine and blood tests

- Dipstick urine for protein and blood; microscopy to look for red blood cells and casts if positive. An active urinary sediment would suggest Wegener's granulomatosis in this context.
- FBC: neutrophilia in bacterial lung abscess.
- Electrolytes and renal function tests: renal function may be impaired in anyone who is acutely ill, and also in Wegener's granulomatosis.

Cultures

- Sputum specimens are required for microscopy, culture, and mycobacterial smear and culture. If the cough is non-productive, sputum production may be induced with nebulized saline. If sputum is unavailable or negative on acid-fast smears, gastric washings and/or bronchoscopy should be performed. (See Section 3.1, p. 150.)
- Blood cultures may yield an organism if an abscess is the result of haematogenous infection.

Imaging

- Chest radiograph: upper zone shadowing with or without cavitation should always put TB in the differential diagnosis (Fig. 8). In addition, pulmonary TB may also present with miliary shadowing (Fig. 9) or with a pleural effusion (Fig. 10).
- CT: provides more detail of the extent of pulmonary involvement and can be particularly useful for the detection of mediastinal lymphadenopathy, assessment of empyema or diagnosis of aspergilloma.

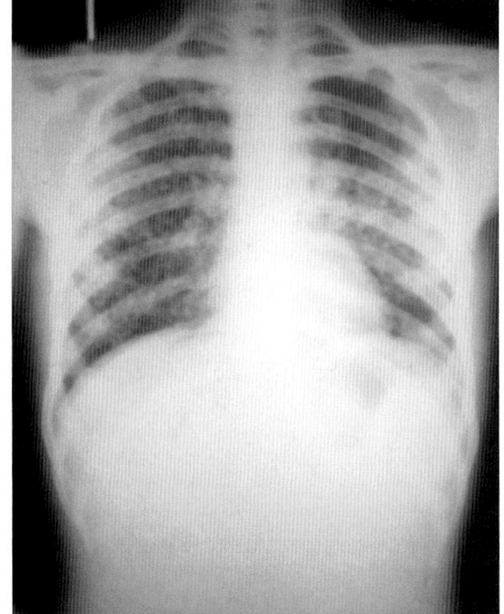

Fig. 9 Miliary tuberculosis.

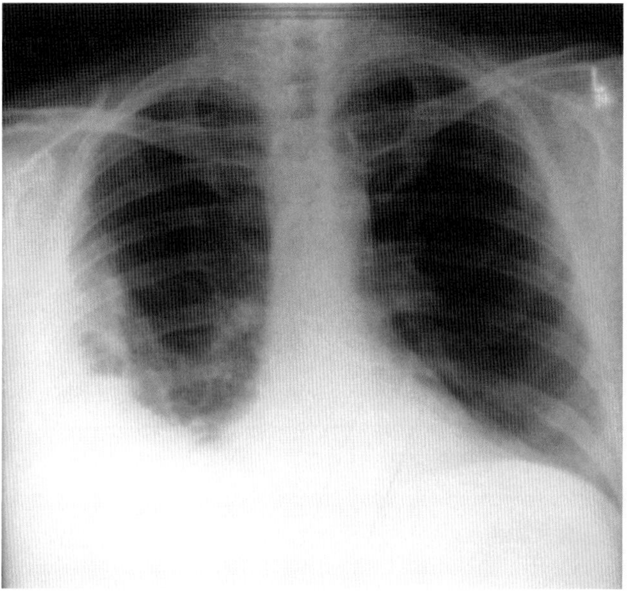

Fig. 10 Right-sided pleural effusion diagnosed as tuberculous on pleural biopsy.

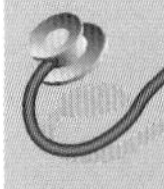

The radiological appearances of pulmonary TB may be atypical in advanced HIV infection. Cavitation is much less common and the appearances may be of focal consolidation or disseminated bronchopneumonia.

Other tests

The following may be required:
• The Mantoux or Heaf test is likely to be positive in active pulmonary TB (see Section 3.2, p. 151), but is commonly negative in the setting of immunosuppression such as HIV.
• Check arterial blood gas if the patient is dyspnoeic or you are considering pulmonary embolus.
• Serological testing, e.g. antineutrophil cytoplasmic antibody (ANCA), for vasculitic disease. (See *Rheumatology and clinical immunology*, Section 3.2.)
• Consider bronchoscopy.
• Pleural biopsy if effusion present.

Management

Pulmonary TB

• Quadruple therapy with oral rifampicin, isoniazid, pyrazinamide and ethambutol for 2 months, followed by 4 months of rifampicin and isoniazid, is recommended for all patients in the UK [1].
• If an organism is found to be resistant to one or more drugs, a combination of drugs based on the sensitivity profile must be commenced, and a physician with an interest in TB should be involved in the case.
• Baseline visual acuity and colour vision testing must be performed *before* commencing ethambutol. Patients must be warned of the small risk of visual deterioration on ethambutol, and stop ethambutol and seek medical advice immediately should they notice any visual problems.
• Be careful of drug-induced hepatitis, particularly in elderly people, people with alcohol problems and those with underlying liver disease [2].
• Compliance with medication is the key to successful treatment; this should be emphasized to all patients.
• All cases of suspected or proven TB must be notified to the local CCDC and this initiates contact tracing. (See Section 1.39, p. 93.)

Multi-drug-resistant TB

Multi-drug-resistant TB (MDR-TB) is defined as resistance to two or more antituberculous drugs, including isoniazid and rifampicin. MDR-TB should be suspected in patients who may have acquired TB abroad, who have a past history of treated TB, who are drug or alcohol abusers, and those co-infected with HIV [3].

People with suspected MDR-TB should be isolated in an appropriate facility with negative-pressure ventilation. Therapy of this group of patients should be guided by a physician with expertise in the management of TB [4]. Polymerase chain reaction (PCR)-based probes can help to identify resistance genes and aid in the choice of antimicrobial therapy.

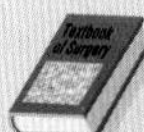

See *Respiratory medicine*, Section 1.9.

British Thoracic Society: www.brit-thoracic.org.uk (the BTS will post updates of the guidelines for the management of tuberculosis on this site).

1 Joint Tuberculosis Committee of the British Thoracic Society. Chemotherapy and management of tuberculosis in the United Kingdom: recommendations 1998. *Thorax* 1998; 53: 536–548.

2 Ormerod LP, Skinner C, Wales J. Hepatotoxicity of antituberculous drugs. *Thorax* 1996; 51: 111–113.

3 Hayward AC, Bennett DE, Herbert J, Watson JM. Risk factors for drug resistance in patients with tuberculosis in England and Wales 1993–4. *Thorax* 1996; 51 (suppl 3): 532.

4 Lazarus A, Sanders J. Management of tuberculosis. Choosing an effective regimen and ensuring compliance. *Postgrad Med* 2000; 108: 71–74.

1.6 Fever, back pain and weak legs

Case history

A 54-year-old Somalian refugee complains of back pain and weak legs. He gives a 3-month history of weight loss and night sweats.

Clinical approach

For any patient who presents with leg weakness and back pain, your first thought must be of spinal cord compression. This is a medical emergency, and an immediate assessment should be made (see *Emergency medicine*, Section 1.23). Weight loss and night sweats make infection or malignancy high on the differential, and the knowledge that the patient is from Somalia suggests TB. However, it is important to consider other possibilities—both infectious (Table 3) and non-infectious—such as trauma, malignancy or a ruptured aortic aneurysm. Do not exclude the possibility of immunocompromise and HIV infection in this patient.

History of the presenting problem

Back pain and weak legs

Detailed description of the symptoms is required:
- The pain: where is it, is there any radiation, how long has it been present, is it constant, is it present at night?
- The weakness: is there true loss of power, or is movement restricted by pain? Was it of sudden or gradual onset? Is it bilateral? What activities are interfered with?
- Associated symptoms: ask specifically about bowel and bladder function. Is there incoordination? Are there associated sensory symptoms?

Other features

A thorough systems enquiry is needed:
- This man has had night sweats: has he measured his temperature or had rigors?
- Weight loss: how much?
- Symptoms in other body systems may point to an additional focus of infection or site of primary/secondary malignancy.

Table 3 Causes of vertebral osteomyelitis and discitis.

Common	*Staphylococcus aureus* >50% pyogenic vertebral osteomyelitis
	Mycobacterium tuberculosis
Less common	Coliforms (risk factors include intravenous drug use, urinary tract infections)
	Streptococci (especially in association with infective endocarditis)
	Brucellosis (consider if relevant travel history)

Relevant past history

Infection

Ask about risk factors for infection:
- How long has he been in the UK?
- Was he well previously or has he had recurrent illness?
- Is there a past history of TB or known contacts?
- HIV? Remember that HIV is essentially a heterosexual disease in Africa and his place of origin is in itself a risk factor. Are there any other features in the history that are suggestive, e.g. chronic diarrhoeal disease, long-standing weight loss, recurrent infections?

Neurological disease and malignancy

Is there any past history of neurological problems or of malignancy?

Examination

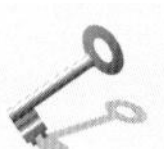

Back pain and weak legs

- Perform a full neurological examination—is there spinal cord compression? Look for increased tone in the legs, weakness, upgoing plantars and a sensory level
- Examine the back
- Look for other septic foci.

Your priority should be to make an assessment of this man's leg weakness. Does he have clinical evidence of cord compression? (see *Emergency medicine*, Section 1.23 and *Neurology*, Section 1.11.)

First impressions are important. If this man is a fat, fit, healthy looking individual moving about the bed, you will think differently than if he were wasted with oral thrush and widespread lymphadenopathy, and unable to move his legs. Examination should include all other systems but specifically the following:
- Examine his back. Is there an obvious deformity? Does he have an area of localized tenderness?
- Are there any features consistent with systemic infection or malignancy? Examine the mouth, feel for lymphadenopathy and hepatosplenomegaly. Do not overlook genital pathology, e.g. testicular masses.
- Listen to the heart and look for features of infective endocarditis.
- Are there abnormal chest signs that might indicate pulmonary TB?

Approach to investigation and management

> **Back pain, fever and weak legs**
>
> • The absence of neurological signs does not mean that there isn't a lesion that needs urgent intervention. The patient may go on to develop cord compression or suffer cord infarction after spinal artery thrombosis in association with a spinal epidural abscess [1].
>
> • Do not be complacent. Aggressive investigation and management before an irreversible neurological event is preferable to waiting for something to happen. If in doubt, always perform urgent spinal imaging and obtain a surgical opinion.

Investigations

Blood tests

Check the following:

• Blood cultures: these are essential, preferably more than one set. (See Section 3.2, p. 151.)

• FBC: is the WCC raised, is the total lymphocyte count abnormally low? A low lymphocyte count is common in disseminated TB or may be a sign of HIV infection.

• Electrolytes, renal and liver function tests.

• Inflammatory markers: CRP and ESR.

• Serum immunoglobulins: myeloma does not seem likely in this context, but it is a bad diagnosis to miss!

Consider checking vitamin B_{12} levels and HIV testing with consent. (See Section 1.24, p. 61.)

Take serum for storage, which can be used later for serology if necessary.

Imaging

Plain radiographs may be of help:

• Chest radiograph: look for evidence of old or active TB, hilar lymphadenopathy and a paraspinal mass, especially if the back pain is thoracic.

• Radiographs of the spine (anteroposterior [AP] and lateral) (Fig. 11a): look for bony destruction, wedge fractures and lytic or sclerotic lesions.

The spine can be imaged with CT (Fig. 11b) and myelography, but magnetic resonance imaging (MRI) is the investigation of choice. MRI can exclude osteomyelitis, a paraspinal mass or abscess, and detect cord compression. (See *Neurology*, Section 3.4.)

Tissue

In the event of a diagnosis of a mass lesion, irrespective of the need for debridement, drainage or decompression, there is a need to get tissue for histology and microbiology.

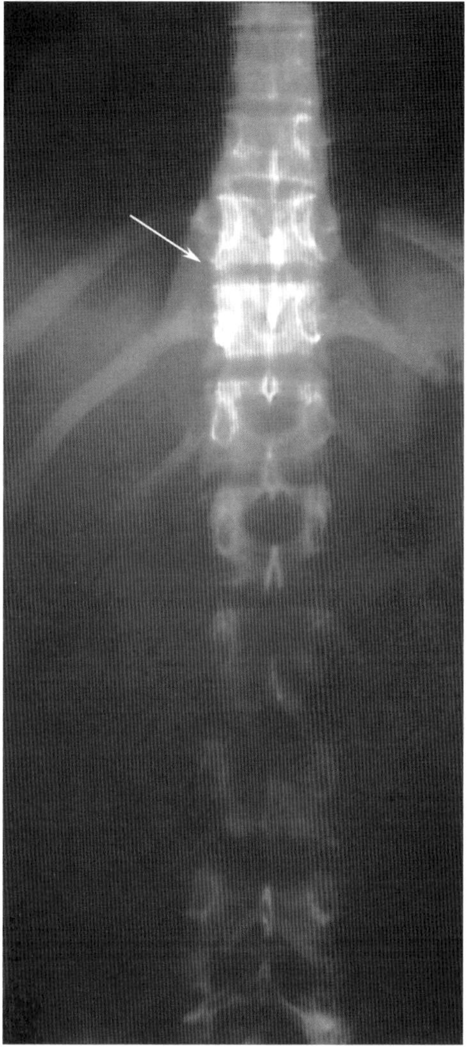

(a)

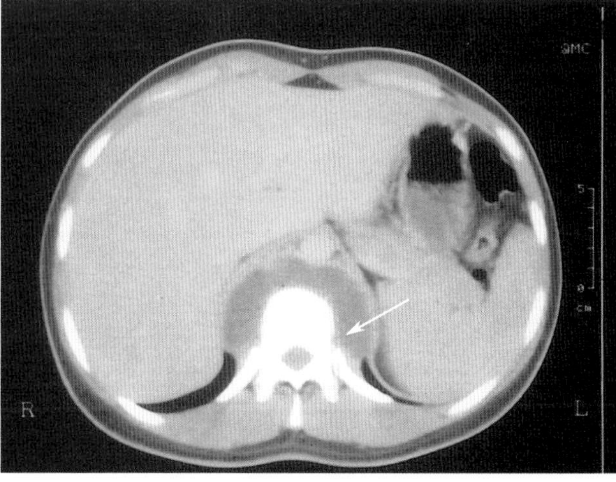

(b)

Fig. 11 (a) Plain radiograph demonstrating a paraspinal soft tissue mass (arrowed). (b) CT scan from the same patient demonstrating a paravertebral collection (arrowed). This was aspirated and confirmed to be tuberculous. (Copyright of Dr C Conlon.)

Others

Do not forget to send sputum and urine for mycobacterial detection and culture.

Management

Management is directed towards the underlying cause and preserving spinal cord function. (See *Emergency medicine*, Section 1.23.)

Vertebral osteomyelitis

- Early surgical intervention is often needed for diagnosis or decompression.
- Tissue/pus should be sent for histology or cytology, and culture for standard bacteria, mycobacteria and brucellosis. If immunocompromised, also request nocardia and fungal culture.
- Consider adjunctive steroids in compressive lesions, especially with TB and malignancy.
- Consider radiotherapy in malignancy.

Paraspinal abscess

Urgent drainage is required, with microscopy, and Gram and auramine staining of pus. Every attempt should be made to get a histological and microbiological diagnosis before commencing antimicrobial therapy. However, if this is not possible, antimicrobial therapy can be started after taking blood cultures. The empirical regimen will depend on the immunological status of patient, but for an immunocompetent individual with a pyogenic abscess give a third-generation cephalosporin plus flucloxacillin and metronidazole. To obtain good penetration into bone, high-dose parenteral antibiotics are required. Antituberculous and antibrucella therapy should be considered where clinically appropriate.

Vertebral osteomyelitis and discitis

A tissue biopsy is essential for a definitive diagnosis and should be obtained before commencing antimicrobial therapy. Debridement and spinal stabilization may be needed. In pyogenic infection, give an initial 4–6 weeks' parenteral antibiotics, followed by a further 6 weeks of oral therapy, guided by the microbiology. Tuberculosis [4] and brucellosis [5] require specific regimens. (See Sections 2.5.2, p. 104 and 2.6.1, p. 110.)

See *Haematology*, Sections 1.15 and 2.2.1.

1 Baker AG, Ojemann RG, Baker RA. To decompress or not to decompress—spinal epidural abscess. *Clin Infect Dis* 1992; 15: 28–29.

2 Bateman JL, Pevzner MM. Spinal osteomyelitis: A review of 10 years' experience. *Orthopaedics* 1995; 18: 561–565.

3 Lew DP, Waldvogel FA. Osteomyelitis. *N Engl J Med* 1997; 336: 999–1007.

4 Fourteenth report of the Medical Research Council Working Party on Tuberculosis of the Spine. Five-year assessment of the controlled trials of short-course chemotherapy regimens of 6, 9 or 18 months' duration for spinal tuberculosis in patients ambulatory from the start or undergoing radical surgery. *Int Orthop* 1999; 23: 73–81.

5 Young E. An overview of human brucellosis. *Clin Infect Dis* 1994; 21: 283–290.

1.7 Fever and lymphadenopathy

Case history

A 57-year-old woman is referred with fever and lymphadenopathy in her neck.

Clinical approach

The wide variety of causes of lymphadenopathy (Table 4) make a structured approach to diagnosis essential. The majority of cases are benign/reactive and secondary to a self-limiting infectious cause [1]. The probability of malignancy increases with age: this is an important diagnosis not to miss, as are infectious causes that need specific treatment, e.g. mycobacterial infection.

History of the presenting problem

What and how long

A detailed description is required:

- How long has she been unwell?
- What did she notice first?
- Has she noticed any other enlarged lymph nodes elsewhere?
- Has she measured her temperature?
- Are there any other systemic features—weight loss, night sweats?
- Are there any other symptoms, e.g. generalized rash, suggesting a viral infection or syphilis or localized symptoms that might indicate malignancy?

Regional lymphadenopathy is usually secondary to a local problem draining to that set of nodes, e.g. pharyngitis with cervical lymphadenopathy, scalp infection with occipital nodes, lower leg cellulitis and inguinal nodes, enlarged axillary nodes and breast carcinoma, supraclavicular nodes and gastrointestinal malignancy. Inguinal lymphadenopathy brings in a new set of possibilities with sexually transmitted disease (STD) and metastatic genital

Table 4 Principal causes of lymphadenopathy.

Category	Cause	Examples
Infectious	Viruses	Common: EBV, CMV, parvovirus, enteroviruses Less common: HIV, hepatitis B, rubella
	Bacteria	Common: *Staph. aureus, Strep. pyogenes* Less common: cat scratch disease (*Bartonella* spp.), syphilis, Lyme disease, rickettsiae
	Mycobacteria	Common: *Mycobacterium tuberculosis* Less common: atypical mycobacteria
	Parasites	*Toxoplasma* spp., trypanosomiasis, leishmaniasis
	Fungi	Sporotrichosis, coccidioidomycosis
Non-infectious	Malignancy	Metastatic disease, lymphoma, chronic lymphatic leukaemia
	Collagen–vascular disorders	SLE, rheumatoid arthritis
	Miscellaneous	Sarcoidosis, Kawasaki's disease, Kikuchi's necrotizing lymphadenitis, Castleman's disease, amyloidosis, histiocytosis X, hypersensitivity reactions

EBV, Epstein–Barr virus; CMV, cytomegalovirus; HIV, human immunodeficiency virus; SLE, systemic lupus erythematosus.

neoplasia. Generalized lymphadenopathy suggests a systemic problem.

Full history

Take a full social, travel and sexual history. Do not forget the obvious, such as her country of origin. Be sure to clarify a travel history because time spent in the tropics widens the differential diagnosis. A 57-year-old woman is still at risk of sexually acquired infection and, if no diagnosis is immediately apparent, a sexual history needs to be taken—this will clearly need to be approached with particular tact and care (see *General clinical issues*, Section 2).

Relevant past history

Has she had previous malignancy, TB, STDs or connective tissue disease?

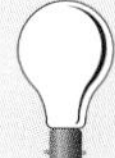

Lymphadenopathy with a travel history

- Tuberculosis: not to be forgotten and a possibility even without a travel history. Suspicion is greater in certain ethnic populations.
- Rickettsial disease: look for an eschar at the site of a tick bite; also regional lymphadenopathy and rash. Patients often complain of headache.
- Trypanosomiasis: African or American. May also have a lesion at the site of the original bite and regional lymphadenopathy.
- Leishmaniasis: can have locally enlarged nodes with the cutaneous form or more widespread with the visceral form.
- Endemic mycoses (coccidioidomycosis, histoplasmosis): is there a history of travel to parts of North and Central America?

Examination

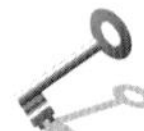

Examination of the patient with lymphadenopathy

- General impression: is he or she unwell?
- Systematic examination of all lymph node groups
- Look for hepatosplenomegaly
- Is there a local abnormality, especially with regional lymphadenopathy? Examine local structures, e.g. breasts.

Do not underestimate your first impressions. A pale, thin, nontoxic, 57-year-old woman with non-tender lymphadenopathy has malignancy until proved otherwise (see *Haematology*, Section 1.16 and *Oncology*, Section 1.1). A flushed and toxic looking 57-year-old woman with a hot swollen toe, lymphangitis and tender inguinal lymphadenopathy probably has group A streptococcal or *Staph. aureus* infection. If the node is fluctuant, infection is much more likely and pus may be aspirated (Fig. 12). Be thorough with your examination: an eschar between

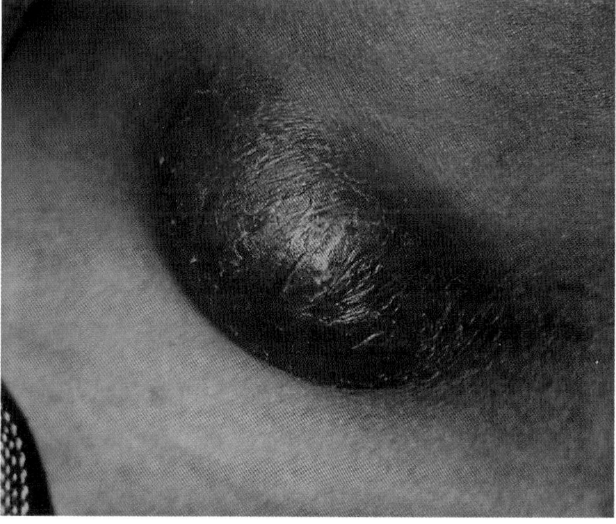

Fig. 12 Suppurative supraclavicular lymphadenopathy, in this case caused by *Mycobacterium tuberculosis*.

the toes in a traveller returned from South Africa or a breast lump can both easily be missed.

Approach to investigation and management

Investigations

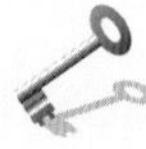

Investigation of fever and lymphadenopathy

- FBC, film, monospot or Paul–Bunnell test for glandular fever
- Chest radiograph
- Blood cultures
- Serum for appropriate serology
- Fine needle aspirate and/or lymph node biopsy (remember cytology and histology, but also routine bacterial and mycobacterial culture).

Blood tests

Check the following:

- FBC and ask for review of a blood film—atypical lymphocytes are commonly seen in viral infections such as Epstein–Barr virus (EBV) and cytomegalovirus (CMV).
- Electrolytes, renal and liver function: is there an associated hepatitis?
- Inflammatory markers (ESR and/or CRP): useful as a baseline.
- Serum sample for storage, which can be used for serological testing (with consent) for other infectious agents: EBV, CMV, *Toxoplasma* spp., *Bartonella* spp., syphilis, HIV, etc.

Chest radiograph

Look closely at the mediastinum. Is there a suggestion of hilar involvement? Look at the lung fields. Other imaging may be needed, such as a CT scan of the thorax, abdomen and pelvis to ascertain the extent of the lymphadenopathy.

Fine needle aspirate/lymph node biopsy

If the diagnosis is not clear, it will almost certainly be important to get tissue. This should be sent for culture, including for mycobacteria, as well as for histology [2].

Management

Management will depend on the cause:

- Viral infections: EBV, CMV, rubella are essentially self-limiting in the immunocompetent.
- Lymphoma and metastatic malignancy: see *Haematology*, Section 2.2 and *Oncology*, Section 1.3.
- Mycobacterial infections: see Section 2.6, p. 110.
- Pyogenic lymphadenopathy: antibiotic therapy, aspiration or drainage if an abscess forms.
- Toxoplasmosis: usually self-limiting and rarely needs specific treatment except reassurance (see Section 2.13.4, p. 144). Be aware of circumstances to ask for specialist advice, e.g. pregnancy, immunosuppression.
- Cat scratch disease: generally self-limiting but may need antimicrobial therapy if associated with systemic symptoms.

1 Rubinstein E, Levi I, Rubinovitch B. Generalized and regional lymphadenopathy. In: Armstrong D, Cohen J (eds) *Infectious Diseases*. London: Mosby, 1999: Section 2, 9.1–9.12.

2 Slap GB, Brooks JS, Schwartz JS. When to perform biopsies of enlarged peripheral lymph nodes in young patients. *JAMA* 1984; 252: 1321–1327.

1.8 Drug user with fever and a murmur

Case history

A 34-year-old intravenous drug user arrives in the A&E department short of breath. On examination he is febrile and has a loud early diastolic murmur in the aortic region.

Clinical approach

The differential diagnosis of infection in intravenous drug users is wide. The cardiac murmur places endocarditis high on the list, but do not be blinkered and miss another obvious focus of infection—for instance, could he have pneumonia and long-standing aortic regurgitation (probably from previous endocarditis)?

History of the presenting problem

Breathlessness

Why is he breathless? The obvious possibilities are endocarditis with aortic valve dysfunction causing pulmonary oedema or pneumonia.

How fast and how bad

Ask the following:

- How long has he been breathless?
- Was it of sudden onset or gradual?

• What makes him breathless? What is he restricted in doing?

Cardiac failure resulting from acute valve rupture secondary to endocarditis will have a sudden onset, whereas the less dramatic development of aortic incompetence or a pneumonic process may have a longer history.

Other features

Note the following:
• Has he had fevers, rigors or night sweats? These could be found in endocarditis or pneumonia, but rigors would be in favour of the latter.
• Are there any respiratory symptoms? Chest pain, productive cough or haemoptysis would suggest pneumonia in this context, as would any history compatible with aspiration.
• Is he more breathless lying down? No one who is severely short of breath will want to lie down, but a clear history of orthopnoea favours pulmonary oedema.

Drug use

Ask about his drug use:
• Is he still injecting?
• Where does he inject and has he had any complications at the injection sites?
• What has he been mixing the drugs with and does he lick the needles? This is a common practice and increases the likelihood of infection with oral organisms.
• Has he ever shared needles? Do not forget the possibility of HIV or hepatitis B or C co-infection.

Relevant past history

It is important to try to establish whether the murmur is old or new.
• Has he had endocarditis in the past?
• Has he ever been admitted to hospital for a long course of antibiotics before?
• Why was that, and where?
• Has he previously been told he has a heart murmur/funny sound?
• Also ask if he has been tested for hepatitis and HIV in the past.

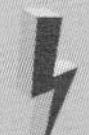

Remember that a past history of endocarditis puts him at greater risk of further episodes and do not gain a false sense of security knowing that the murmur has been noted before.

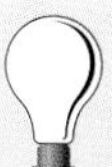

In the febrile, breathless intravenous drug user consider the following:
• Endocarditis: intravenous drug use puts them at high risk of endocarditis, most commonly right sided (see *Cardiology*, Section 1.13).
• Cardiac failure: he could have cardiac failure secondary to valvular incompetence.
• Pneumonia: he may have severe community-acquired pneumonia and drug use places him at increased risk of aspiration pneumonia.
• Pulmonary emboli: either septic emboli in association with right-sided endocarditis or secondary to a venous thrombosis. Femoral injection increases the risk of thrombosis, infected or otherwise.
• Immunosuppression: intravenous drug use is a risk factor for HIV. Is he known to be HIV positive? (See Section 1.26, p. 65.)

Examination

Is the man well, ill, very ill or nearly dead? Does he need immediate resuscitation? See Section 1.2, p. 5 and *Emergency medicine*, Section 1.5 for details of the approach to the patient who is very ill or worse.

A full physical examination is required, concentrating on the following:
• Check vital signs: pulse, BP, respiratory rate, temperature
• Check peripheral perfusion
• Is he cyanosed? Check pulse oximetry
• Has he got stigmata of endocarditis?
• What are the murmurs?
• Is there pulmonary oedema?
• Is there pneumonia?
• Is there splenomegaly?
• Inspect injection sites—there may be an abscess
• Look for signs suggestive of HIV infection (see Sections 1.24, p. 61 and 1.28, p. 70)
• Examine the legs for evidence of DVT and/or septic thrombophlebitis

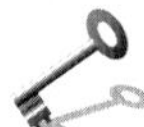

Peripheral stigmata of endocarditis

• Splinter haemorrhages
• Janeway's lesions: transient, non-tender, macular patches on the palms or soles (very rare)
• Osler's nodes: indurated, red, tender lesions, usually in pulps of fingers or toes
• Peripheral emboli
• Conjunctival petechial haemorrhages (Fig. 13)
• Infective endophthalmitis
• Roth's spots: fundal haemorrhages with pale central area
• Microscopic haematuria.
Remember that peripheral signs are not present in all cases, particularly if the valve lesion is right sided.

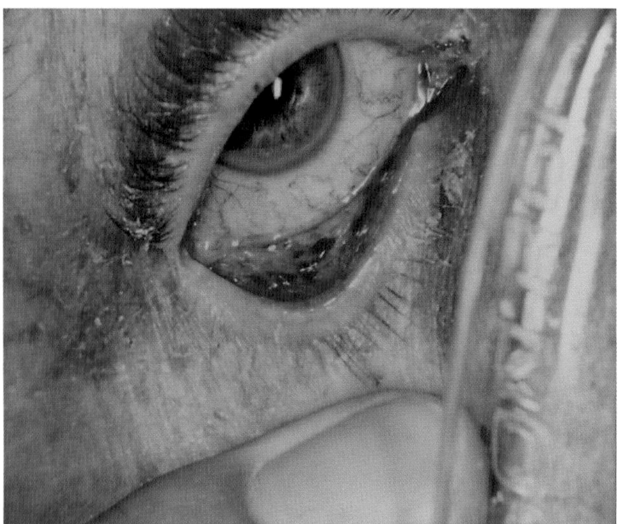

Fig. 13 Peripheral stigmata of endocarditis: subconjunctival haemorrhages.

Table 5 Aetiological agents in infective endocarditis.

Native valve	Common	Viridans streptococci *Staphylococcus aureus*
	Less common	Enterococci HACEK group of organisms β-Haemolytic streptococci Coliforms, pneumococci, fungi, *Brucella* spp., *Bartonella* spp., *Coxiella* spp. (Q fever), *Chlamydia* spp.
Prosthetic valve	Early after surgery	*Staphylococcus epidermidis* *Staphylococcus aureus*
	Late, i.e. >1 year postoperatively	As with native valve
Intravenous drug users	Common	*Staphylococcus aureus*
	Less common	Gram-negative bacilli, *Haemophilus* spp., *Bacillus* spp., *Corynebacterium* spp., fungi

HACEK, *Haemophilus* spp., *Actinobacillus* spp., *Cardiobacterium* spp., *Eikenella* spp. and *Kingella* spp.

Approach to investigation and management

If cardiac failure has developed in the context of an early diastolic murmur, this suggests acute aortic valve insufficiency. This is a medical emergency and the patient should be immediately referred for a cardiothoracic surgical opinion. (See *Cardiology*, Section 1.13.)

Treat hypotension and heart failure urgently (see *Emergency medicine*, Sections 1.2 and 1.5), then establish whether endocarditis is present and treat.

Investigations

Blood tests

FBC, electrolytes, renal and liver function, CRP, ESR and arterial blood gases are essential. You may wish to test for HIV and hepatitis B and C with consent from the patient.

Blood cultures

These must be taken before antibiotic therapy: ideally three sets separated in space and time (see Section 3.2, p. 151). The isolation of the aetiological agent (Table 5) is the key to managing infective endocarditis because it helps to guide therapy.

Imaging

Is there obvious pneumonia on the chest radiograph? Diffuse patchy changes or abscesses would be in keeping with septic emboli secondary to right-sided endocarditis. Look at the apices and remember TB in this population. If the chest radiograph is normal, think of pulmonary emboli and consider proceeding to spiral CT or ventilation–perfusion scanning. (See *Respiratory medicine*, Section 3.6.5 and *Cardiology*, Section 3.10.)

ECG

Particularly note conduction abnormalities, e.g. long PR interval, because this is associated with aortic root abscess. Look for right heart strain in pulmonary embolism.

Echocardiography

This is an essential investigation to assess valve function and look for supportive evidence of endocarditis (Figs 14 and 15). However, remember that:

- echocardiography cannot exclude endocarditis
- the transthoracic approach is less sensitive than the transoesophageal, particularly when looking at the right side of the heart and the aortic root

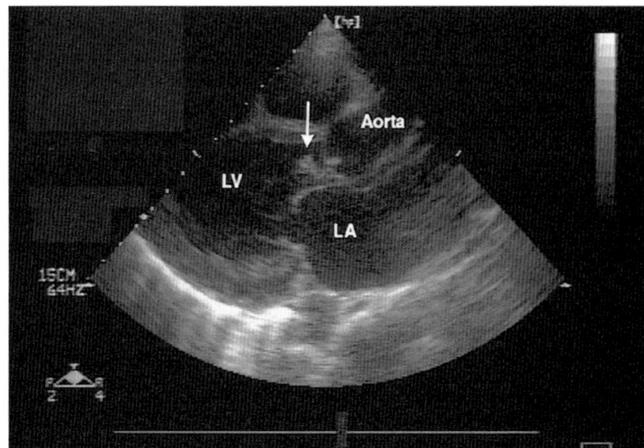

Fig. 14 Transthoracic echocardiogram showing a vegetation on the aortic valve.

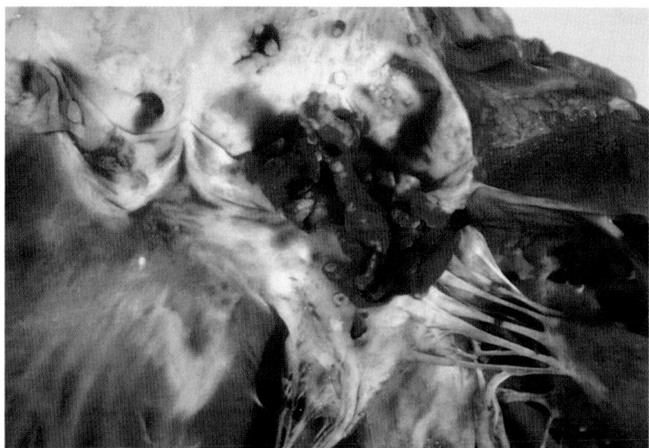

Fig. 15 Pathology specimen showing a vegetation on the aortic valve.

Table 6 The Duke criteria for the diagnosis of endocarditis. Definite diagnosis requires two major, or one major and three minor, or five minor criteria.

Major	Positive blood culture:
	2 with a typical organism, e.g. *Staphylococcus aureus,* viridans streptococci
	Persistently positive cultures (2 12 h apart, or 3 over >1 h) with compatible organism
	Endocardial involvement
	New regurgitant murmur
	Positive echocardiogram
Minor	Predisposing cardiac lesion or intravenous drug use
	Fever
	Vascular phenomena: petechiae, emboli, mycotic aneurysms
	Immunological phenomena: glomerulonephritis, Roth's spots, etc.
	Echocardiogram consistent with infective endocarditis, but not meeting major criteria
	Positive blood cultures but not meeting major criteria or serological evidence of active infection with plausible organism

• serial echocardiography may detect complications such as valve destruction and intramyocardial abscess formation requiring surgical intervention.

Management

The management of pneumonia (see Section 1.4, p. 10) and severe bacterial sepsis (see Section 1.2, p. 5) is covered elsewhere.

Endocarditis

The diagnosis of infective endocarditis is clinical and based on the combination of cardiac, embolic and infective features, along with isolation of an appropriate organism from the blood, as shown in Table 6 [1].

The aim of antimicrobial treatment is to eradicate valvular infection, which requires prolonged intravenous bactericidal therapy [2,3] (see *Cardiology*, Section 1.13). Combination therapy, with two drugs for synergy, has been proved to be better than monotherapy for streptococci. Close liaison with diagnostic microbiology is essential. In addition to standard antimicrobial susceptibility testing, the minimal inhibitory concentration (MIC) of the infecting organism should be measured to guide treatment options and length of therapy (Table 7). Culture negative endocarditis poses a particular therapeutic challenge [4]. Initial therapy should be based on the clinical picture with specialist advice.

Surgical intervention is indicated for failure of medical therapy, severe valve damage or intracardiac abscess formation, and where systemic emboli continue despite adequate medical therapy. Surgical removal of the valve is more often required in endocarditis on a prosthetic valve or in infection resulting from fungi or *Brucella* spp., or in Q fever.

Table 7 Antimicrobial therapy of common causes of endocarditis.

Organism	Therapeutic options	Duration (weeks)
Viridans streptococci: highly susceptible to penicillin	Benzylpenicillin 12–16 g/day	4
	Benzylpenicillin + gentamicin 3 mg/kg per day*	2
	Vancomycin 15 mg/kg twice daily*	4
Viridans streptococci and *Strep. bovis.* Partially penicillin resistant MIC >0.1 mg/L	Benzylpenicillin + gentamicin*	4, stopping gentamicin after first 2
Enterococci	Vancomycin*	4
	Ampicillin or benzylpenicillin + gentamicin	4–6†
	Vancomycin + gentamicin	4–6†
Vancomycin-resistant enterococci (VRE)	Seek specialist advice urgently	
Staphylococcus aureus: sensitive to flucloxacillin	Flucloxacillin 8–16 g/day; consider adding a second agent	4–6
Methicillin-resistant *Staphylococcus aureus* (MRSA)	Vancomycin*	4–6

*Monitor therapeutic drug levels. (See Section 1.37, p. 89.)
†Increased risk of renal and ototoxicity.
MIC, minimal inhibitory concentration.

Septic thrombophlebitis

Incise and drain any collections. Anticoagulation and prolonged antibiotic therapy may be required for infected thrombus. Rarely, surgical intervention is required for prolonged sepsis and embolization.

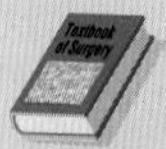

See *Cardiology*, Section 1.13.

1 Durack DT, Lukes AS, Bright DK *et al.* New criteria for diagnosis of infective endocarditis: utilization of specific echocardiographic findings. *Am J Med* 1994; 96: 200–209.
2 Wilson WR, Karchmer AW, Dajani AS *et al.* Antibiotic treatment of adults with infective endocarditis due to streptococci, enterococci, staphylococci and HACEK organisms. 1995 *JAMA*; 274: 1706–1713.
3 Kaye D. Treatment of infective endocarditis. *Ann Intern Med* 1996; 124: 606–608.
4 Barnes PD, Crook DWM. Culture negative endocarditis. *J Infect* 1997; 35: 209–213.

1.9 Fever and heart failure

Case history

A 19-year-old woman has a 'flu-like illness followed by breathlessness and chest pain. On examination, there is a scratchy pericardial rub and evidence of biventricular failure.

Clinical approach

When dealing with any patient presenting with chest pain, it is essential quickly to exclude life-threatening causes such as myocardial infarction, aortic dissection and pulmonary embolism. Both myocardial infarction and aortic dissection would be extremely improbable in a woman of this age. Pulmonary embolism would be more likely, but in this patient the presumptive diagnosis is viral myocarditis [1]. This, however, is a difficult diagnosis to prove definitively, so the priority must be to exclude other treatable causes.

History of the presenting problem

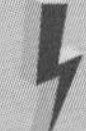

Chest pain in a young woman

- Acute myocardial infarction is unlikely but can present at this age as a result of either inherited lipid disorders or major thrombophilic states such as those that may complicate systemic lupus erythematosus (SLE) or Behçet's disease.
- Consider aortic dissection if features of Marfan's syndrome are present.

When taking the history, consider other causes of chest pain (see *Emergency medicine*, Section 1.3 and *Cardiology*, Section 1.5), but bear in mind the causes of myocarditis (Table 8). It is very important to establish when the disease started—this is important in interpreting serology and helps put progression into context, which is important for identifying those with a poor prognosis.

Symptoms relating to diagnosis

Systemic symptoms such as fever, rigors, weight loss and lethargy suggest an infectious aetiology. Ask about other features of viral infection, including rash, sore throat, headache and diarrhoea, although these features are clearly very non-specific. Joint pains are common, but arthritis is more suggestive of connective tissue disease. Severe muscle pain or marked weakness may be the result of infective myositis, but consider primary muscle disease.

Could this woman have had a pulmonary embolus? Ask about risk factors, pleuritic chest pain (which can be difficult

Table 8 Causes of myocarditis.

Type		Examples
Infectious	Viral	Common: enteroviruses e.g. Coxsackie A and B, polio and echo viruses Less common: influenza, CMV, EBV, hepatitis B, HIV
	Bacterial	Lyme disease. Myocarditis can rarely complicate systemic staphylococcal, streptococcal, meningococcal, mycoplasma and rickettsial infections Bacterial toxin-mediated, e.g. diphtheria
	Parasitic	Toxoplasmosis (immunocompromised host), American trypanosomiasis (Chagas' disease), trichinosis
	Fungal	Histoplasmosis, disseminated fungal infections in immunocompromised host
Non-infectious	Connective tissue diseases	Systemic lupus erythematosus (SLE), dermatomyositis, rheumatoid arthritis
	Idiopathic	Sarcoidosis, Kawasaki's disease, giant cell myocarditis
	Toxins	Scorpion bite
	Drugs	Alcohol, cocaine, daunorubicin, cyclophosphamide, doxorubicin
	Endocrine	Thyrotoxicosis, phaeochromocytoma

CMV; cytomegalovirus; EBV, Epstein–Barr virus; HIV, human immunodeficiency virus.

or impossible to distinguish from pericarditic pain), haemoptysis and leg pain/swelling. (See *Cardiology*, Section 1.9.)

Symptoms relating to cardiac failure

The fever and chest pain could be the result of uncomplicated pericarditis (see *Cardiology*, Section 1.14), but the development of heart failure indicates probable myocardial involvement. It is therefore important to document these symptoms, to confirm the diagnosis and to form a baseline against which to judge disease progression. Ask about breathlessness, orthopnoea, palpitations, ankle swelling and syncope. (See *Cardiology*, Section 1.6.)

Other history

Take note of the following:
• Family history, particularly of muscle and connective tissue diseases
• Alcohol and recreational drugs, particularly cocaine, which can lead to cardiac failure
• Travel history is essential: a number of unusual infections can lead to myocarditis (see Table 8)
• HIV risk factors: see Section 1.24, p. 61
• Risk factors for coronary artery disease.

Relevant past history

Previous cancer treatment, both chemotherapy and radiotherapy, can lead to delayed cardiomyopathy, but fever would be unusual. Current and past drug therapy are also important.

Examination

The aim here is twofold:
1 Assess the degree of cardiac impairment
2 Seek clues as to the precipitating cause.

Cardiovascular system

Note the following:
• Tachycardia that may be out of proportion to the degree of fever
• Signs of cardiac tamponade, e.g. very high JVP, pulsus paradoxus (see *Cardiology*, Sections 1.8 and 2.6.2)
• Signs of heart failure (see *Cardiology* Section 1.6)
• Listen for a pericardial friction rub and cardiac murmurs—functional valvular regurgitation is common in myocardial failure.

Systemic examination

A full physical examination is required, with particular attention to the following:
• Throat: inflammation suggests a viral aetiology (e.g. Coxsackie virus)
• Lymph nodes/liver/spleen
• Joints: looking for synovitis
• Features of acute rheumatic fever.

Approach to investigation and management

The aim is to assess and treat myocardial dysfunction while looking for treatable underlying diseases. For most of the infectious causes of myocarditis, no specific antimicrobial therapy is available.

Investigations

Blood tests

• FBC, electrolytes, renal and liver function, inflammatory markers (ESR, CRP). Most viral infections will show modest lymphocytosis with mild-to-modest elevation of the CRP. A high ESR points to an inflammatory process but is very non-specific. Renal impairment indicates a poor prognosis.
• Cardiac enzymes may be elevated and mimic myocardial infarction. Furthermore, skeletal muscle involvement may increase total creatine phosphokinase (CPK) in the absence of myocardial disease. Thus, ask for myocardial specific tests such as the creatine kinase fraction CK-MB or troponin T, and follow sequential measurements; in myocarditis, the enzymes will tend to remain elevated or rise, whereas in myo-cardial infarction the enzymes will fall after the acute event.
• Autoantibodies such as antinuclear antibody (ANA), double-stranded DNA (dsDNA) and ANCA as appropriate. (See *Rheumatology and clinical immunology*, Section 3.2.)

Cultures and serology

• Blood cultures in all cases, along with culture of pleural or pericardial fluid if available.
• Serology: take an acute sample and make sure the date of onset is clear to the lab. Single elevated titres may be indicative of Coxsackie virus or influenza. IgM tests are available for CMV and EBV. Rickettsial infection (in the appropriate setting of foreign travel) can be diagnosed with IgM, although this test will not be available immediately in most hospitals in the UK. Make sure that arrangements are in place to take a follow-up sample after 10–14 days to confirm a rise in titre.

ECG

There may be widespread ST segment changes (see *Cardiology*, Section 1.14), with T-wave inversion. These do not follow the normal evolution of changes seen in myocardial ischaemia and may last for weeks.

Imaging

• Chest radiograph may reveal a large heart, resulting either from dilatation or from pericardial effusion, and pulmonary congestion/oedema.
• Echocardiogram should be obtained urgently to assess the degree of ventricular dilatation and dysfunction, and also to look for a pericardial effusion. Serial echocardiography can follow disease progression and response to therapy [2].
• If there is clinical suspicion of pulmonary embolism, ventilation–perfusion scanning or CT angiography will be required.

Histology

The gold standard for diagnosis of myocarditis is an endomyocardial biopsy, but this is very rarely performed. Histology may reveal inflammatory changes accompanied by lymphocytic infiltration (Fig. 16) and can also be used to provide tissue for analysis for viral genome by PCR or *in situ* hybridization (see *Genetics and molecular medicine*, Sections 3 and 4).

Management

In viral myocarditis the treatment is supportive. The treatment of ventricular failure will depend on its severity (see *Cardiology*, Section 1.6). No antiviral therapy has been shown to be effective. The use of corticosteroids is controversial. There are no clear data showing efficacy and, in acute viral myocarditis, corticosteroids may accelerate disease progression. Most cases will resolve spontaneously over weeks or months, but a minority may progress to severe cardiac failure and death unless heart transplantation is considered. Long-term prognosis following fulminant myocarditis is generally good and aggressive supportive care is justified [3]. Some patients develop a chronic dilated cardiomyopathy, but although this has an inflammatory basis there is no benefit shown from trials of immunosuppression [4].

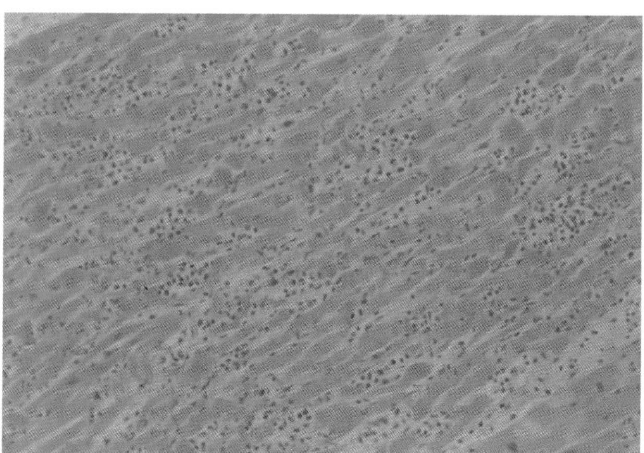

Fig. 16 Cardiac histology from a fatal case of viral myocarditis in a 48-year-old man. High power view showing disordered and apoptotic myocytes with a marked lymphocytic infiltrate. (Courtesy of Dr M Falzon, Ealing Hospital.)

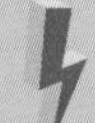

Do not miss rare cases of autoimmune myocarditis. Always consider this diagnosis and investigate accordingly because immunosuppression may reverse the condition or prevent further deterioration [5].

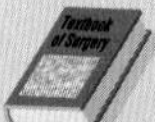

See *Cardiology*, Section 1.14.

1 Dec GW Jr, Palacios IF, Fallon JT *et al.* Active myocarditis in the spectrum of acute dilated cardiomyopathies. Clinical features, histological correlates, and clinical outcome. *N Engl J Med* 1985; 312: 885–890.
2 Felker GM, Boehmer JP, Hruban RH *et al.* Echocardiographic findings in fulminant and acute myocarditis. *J Am Coll Cardiol* 2000; 36: 227–232.
3 Lange LG, Schreiner GF. Immune mechanisms of cardiac disease. *N Engl J Med* 1994; 330: 1129–1135.
4 McCarthy RE III, Boehmer JP, Hruban RH *et al.* Long-term outcome of fulminant myocarditis as compared with acute (non-fulminant) myocarditis *N Engl J Med* 2000; 342: 690–695.
5 Mason JW, O'Connell JB, Herskowitz A *et al.* Clinical trial of immunosuppressive therapy for myocarditis. *N Engl J Med* 1995; 333: 269.

1.10 Still feverish after 6 weeks

Case history

You are referred a 49-year-old teacher with persistent fever. Symptoms started 6 weeks earlier; no cause has been found despite investigation by the GP.

Clinical approach

For practical purposes, the term 'pyrexia of unknown origin' (PUO) can be applied to patients with documented fever for which no cause has been found after a period of investigation [1]. A systematic approach to the problem is required: the clinical scenario will alter the likely aetiology, e.g. infection is much the likeliest cause in the returning traveller, the immunocompromised host or when the fever has developed within the hospital [2–4]. Endocarditis, extrapulmonary TB and occult abscesses (commonly intra-abdominal) need careful consideration, but non-infectious causes of fever must not be neglected (Table 9).

Table 9 Some non-infectious causes of fever.

Non-infectious cause	Common or important examples
Malignancies	Lymphoma Renal cell carcinoma Hepatoma Atrial myxoma
Autoimmune rheumatic disorders	Systemic lupus erythematosus, polyarteritis nodosa Adult Still's disease
Granulomatous diseases	Granulomatous hepatitis Sarcoidosis Crohn's disease Giant cell arteritis/polymyalgia rheumatica
Hyperthermia	Malignant neuroleptic syndrome
Drugs	Phenytoin, rifampicin, azathioprine
Inherited disorders	Familial Mediterranean fever
Factitious	Munchhausen's syndrome
Other	Thromboembolic disease

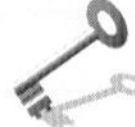

Pyrexia of unknown origin

- Confirm that the patient really has a fever
- A thorough review of the history is essential—occupation, travel history, pets, contacts (e.g. TB), medication, recreational drug use, past history and family history
- Detailed clinical examination
- Careful analysis of the results of investigations.

History of the presenting problem

A detailed history is required:
- Has pyrexia been documented? (See Section 1.1, p. 3.)
- For how long have the symptoms been present? In general, the longer the duration of symptoms the less likely infection is.
- Periodicity of fever? Intermittent attacks suggest a non-infectious inflammatory process, e.g. familial Mediterranean fever or cyclical neutropenia.
- Weight loss should always be taken seriously and usually indicates serious infection or malignancy.
- Detailed systems enquiry is needed because specific symptoms may point to a focus of infection or abnormal organ system, e.g. cough, headache, rash, arthralgia, diarrhoea, dysuria, urethral discharge.

Exposure

Occupation

- Vets and farmers: Q fever, brucellosis
- Sewer workers: leptospirosis.

Travel history

- Where? Think of malaria and visceral leishmaniasis if the patient has recently travelled to the tropics. (See Section 1.20, p. 52.)
- When? Need to know incubation periods.
- What was he exposed to? If unpasteurized milk, think of brucellosis; if freshwater exposure, think of schistosomiasis.

Pets

- Cats: toxoplasmosis, cat scratch disease (*Bartonella henselae*)
- Parrots: psittacosis.

Additional clues

- Medication: drug fever.
- 'Foreign bodies': does the patient have any indwelling prostheses, e.g. heart valves, joint replacements or metalwork from previous surgery?
- Age: neoplasia and giant cell arteritis/polymyalgia rheumatica are more common in elderly people.

Relevant past history

Immunocompromise, previous surgery and previous illnesses may be relevant.

Examination

A thorough examination is essential. Take particular note of the following:
- Temperature: is there really a fever? If the patient is an outpatient, give him a temperature chart and show him how to fill it in.
- Rash, e.g. erythema chronicum migrans in Lyme disease, evanescent macular rash of Still's disease.
- Mouth: check for signs of dental disease, systemic illness (Fig. 17) or immunosuppression.
- Ears, throat and sinuses for evidence of infection.
- Lungs for evidence of infection or neoplasm.
- Cardiac murmurs and signs of infective endocarditis. (See Section 1.8, p. 20.)
- Hepatosplenomegaly or any abdominal masses.
- Lymphadenopathy: lymphoma, TB, glandular fever.
- Joints for evidence of arthritis: connective tissue disease.
- Genitourinary examination: see Sections 1.31, p. 76 and 1.33, p. 81. TB may cause epididymo-orchitis. A tender prostate suggests prostatitis. In women, pelvic infection is often overlooked.
- Fundoscopy with dilated pupils looking for retinitis, ophthalmitis, Roth's spots or choroidal tubercles.

Approach to investigation and management

Almost by definition, patients with PUO do not have an obvious focus of infection, but you should not and cannot simply perform every available investigation. The history,

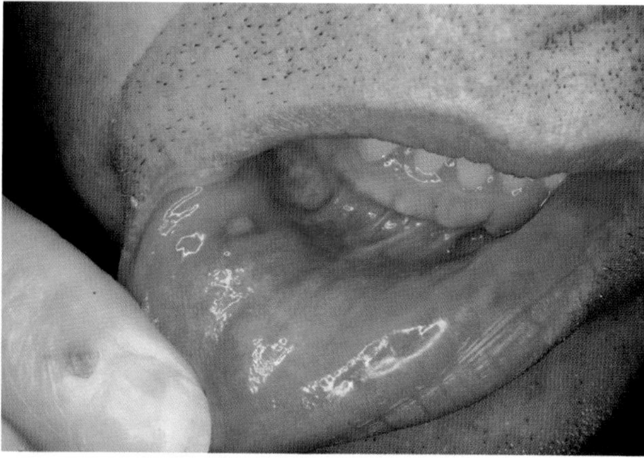

(a)

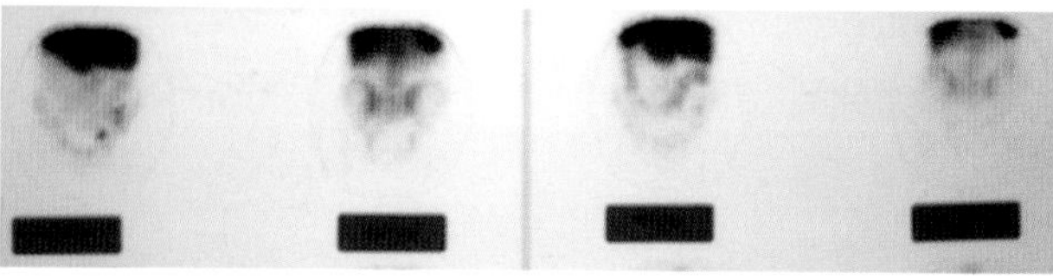

(b)

Fig. 17 (a) A 58-year-old man with a 17-year history of fever, fatigue and aphthous mouth ulcers as shown. Many investigations had been negative until he developed right iliac fossa pain. (b) Indium-111-labelled white blood cell scan showing increased uptake in the area of the caecum. A subsequent barium study suggested Crohn's disease, which was confirmed at laparotomy.

examination and initial investigations should be used as pieces of a jigsaw puzzle to direct you towards an area in which to focus your diagnostic efforts. If the patient is generally well, investigation can be undertaken as an outpatient, but admission may be required for invasive procedures or, on occasion, to document the fever.

Investigations

Blood tests

- FBC and review of a blood film.
- Urea and renal function tests.
- Liver function tests: some causes of hepatitis may present with PUO; in addition, liver function tests can provide a clue to occult biliary sepsis or hepatic infiltration with infection or malignancy.
- Thyroid function tests: may be abnormal in subacute thyroiditis. Hyperthyroidism is not associated with pyrexia but patients often complain of 'fever'.
- ESR or CRP: relatively non-specific markers of inflammation but, if abnormal, can be followed sequentially. In acute SLE, the CRP is often normal with a markedly elevated ESR. The CRP is raised during attacks of familial Mediterranean fever.
- Autoimmune screen where clinically indicated. (See *Rheumatology and clinical immunology*, Section 3.2.)
- Protein electrophoresis: tumour markers as clinically indicated.
- Serum angiotensin-converting enzyme (ACE) is elevated in granulomatous disorders, but is non-specific and may be raised in TB and lymphoma as well as sarcoidosis.

Cultures and serology

- Blood cultures: essential in all cases. (See Section 3.2, p. 151.)
- Urine dipstick, microscopy and bacterial culture: the presence of proteinuria and/or haematuria might indicate renal inflammation and support a diagnosis of autoimmune or vasculitic illness, but would also be consistent with glomerulonephritis associated with infection, particularly endocarditis. Consider three early morning urine samples for TB smear and culture if white cells are present in urine with no bacterial growth.
- Bacterial, TB and fungal culture of any biopsy specimens.
- Culture any wounds and other body fluids, e.g. cerebrospinal fluid (CSF), as clinically indicated.
- Serology: acute and convalescent samples as clinically indicated for EBV, CMV, HIV, *Coxiella burnetii*, *Mycoplasma pneumoniae*, toxoplasmosis, brucellosis, *Borrelia burgdorferi*.

Imaging

- Chest radiograph: look for evidence of infection, TB, lymphadenopathy or neoplasia.
- Ultrasonography, CT or MRI: look for occult abscesses, neoplasms or intra-abdominal lymphadenopathy. Chest and abdominal CT should be considered where lymphoma is suspected.
- Echocardiography: where endocarditis is suspected; it may also detect atrial myxoma. Low yield if the cardiac examination is normal.
- Ventilation–perfusion scanning or phlebography, where thromboembolic disease is suspected
- Nuclear medicine imaging may be helpful in selected cases. Radiolabelled white cell scans may detect focal bacterial infection and inflammatory bowel disease (see Fig. 17). Gallium-67 injection labels macrophages and can detect chronic inflammatory lesions and granulomatous diseases.

Invasive procedures

Use in a targeted manner in response to finding an abnormality. Biopsy of lymph node, liver, skin lesions, bone marrow and an intra-abdominal or thoracic mass are most commonly performed. Always request both histology and culture (including TB) of biopsy specimens.

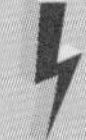

Before performing invasive tests, such as CSF analysis or tissue biopsies, check exactly what material is required in the laboratory. You do not want to have to repeat an investigation because the specimen was not handled properly.

Other tests

• Mantoux or Heaf test (see Section 3.2, p. 151).

Management

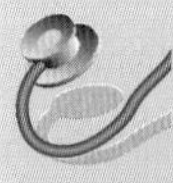

Therapeutic trials

The temptation to commence the patient with PUO on empirical antibiotic therapy should be resisted unless they are severely ill. However, once a reasonably secure clinical diagnosis has been established, there may be a place for judicious trials of appropriate therapy.

Specific treatment of the patient with PUO depends on identifying the diagnosis and targeting therapy appropriately. Therapeutic trials should be avoided unless all other approaches have failed. It is important to recognize that a significant proportion of patients remain undiagnosed. Warn the patient of this at the onset of investigations. If this happens, fully review the case; if the patient is stable it is often best to stop investigations and carefully follow his or her progress. In general, the prognosis for prolonged PUO is good because infection and malignancy will usually declare themselves within a relatively short period of time.

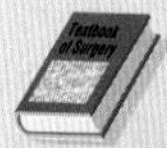

See *Rheumatology and clinical immunology*, Section 1.16.

1 Arnow PM, Flaherty JP. Fever of unknown origin. *Lancet* 1997; 350: 575–580.
2 Larson EB, Featherstone HJ, Petersdorf. Fever of undetermined origin: diagnosis and follow-up of 105 cases, 1970–80. *Medicine (Baltimore)* 1982; 61: 269–292.
3 Marik PE. Fever in the ICU. *Chest* 2000; 117: 855–869.
4 Armstrong WS, Katz JT, Kazanjian PH. Human immunodeficiency virus-associated fever of unknown origin: a study of 70 patients in the United States and review. *Clin Infect Dis* 1999; 28: 341–345.

1.11 Persistent fever in the ICU

Case history

You are asked to see a 20-year-old man who is being ventilated on the ICU. He was involved in a severe road traffic accident 4 weeks earlier and now has a persistent fever and elevated WCC.

Clinical approach

Infection will be the most likely cause of fever and leucocytosis, but do not ignore non-infectious problems such as gut ischaemia or adverse drug reactions. The 'EPIC' one-day snapshot of European ICUs revealed a point prevalence of infection of 60% [1]. The challenge when managing these patients is to locate and treat serious infection, while not overusing empirical broad-spectrum antimicrobial agents that increase the risk of antibiotic resistance and fungal superinfection [2].

History of the presenting problem

History-taking in this situation is very different to the usual practice: most patients are unconscious and most of the relevant information comes from events that have happened after hospitalization. As you look for clues, consider the following possibilities:

• Nosocomial pneumonia: hospital-acquired pneumonia is a common cause of fever in the ventilated patient. Organisms include *Strep. pneumoniae*, *Staph. aureus*, Enterobacteriaceae and *Pseudomonas aeruginosa*.
• Nosocomial UTI: *Escherichia coli* is the most common associated organism, but infection with *Proteus* spp., enterococci, *Klebsiella* spp. and *Pseudomonas* spp., and *Candida* spp. also occurs.
• Wound infection: you may well be the only person to take the trouble to uncover the wound.
• Intravascular line infection: multiple cannulae are used in intensive care and are a common source of fever in the ICU (Fig. 18). Organisms include *Staph. aureus* and *Staph. epidermidis* [3,4].
• Infection of a prosthesis: any foreign body is at risk of infection.
• Sinusitis: this may complicate nasogastric tube feeding.
• Fungal infection: persistent fever and deterioration despite broad-spectrum antibiotics.
• Thromboembolic disease: DVT or pulmonary emboli may occur in an immobilized patient despite prophylaxis.
• Drug fever.

Finding the information

Medical records

Thoroughly review the medical notes, intensive care charts and investigation results. These will tell you how long the fever has been present and give important information regarding procedures and complications, e.g. in this case you may discover that the patient had a base of skull fracture and may have meningitis or that blood transfusion-related infections must be considered.

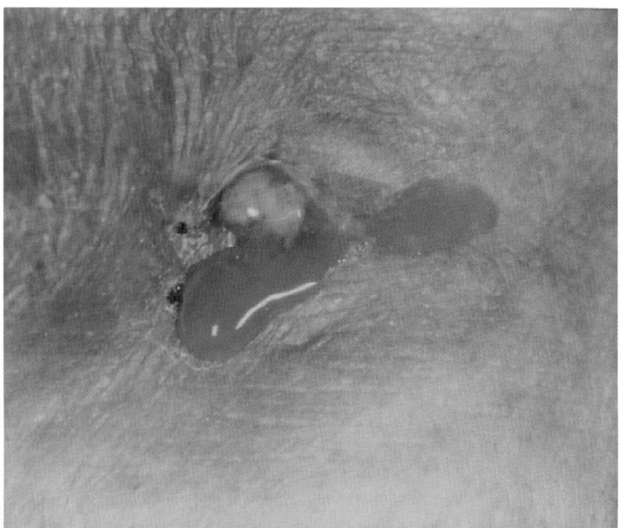

Fig. 18 Pus coming from a peripheral venous cannula site when the cannula was removed. The patient had been admitted with epilepsy and developed fever as he was discharged from intensive care to the ward. Methicillin-resistant *Staphylococcus aureus* (MRSA) was cultured.

Other staff

Talk to the nurses looking after the patient and ask specifically about changes in the skin (it is easy to miss the pressure areas), diarrhoea (*Clostridium difficile*) and the quantity/quality of the sputum. When were his various invasive lines placed or last changed? Also ask whether there have been any recent outbreaks of infection within the unit. If necessary, track down the various medical and surgical teams involved in his care because important information is often not in the notes.

Relevant past history

Previous medical/surgical conditions and severe immunocompromise can be relevant. You may need to talk to a family member or phone the patient's general practitioner.

Examination

General

If the patient is shocked, resuscitation and treatment are the priority, followed by a more detailed evaluation. As full a physical examination as possible is required: this will often have been omitted by your colleagues on the ICU, perhaps in the erroneous belief that all of the monitoring paraphernalia render it unnecessary, yet no monitor has been devised that will detect an abscess on someone's buttock. Take careful note of the following:

- Skin: for cellulitis around lines; check all wounds and pressure areas
- Lungs: for consolidation or pleural fluid
- Heart: for new murmurs suggesting endocarditis
- Legs: swelling suggestive of DVT
- Abdomen: new-onset ileus can indicate gut ischaemia or infective colitis; a palpable gall bladder suggests acalculous cholecystitis
- Ears, throat and sinuses: evidence of infection
- Fundoscopy, preferably with dilated pupils: may reveal candida endophthalmitis
- Urine: if cloudy, consider catheter-associated urinary tract infection.

Approach to investigation and management

Consider the 'usual suspects': infection of the respiratory tract, urinary tract, pressure areas and sites of surgery. If there is no apparent focus of infection and the patient is not haemodynamically compromised, stop all antibiotics with a view to reculturing.

Investigations

In many ways the process is similar to that described for the patient with PUO in Section 1.10, p. 26, with investigations looking for areas of abnormality to focus imaging and other diagnostic tests. The care of patients on the ICU should always be multidisciplinary, with review of the results of investigations with the relevant specialists.

Routine blood tests

These will often be persistently abnormal in intensive care, so concentrate on newly abnormal results and look for trends. This is a complicated situation and there may be many explanations for an abnormal value, e.g. a rising alkaline phosphatase may be the result of acalculous cholecystitis, cholangitis, liver abscess or transfusion-acquired viral infections, or simply be caused by drug-related cholestasis and be unrelated to the fever. Monitor organ function and acidosis because these will indicate the development of severe sepsis that requires urgent therapy.

Cultures

Ask the microbiology department to process all specimens urgently, and if possible review all of the culture results from this admission with the microbiologist.

- Blood cultures: essential in all cases. If a central line is *in situ*, take a set through the line and a further set peripherally (see Section 3.2, p. 151). Consider specific fungal blood cultures.
- Lower respiratory samples can be obtained by endotracheal aspiration or bronchoscopy in the ventilated patient. Such patients are usually colonized with bacteria, hence the results must be interpreted with caution. Do not forget TB which can reactivate in debilitated intensive care patients.

• Urinary microscopy and culture, but do not assume that simply because the urine culture is positive this is the cause of the fever.
• Take swabs from any wounds that appear infected.
• Culture any drain fluid and other body fluids as indicated.
• Culture any line tips that are removed.

Tranfusion-acquired infection

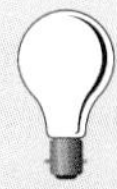

Trauma patients often receive multiple blood products. These can transmit CMV and parvovirus as well as hepatitis. Consider this possibility in persistent unexplained fever, particularly where the patient is leucopenic or has evidence of hepatitis.

Imaging

• Chest radiographs can be very difficult to interpret, particularly if the patient has ARDS, but any change from previous films should be taken seriously.
• Abdominal ultrasonography is technically difficult in intensive care but may detect cholecystitis and occult abscesses.
• CT of the chest and abdomen is increasingly used in intensive care to detect infectious foci.
• Echocardiography is used if endocarditis is suspected, but this will only help to confirm a clinical diagnosis and cannot exclude the condition. (See Section 1.8, p. 20.)

Management

This will depend on how unwell the patient is:
• If stable and no focus of infection is obvious, stop all antibiotics with a view to reculturing blood, urine and endotracheal aspirates. Remove all unnecessary intravascular lines and change others if possible (often line-related fever will abate).
• If clinically unstable and developing severe sepsis, you will need to consider empirical antibiotics. The choice is difficult and needs to be made in the light of the suspected site of infection, past and current therapy, local antibiotic policies and antimicrobial resistance patterns. Always take advice from the local microbiology laboratory.
• Fungal infection is being encountered more commonly in intensive care and adding empirical antifungal therapy, with amphotericin B, should be considered where the patient is deteriorating despite appropriate antibacterial therapy.

Need for surgical intervention

Deep-seated abscesses are unlikely to resolve without drainage either percutaneously or operatively. When such a patient is deteriorating despite antibiotics, you may need to push for surgical intervention. Do not accept the argument that 'they are too sick for an operation'—they are more likely to die without one if they have an undrained collection.

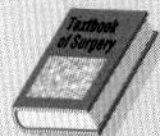

1 Vincent JL, Bihari DH, Suter PM *et al.* The prevalence of nosocomial infection in the intensive care units in Europe. Results of the EPIC study. *JAMA* 1995; 274: 639–644.
2 Rabinowitz RP, Fiore AE, Joshi M, Caplan ES. Multiple trauma. In: Mandell GL, Bennett JE, Dolin R (eds) *Principles and Practice of Infectious Diseases* (5th edn). Philadelphia: Churchill Livingstone, 2000: 3191–3197.
3 Oppenheim BA. Optimal management of central venous catheter-related infections—what is the evidence? *J Infect* 2000; 40: 26–30.
4 Marik PE. Fever in the ICU. *Chest* 2000; 117: 855–869.

1.12 Pyelonephritis

Case history

A GP asks you to review a young woman with high fever, rigors and loin pain.

Clinical approach

The presence of loin pain points to a diagnosis of pyelonephritis [1]. However, care must be taken to exclude other intra-abdominal and retroperitoneal pathologies. This may require investigation but, if the patient is unwell with presumed bacterial sepsis, 'blind' antimicrobial therapy is essential.

History of the presenting problem

Urinary tract infection

A history of typical urinary symptoms (frequency, dysuria, change in smell, urgency) is clearly a useful pointer here, but these are not always present, particularly in older patients, people with diabetes or those who have been partially treated. Urinary tract infections may be related to sexual activity, particularly in women [2], and tactful history-taking is required. (See Section 1.31, p. 76.)

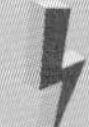

Patients with symptoms of lower urinary tract infection may also have infection of the upper urinary tract.

How sick is the patient?

This is a key question in determining the intensity of investigation and treatment. Were these true rigors where the patient could not control the shaking? Is there confusion or cardiovascular collapse, likely to indicate bacteraemia in this context? Nausea and vomiting are common features of any infection and may preclude oral therapy.

Type of pain

Site, type, radiation and intensity are essential features. Although described as loin pain, is this really the case? The strong presumption from the details given is that it is coming from the kidney, but pain in the general area of the loin could be the result of bony pain, superficial pain in the skin or soft tissue, radiated pain from the retroperitoneum or even a basal pneumonia. Colicky pain could be caused by a renal stone, or bowel or biliary tract disease.

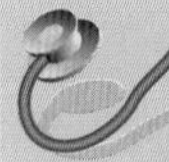

Do not forget shingles as a cause of unilateral pain starting in the back and radiating forward. The pain usually precedes the rash.

Other sources for the fever

Intra-abdominal sources may be suggested by a history of gastrointestinal disturbance, or features suggesting pancreatitis.

Pregnancy

The consequences of urinary tract infection are more significant in pregnant women, and the issue also has implications for radiological investigations and antibiotic therapy.

Relevant past history

The important aspects to cover are previous urinary or abdominal problems. Has the woman had previous urinary tract infections, renal stones, instrumentation of the urinary tract, or trauma and neurological diseases that may affect bladder function? Ask about diabetes and renal disease. Prior antibiotic use may increase the risk of antibiotic resistance. Allergies must not be forgotten.

Examination

General

Is the patient shocked, breathless or confused? These are all signs of severe sepsis that can complicate focal urinary infection or bacteraemia. Check pulse, BP, peripheral perfusion and respiratory rate. For details of the management of the patient with profound hypotension/septicaemia, see Section 1.2, p. 3 (see also *Emergency medicine*, Sections 1.2 and 1.28).

The back

As the complaint is of loin pain, sit the patient up and examine the renal angle and back:

- Is the pain in the renal angle?
- Is there bony tenderness?
- Is there swelling or erythema (suggesting local soft tissue swelling)?
- Is there a rash (e.g. the vesicles of shingles)?

The abdomen

- Look for scars and swellings
- Listen for bowel sounds
- Examine for local tenderness—is there peritonism?
- Is there hepatosplenomegaly?

Genitourinary examination

This is described in Sections 1.31, p. 78 and 1.33, p. 82. In all men with possible urinary tract infection (UTI), digital evaluation of the prostate is mandatory.

Do not miss a basal pneumonia and look for signs of endocarditis because a renal embolus may mimic pyelonephritis. This is extremely unlikely, but you'll never make the diagnosis unless you consider it.

Approach to investigation and management

Investigations

Blood tests

Check the FBC, electrolytes, renal and liver function tests, glucose and inflammatory markers (CRP). Impairment of renal function may be the result of chronic disease or severe bacterial sepsis. Check serum amylase if pancreatitis is possible.

Cultures

Take cultures of urine and blood (see Section 3.2, p. 151). Dipstick the urine, looking for urinary nitrites and leucocytes; these tests are specific and sensitive and should be positive in most cases of pyelonephritis. Send a midstream urine (MSU) specimen for microscopy and culture before antimicrobial therapy is started, except in those with severe sepsis in whom therapy is urgent.

Imaging

Imaging is not required immediately in uncomplicated pyelonephritis but should be performed urgently if there is renal impairment, or the patient is severely unwell or not responding to therapy. A plain radiograph may reveal a renal stone or rarely gas around the kidney (Fig. 19), but renal tract ultrasonography is the first-line modality. In suspected perinephric abscess, CT may provide more detail. A chest radiograph may be needed to avoid missing a lower lobe pneumonia.

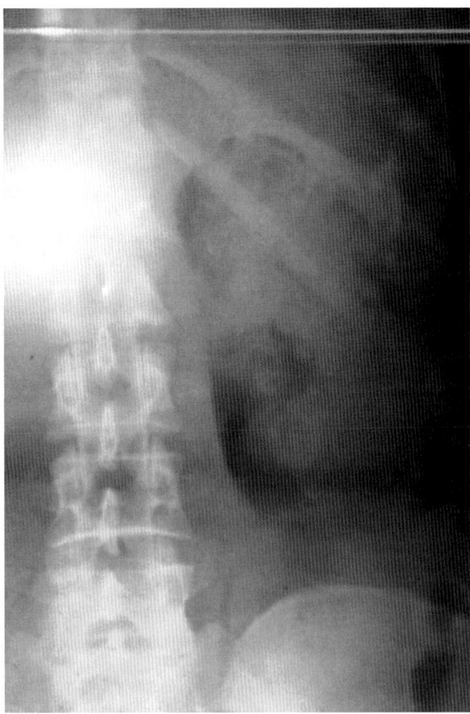

Fig. 19 Plain radiograph showing gas in and around the left kidney as a result of emphysematous pyelonephritis in a 43-year-old woman with diabetes. *Escherichia coli* was isolated from the blood and urine, and a left nephrectomy was required despite attempts to conserve the kidney.

Management

Most patients with pyelonephritis will need hospital admission, intravenous rehydration and intravenous antibiotics. Initial therapy will usually be given blind, unless there is a culture result available from a recent urine sample. Antibiotic regimens will vary according to local policies but consider the following [3].

Uncomplicated UTI

• Commonly *E. coli*, less commonly other Gram-negative organisms, enterococci and staphylococci.
• Keep duration of therapy (e.g. with trimethoprim 200 mg b.d. p.o.) to a minimum, i.e. 3 days in women, 7 days in men. Longer therapy is indicated in diabetes.

Pyelonephritis

• Commonly *E. coli* and occasionally other Gram-negative bacilli.
• Treat (e.g. with trimethoprim 200 mg b.d. p.o. or i.v., or ciprofloxacin 250–500 mg b.d. p.o. or 100–200 mg b.d. i.v.) for 10–14 days.

Structural renal tract abnormality

Escherichia coli is still common but there is an increased incidence of other enteric Gram-negative bacilli, *Pseudomonas aeruginosa* and enterococci. Treat for a minimum of 14 days.

Urinary catheter *in situ*

Escherichia coli is still common but the incidence of other enteric Gram-negative bacilli, *Ps. aeruginosa* and enterococci is higher. Treat for a minimum of 5 days unless there is evidence of upper tract disease.

Recurrent UTI

Suspect antimicrobial resistance. Evaluate for underlying diabetes or a renal tract abnormality.

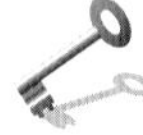

Renal obstruction with infection

• This is a medical emergency
• Urgent relief of obstruction is essential
• Anterograde nephrostomy is usually the preferred technique.

Ampicillin is a poor choice for blind therapy of UTI/pyelonephritis, as the prevalence of resistance among *E. coli* in the community is very high.

Symptoms should resolve rapidly. If they do not there may be antibiotic failure (this will be guided by the MSU which you took at presentation), local abscess formation or an obstructed kidney [4]. Priorities then are to reculture blood and urine and arrange for urgent ultrasonography or CT.

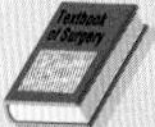

1 Hooton TM. Pathogenesis of urinary tract infections: an update. *J Antimicrob Chemother* 2000; 46(suppl A): 1–7.
2 Hooton TM, Scholes D, Hughes JP *et al.* A prospective study of risk factors for symptomatic urinary tract infection in young women. *N Engl J Med* 1996; 335: 468–474.
3 Warren JW; Abrutyn E; Hebel JR *et al.* Guidelines for antimicrobial treatment of uncomplicated acute bacterial cystitis and acute pyelonephritis in women. *Clin Infect Dis* 1999; 29: 745–758.
4 Fowler JE Jr, Perkins T. Presentation, diagnosis and treatment of renal abscesses: 1972–88. *J Urol* 1994; 151: 847–851.

1.13 A sore throat

Case history

A 32-year-old man developed a sore throat for which he took simple analgesia. The pain worsened over the next 2 days and he consults you requesting antibiotics.

Clinical approach

The differential diagnosis lies between bacterial and viral infections (Fig. 20). These may be distinguished clinically,

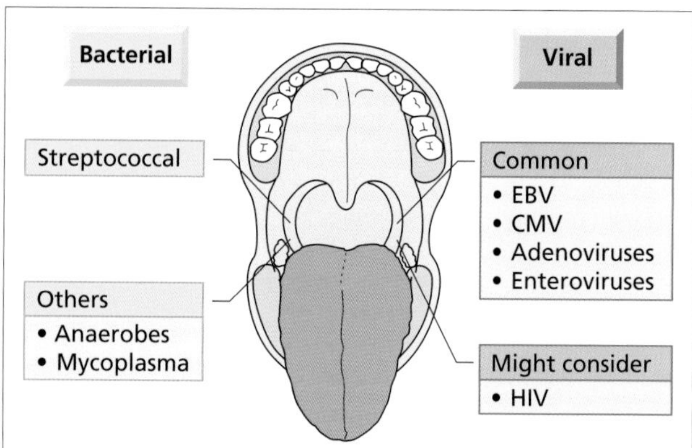

Fig. 20 Differential diagnosis of sore throat. EBV, Epstein–Barr virus; CMV, cytomegalovirus; HIV, human immunodeficiency virus.

but overlap substantially, and culture or serology is really required to make a definitive diagnosis. Throat infections are often trivial and settle spontaneously, but more serious conditions, including pharyngeal abscess [1], epiglottitis and neutropenic sepsis, need to be considered.

History of the presenting problem

Assessing the severity

This is important not only for diagnosis and in guiding treatment, but also for basic supportive measures. With increasing tonsillar and local tissue swelling, some patients may become unable to eat or drink, finally developing stridor and even requiring tracheostomy in extreme cases.

Local problem

Most patients with a sore throat will have a fever. Marked systemic symptoms with myalgia and neck pain are common in streptococcal throat infections. Viral infections are commonly associated with systemic symptoms, including those related to hepatitis (nausea, lethargy), or rarely neurological symptoms.

Likely source

There may be no obvious source despite the fact that the common viral infections are passed from person to person by saliva. CMV and EBV are often asymptomatic if acquired young but associated with local and systemic disease if in adulthood. HIV seroconversion may present with sore throat (see Section 1.24, p. 61). Coxsackie virus infections may occur in outbreaks.

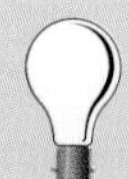

Sexually transmitted infection

Neisseria gonorrhoeae can present with a sore throat and exudative pharyngitis.

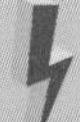

Diphtheria

- Consider if there has been recent travel from eastern Europe or a developing country
- Look for a grey pseudomembrane in the posterior pharynx.

Relevant past history

Some patients have recurrent bacterial throat infections and this may simply be another presentation of the same syndrome. A past history of 'glandular fever' might make EBV unlikely, although in the absence of documented serology you should not be put off this diagnosis.

Examination

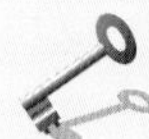

Examine the whole patient, not just the throat. A corollary of this is not to forget to examine the throat carefully in patients with systemic disease.

Assess level of illness

The most important aspects are the following:
- Check vital signs: temperature, pulse, BP, respiration.
- Check the airway: is there stridor? Is the patient able to swallow? Is he or she dribbling? If so, get urgent assistance from an ENT specialist or anaesthetist. (See *Respiratory medicine*, Section 1.14.)

The throat

Pharyngitis is very non-specific. Pus or exudate does not reliably differentiate between viral and bacterial infections. Severe unilateral tonsillar swelling with a pointing lesion ('quinsy') suggests local bacterial infection. The presence of small petechiae on the palate may indicate viral infection, as do vesicular lesions that are typical of 'herpangina' caused by Coxsackie viruses. White plaques suggest candidiasis. Oral candida infection is not associated with fever, but is a sign of underlying immunodeficiency and needs to be taken very seriously in this context (see Section 1.28, p. 70).

Local disease

Feel for local lymph nodes and note their size and tenderness. Look for a tender swelling associated with internal jugular vein thrombosis in Lemierre's syndrome.

Systemic disease

Epstein–Barr virus is associated with a number of clinical syndromes (see Section 2.10.4, p. 129). Look for hepatic, neurological and haematological complications, and in particular, feel for a spleen. CMV may produce a similar

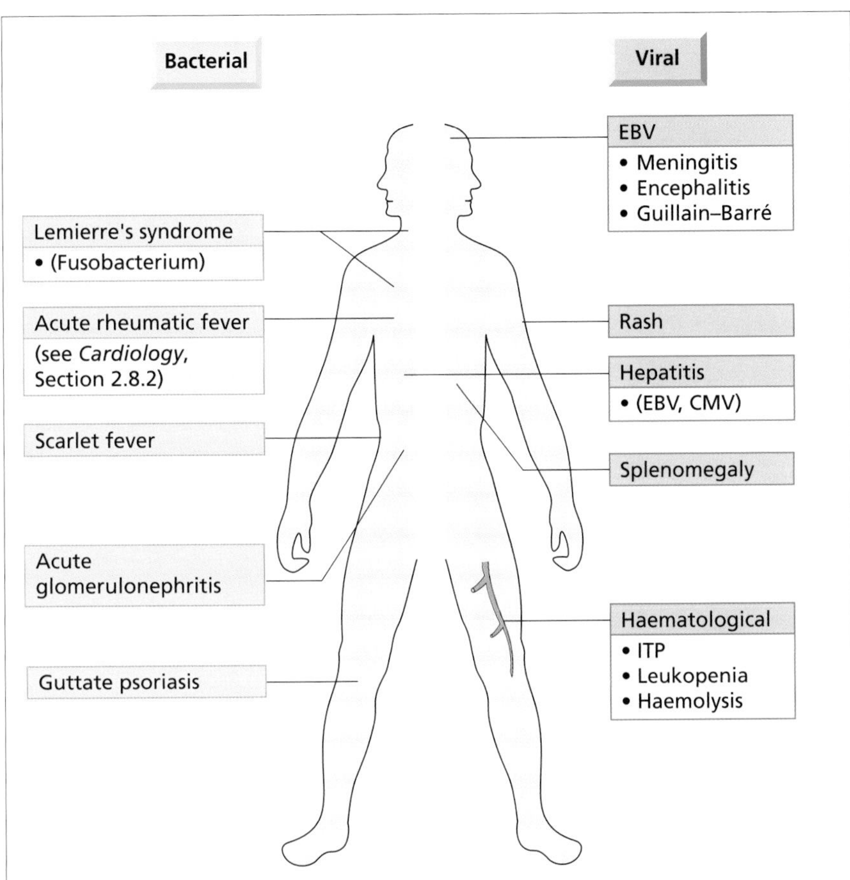

Fig. 21 Systemic complications of throat infections. CMV, cytomegalovirus; EBV, Epstein–Barr virus; ITP, idiopathic thrombocytopenic purpura.

pattern. The systemic consequences of group A streptococcal (GAS) disease include scarlet fever, acute glomerulonephritis, acute rheumatic fever and guttate psoriasis (Fig. 21).

Rash

Streptococcal infections may be associated with the rash of 'scarlet fever' (fine erythematous macules mainly over the body, associated with circumoral pallor and a coated 'strawberry' tongue). CMV and EBV may produce a fine macular rash, although the most striking rash associated with EBV is that produced after amoxicillin therapy, which for this reason should never be given as treatment for a sore throat. This is not associated with allergy to other penicillins.

Lemierre's disease is caused by polymicrobial infection of the posterior pharyngeal space and characterized by the isolation of *Fusobacterium necrophorum*. Local throat disease is associated with thrombosis of the internal jugular vein and metastatic spread of infection, particularly to the lungs.

Approach to investigation and management

Investigations

The intensity of investigation will largely depend on how unwell the patient is, but also to some degree on his or her desire to obtain an accurate diagnosis. The following tests should be considered.

Blood tests

• FBC: revealing neutrophilia in bacterial infections, and atypical lymphocytes in acute EBV or CMV infection. Haemolysis may complicate EBV.
• Inflammatory markers: a high CRP is most consistent with bacterial infection.
• Liver function tests: may show a hepatitic picture with EBV and CMV.
• Monospot and Paul–Bunnell tests: these can rapidly diagnose EBV infection. Positives may also occur with other viral infections, including CMV and hepatitis B. Serology is essential if the diagnosis is not clearly bacterial (Table 10).

Cultures

Send throat swab for bacterial culture (see Section 3.1, p. 150). Routine viral swabs are not performed but can yield entero-viruses, and viral culture is important when mouth ulcers are present to detect herpes viruses. Blood cultures are required if there are severe systemic symptoms or if neutropenia is present.

Table 10 Serological investigations of use in pharyngitis.

Organism	Test	Interpretation
Streptococci	ASOT	Titres >1 : 800 significant. May be higher in children
	DNAase	Less commonly positive in pharyngeal infection.
Epstein–Barr virus	GF test	Positive in acute EBV
	EBNA	Suggests past infection
	EBV IgM*	Positive in acute EBV
Cytomegalovirus	CMV IgM*	Positive in acute CMV

*Occasional crossreactivity.
ASOT, anti-streptolysin O titre; GF, glandular fever; EBNA, Epstein–Barr nuclear antigen; EBV, Epstein–Barr virus; CMV, cytomegalovirus.

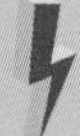

Neutropenic sepsis often presents with fever and a sore throat and should be considered in all cases. Has the patient recently been started on a new medication? See *Haematology*, Sections 1.6 and 1.7.

Imaging

This is only necessary when stridor, severe dysphagia or marked neck swelling is present. A lateral neck radiograph can assess the epiglottis and detect retropharyngeal swelling. CT or MRI of the neck is indicated to assess retropharyngeal abscess or Lemierre's syndrome [2].

Management

In uncomplicated viral or bacterial pharyngitis, there is little evidence that antimicrobial therapy is of more than modest benefit and over-prescribing encourages antibiotic resistance. The patient should be given symptomatic advice and warned to return if his condition deteriorates [3].

Antibiotics are indicated for marked local disease with proven or suspected streptococcal infection. Ampicillin should be avoided in empirical therapy. Phenoxymethylpenicillin 250 mg four times daily for 10 days would be the standard treatment, with erythromycin or clindamycin as alternatives in penicillin allergy [4].

Retropharyngeal abscess and Lemierre's disease are treated with broad-spectrum antibiotics including metronidazole. Surgical intervention may be required.

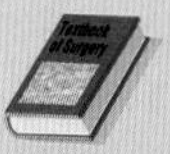

1 Goldenberg D, Golz A, Joachims HZ. Retropharyngeal abscess: a clinical review. *J Laryngol Otol* 1997; 111: 546–550.
2 Boucher C, Dorion D, Fisch C. Retropharyngeal abscesses: a clinical and radiologic correlation. *J Otolaryngol* 1999; 28: 134–137.
3 Del Mar CB, Glasziou PP, Spinks AB. Antibiotics for sore throat. *Cochrane Database Syst Rev* 2000; (2): CD000023.
4 Zwart S, Sachs APE, Ruijs GJHM *et al.* Penicillin for acute sore throat: randomised double blind trial of seven days vs. three days treatment or placebo in adults. *BMJ* 2000; 320: 150–154.

1.14 Fever and headache

Case history

A 23-year-old woman presents with a 12-h history of fever, headache and photophobia.

Clinical approach

This is a medical emergency: you must act quickly. Your main concern is whether she has meningitis, and, if so, what is the causative organism (Table 11)?

You must also do the following:

- Look for signs of shock because she may develop fulminant sepsis (see Section 1.2, p. 5)
- Consider other common possibilities such as subarachnoid haemorrhage and migraine.

History of the presenting problem

You want to look for symptoms of meningitis and search for underlying risk factors and exposure to pathogens. If the patient cannot give a lucid history because he or she is extremely unwell or drowsy, it is extremely important to seek information from relatives or friends.

Headache and fever

Ask the following:

- When did the symptoms start? If more than 5–7 days previously, consider causes of chronic meningitis such as TB, Lyme disease and fungi, and non-infectious conditions such as sarcoidosis.

Table 11 Infective causes of meningitis in adults.

Type of infection	Frequency	Examples
Viral	Common	Enteroviruses
	Less common	Mumps, adenoviruses HSV, VZV and HIV
Bacterial	Common	*Neisseria meningitidis* *Streptococcus pneumoniae*
	Less common	*Staphylococcus aureus* *Listeria monocytogenes* *Mycobacterium tuberculosis* Leptospirosis *Borrelia burgdorferi*
Rickettsial	Uncommon	Rocky Mountain spotted fever
Fungal	Rare unless immunocompromised	*Cryptococcus neoformans* Coccidioidomycosis

HSV, herpes simplex virus; VZV, varicella-zoster virus; HIV, human immunodeficiency virus.

• Where is the headache and how did it start? Sudden-onset headache, particularly during physical exertion, means that subarachnoid haemorrhage (SAH) must be excluded, but the headache of meningitis can also have an abrupt onset. SAH typically causes occipital headache.

Associated symptoms

Ask about the following:
• Rash: supports the diagnosis of meningococcal meningitis.
• Nausea and/or vomiting: common but non-specific because it occurs with meningitis, SAH and migraine.
• Associated earache, sinusitis or cough: these make pneumococci more likely as the aetiological agent.
• Any focal weakness, confusion or diplopia? If so, need to consider cerebral oedema, encephalitis, brain abscess and TB.

History of specific exposure

Are any of the following relevant in this case?
• Recent contact with anyone suffering from meningitis, particularly meningococcal.
• Contact with fresh water or working as a farmer—consider leptospirosis.
• Tick bite or camping trip to an endemic area—consider Lyme disease.
• Travel: coccidioidomycosis is endemic in the western USA.
• Unpasteurized dairy products: consider *Listeria* and *Brucella* spp.

Additional clues

• Is she pregnant? Consider *Listeria* spp. in pregnancy and in immunocompromised individuals.
• Season: meningococcal disease is more common during winter and enteroviral outbreaks are more common in the spring and summer.
• Is there a local outbreak, particularly of meningococcal infection?

Relevant past history

• Previous history of meningitis? Recurrent pneumococcal meningitis may occur as a result of a persistent CSF leak. Mollaret's meningitis is a rare recurrent condition caused by herpes simplex virus 2 (HSV-2). Deficiency in complement increases risk of meningococcal disease. (See *Rheumatology and clinical immunology*, Section 1.2.)
• History of neurosurgery, a ventriculoperitoneal shunt or head trauma?
• Immunocompromise: much broader differential, including cryptococcal meningitis.
• Congenital heart disease or suppurative pulmonary disease increases the risk of pyogenic brain abscess.

Examination

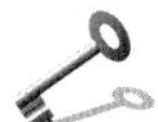

Fever and headache

• Look thoroughly for a petechial/purpuric rash (see Section 1.2, p. 5). In meningitis in the UK, this is virtually pathognomonic of meningococcal infection.
• Treatment must be instituted without delay in bacterial meningitis.

A full physical examination is required, but take particularly careful note of the following:
• Vital signs: temperature, pulse, BP and respiratory rate for evidence of septic shock. Hypertension with bradycardia suggests raised intracranial pressure.
• Level of consciousness (Glasgow Coma Score) and Mini-Mental Test Score.
• Neck stiffness or positive Kernig's sign, indicating meningism.
• Rash: look very carefully over the whole body, including the conjunctivae and buttocks, for the petechial/purpuric rash of meningococcal disease, which may be maculopapular at an early stage.
• Detailed neurological examination looking for focal neurological signs and evidence of raised intracranial pressure.
• Otitis media or pneumonia: these make *Strep. pneumoniae* infection more likely.
• Evidence of infective endocarditis: septic emboli can enter the cerebral circulation.

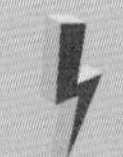

Meningitis is deadly. Even if the patient looks reasonably well, meningitis is potentially life threatening and can progress at frightening speed.

Approach to investigation and management

'Shoot first, ask questions later'

• You cannot reliably differentiate viral from bacterial meningitis on clinical grounds alone—lumbar puncture is essential unless there are contraindications or the patient has a petechial/purpuric rash (in which case the agent is almost certainly *Neisseria meningitidis*).
• Do not delay antimicrobial therapy while awaiting investigation results.

Investigations

Cultures

• Lumbar puncture: CSF analysis (Table 12) is the only way to establish a secure diagnosis and should be performed unless there are contraindications or if the patient has a petechial/purpuric rash. CT is essential before LP if there is decreased consciousness, focal neurological signs or any suspicion of elevated intracranial pressure.

Table 12 Interpretation of CSF findings in meningitis.

Condition	CSF	Cells/μL	Protein (g/L)	Glucose	Microbiology tests
Normal	Clear	0–5 lymphocytes	0.15–0.45	60% of plasma	–
Bacterial	Cloudy, purulent or clear	500–2000 mainly polymorphs	0.5–3.0	Low	Gram stain, culture Bacterial antigen detection for common pathogens PCR for meningococci
Viral	Clear	15–500 mainly lymphocytes	0.15–1.0	Normal	PCR available for enteroviruses and herpes viruses
Fungal	Clear or cloudy	0–500 lymphocytes Absent in severe immunocompromise	0.5–3.0	Low	India ink stain and cryptococcal antigen
Tuberculous	Clear	30–500 mixed lymphocytes + polymorphs	1.0–6.0	Low	Ziehl–Neelsen smear positive in <5% and PCR in 30–40% of TB meningitis

CSF, cerebrospinal fluid; PCR, polymerase chain reaction; TB, tuberculosis.

• Blood culture.
• Throat swab and stool for viral culture: these have a higher yield than CSF culture.
• Throat swab for bacterial culture: particularly important for detecting meningococci.
• If a petechial rash is present, disrupt a lesion for Gram stain and culture.

Blood tests

• FBC and film: neutrophilia suggests bacterial infection but fulminant meningococcal disease may present with leucopenia and thrombocytopenia. Reactive lymphocytes may be seen in viral meningitis.
• Coagulation screen in patients with suspected meningococcal disease.
• Save an ethylenediamine tetraacetic acid (EDTA) blood specimen for bacterial PCR. This is useful in culture-negative cases and where lumbar puncture cannot be performed.
• Electrolytes, renal and liver function tests, glucose and (possibly) arterial blood gases will also be required in any patient presenting with meningitis.

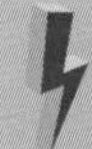

Contraindications to lumbar puncture

• Symptoms or signs suggestive of raised intracranial pressure: the absence of papilloedema does not exclude this
• Local infection around the lumbar puncture site
• Septic shock
• Coagulopathy.

Imaging

• Chest radiograph: primarily to exclude pneumonia
• Sinus radiographs: may be abnormal in pneumococcal infection (Fig. 22)
• CT or MRI of brain (before lumbar puncture when needed): this may also detect brain abscess and sinusitis.

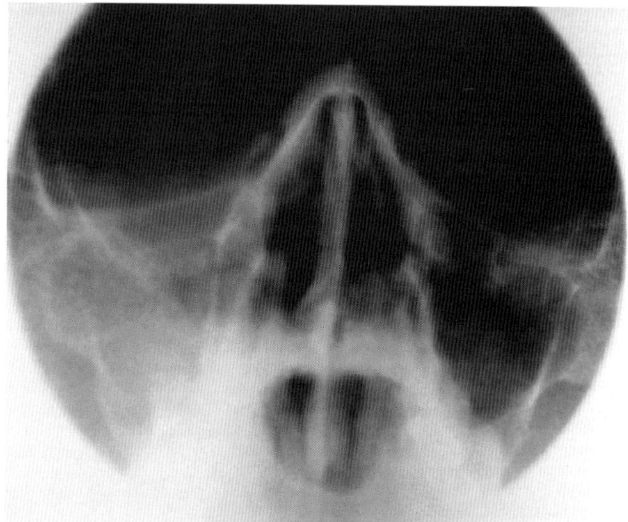

Fig. 22 Right maxillary sinusitis in a patient with pneumococcal meningitis.

Management

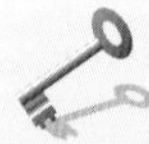

Meningitis

Telephone advice to GP:
• Benzylpenicillin 1200 mg (2 MU) i.v. or i.m. immediately in suspected meningococcal disease
• Cefotaxime (or ceftriaxone) 1 g if history of anaphylaxis to penicillin [1].

If there is circulatory compromise, resuscitation must begin immediately, while the history and examination are completed (see Section 1.2, p. 5). The following are key aspects:
• Check airway, breathing, circulation
• Ensure airway and give high-flow oxygen
• Obtain venous access
• Give colloid/0.9% saline i.v. rapidly until BP restored or JVP clearly visible
• Call for help from the ICU sooner rather than later.

Empirical antibiotics

These will depend on the clinical context:

• If meningococcal meningitis suspected (typical rash or shocked), immediately administer high-dose intravenous cefotaxime or ceftriaxone, but take blood cultures first [1,2].

• If recent head injury, neurosurgery or a ventricular shunt is present, add flucloxacillin to cover *Staph. aureus*.

• If the patient is pregnant, aged over 50 or moderately immunocompromised—add ampicillin to cover *Listeria* spp.

• Consider adding aciclovir if there are features of encephalitis (see Section 1.15, p. 39).

• If severely immunocompromised, seek expert advice (see Section 2.11, p. 134).

Antibiotic resistance to meningitis

In 1997, 7% of blood and CSF isolates of *Strep. pneumoniae* were penicillin resistant in England and Wales. In southern Europe and the USA, this figure is much higher and a proportion are also cephalosporin resistant.

Meningitis: no pathogen identified and not responding

- Wrong empirical therapy, e.g. unusual organism
- Parameningeal focus, e.g. epidural abscess
- Antibiotic resistance
- Non-infectious cause, e.g. sarcoidosis or malignancy.

Specific antimicrobial therapy

• *Neisseria meningitidis*, *H. influenzae* or *Strep. pneumoniae*: intravenous cefotaxime 2 g 4-hourly or ceftriaxone 2 g 12-hourly. High-dose penicillin or ampicillin can be substituted when sensitivities are available. Duration of treatment is 7 days for *N. meningitidis* and *H. influenzae*, but 14 days for *Strep. pneumoniae*.

• *Listeria monocytogenes*: intravenous ampicillin 2 g 4-hourly for 14–21 days; consider adding gentamicin.

• Tuberculous: rifampicin, isoniazid, pyrazinamide and ethambutol for 2 months, followed by rifampicin and isoniazid for a further 10 months [3]. Consider adjunctive corticosteroids.

• Aseptic meningitis: conservative treatment.

Contacts

Meningitis is a notifiable disease. If meningococcal infection is confirmed or likely, notify your microbiologist and the local CCDC by phone immediately. Ensure that appropriate prophylaxis is instituted. (See Section 1.38, p. 91.)

Long term

• After any bacterial meningitis, perform audiometry during follow up.

• In recurrent meningococcal meningitis, or if there is family history, measure complement levels, immunoglobulins and IgG subclasses. Immunize with ACYW135 meningococcal vaccine. (see *Rheumatology and clinical immunology*, Section 1.2).

• In recurrent pneumococcal meningitis, investigate for a CSF leak.

See *Emergency medicine*, Section 1.22

1 Begg N, Cartwright KAV, Cohen J *et al.* Consensus statement on diagnosis, investigation, treatment and prevention of acute bacterial meningitis in immunocompetent adults. *J Infect* 1999; 39: 1–15.

2 Wood AJJ, Quagliarello VJ, Scheld WM. Treatment of bacterial meningitis—Review article. *N Engl J Med* 1997; 336: 708–716.

3 Joint tuberculosis committee of the British Thoracic Society. Chemotherapy and management of tuberculosis in the United Kingdom: recommendations 1998. *Thorax* 1998; 53: 536–548.

1.15 Fever with reduced conscious level

Case history

You are asked to see a 29-year-old man who has been admitted under a psychiatric section, having been found wandering in the street. On admission, he was found to have a temperature of 39°C and his conscious level has fallen since admission.

Clinical approach

The differential diagnosis for this scenario is broad and the falling level of consciousness requires urgent action. The airway must be protected, high-flow oxygen given and readily treatable causes of impaired consciousness excluded immediately, e.g. hypoglycaemia, drug (opiate) intoxication (see *Emergency medicine*, Section 1.26). The patient will not be able to give a useful history: obtain as much information as possible from friends, relatives or observers. Given the high fever, it is critically important to consider infection, particularly meningitis, encephalitis (Table 13) and brain abscess. Less common travel-related infections include rickettsial infections, malaria, African trypanosomiasis and typhoid. Remember that confusion may complicate severe sepsis.

History of the presenting problem

The history, if available, will be from a friend or relative:

• Duration of illness: was there any prodromal illness suggestive of a viral infection?

Table 13 Aetiological agents of acute encephalitis.

Scenario	Organisms
Immunocompetent adult	HSV* Enteroviruses Influenza EBV HIV seroconversion* *Mycoplasma pneumoniae** *Legionella pneumophila**
Travel related	Japanese B encephalitis Tick-borne encephalitis Various flaviviruses (e.g. West Nile virus)
Severe immunocompromise	VZV*, CMV* (HSV* less common) HIV* Toxoplasmosis*

*Treatable causes.
EBV, Epstein–Barr virus; VZV, varicella-zoster virus; CMV, cytomegalovirus; HSV, herpes simplex virus; HIV, human immunodeficiency virus.

• Has he experienced headache, neck pain or photophobia suggestive of meningitis? (See Section 1.14, p. 36.)
• What has his behaviour been like? Typically, in encephalitis patients start acting strangely, become confused and then develop coma.
• Is there a possibility of trauma?
• Has he had a fit or convulsion?
• Does he suffer from any medical conditions?
• Ask about his premorbid mental state, drug and alcohol use. Is there any possibility of an overdose?

Travel history

Recent travel raises the possibility of exposure to many organisms (see Section 1.20, p. 52). If relevant, obtain precise details of the area involved and seek expert advice on possible exposure. Consider the following:
• Malaria, typhoid, trypanosomiasis.
• Specific encephalitis viruses, e.g. Japanese B encephalitis in south-east Asia, eastern equine encephalitis in North America, tick-borne encephalitis in eastern Europe (in summer) [1–3].

Relevant past history

• Diabetes mellitus (hypo- or hyperglycaemia)?
• Drug overdose or depression?
• Use of alcohol or recreational drugs?
• Regular medication such as neuroleptics?
• Immunocompromise such as HIV infection or recent chemotherapy?

Confusion may occur in any severe systemic infection, particularly in elderly people. Always consider encephalitis and meningitis and, if in doubt, perform a CT scan and lumbar puncture.

Examination

Take particular note of the following:
• Vital signs: pulse, BP, respiratory rate.
• Glasgow Coma Score and Mini-Mental Test Score: follow these over time as falling consciousness requires immediate review.
• Look for signs of trauma.
• Look for a Medic-Alert bracelet or other useful 'clues', e.g. medication (insulin, anticonvulsants).
• Neck stiffness: signs of meningism are usually absent in encephalitis, but remember that the distinction is not always absolutely clear and meningoencephalitis may be present.
• Skin: an erythematous maculopapular rash is non-specific, occurring in mycoplasma and enteroviral infection. Is there a meningococcal rash (see Section 1.2, p. 5)? In travellers hunt for an eschar or tick.
• Ocular fundi: papilloedema indicates raised intracranial pressure in this context, although its absence does not exclude it. In advanced HIV infection, CMV retinitis may indicate coexistent CMV encephalitis. (See Section 1.27, p. 68.)
• Focal neurological signs: these may occur in viral encephalitis, but consider cerebral abscess and other space-occupying lesions.
• Muscle rigidity: present in neuroleptic malignant syndrome.
• Cardiac murmurs: consider infectious endocarditis with septic embolus to the brain.

Approach to investigation and management

Investigations

Blood tests

Check the FBC, electrolytes, renal and liver function, glucose and arterial blood gases to exclude metabolic causes, along with creatine kinase if neuroleptic malignant syndrome is possible and a toxicology screen. Check thick and thin malaria films if the patient has travelled to an endemic area within the last month.

Cultures and serology

Carry out blood cultures and CSF analysis (if safe), as in Section 1.14, p. 36. In encephalitis the opening pressure is commonly raised (>200 mm CSF); the CSF itself may be normal but a mild lymphocytosis is common. PCR is now the gold standard for recognizing the infectious agent, i.e. enteroviruses, herpes simplex, EBV, CMV, varicellazoster virus (VZV) [4], mumps and *Mycoplasma* spp. (Fig. 23) (see *Genetics and molecular medicine*, Section 4).

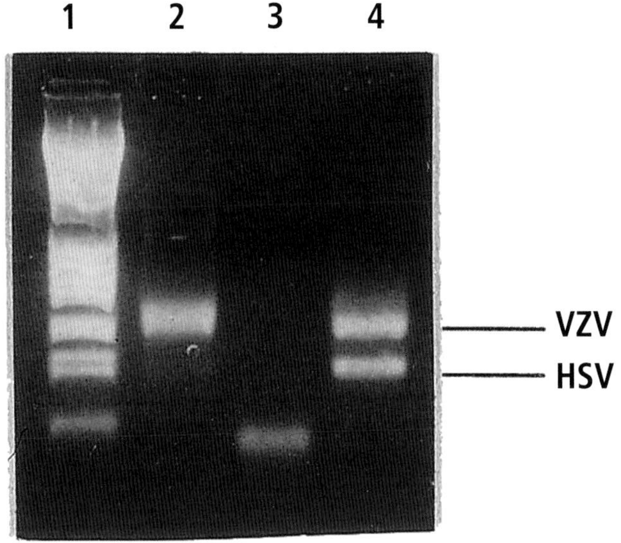

Fig. 23 PCR of CSF from a patient with AIDS revealing varicella-zoster virus (VZV) DNA. Lane 1, DNA ladder; lane 2, CSF from patient; lane 3, negative control; lane 4, positive control. HSV, herpes simplex virus. (Courtesy of Dr C Bangham.)

Acute serology should be saved for paired testing later. Consider an HIV test if risk factors for HIV infection are present—this may be performed in an incompetent patient without consent if you believe that the result will benefit the patient. (See Section 1.24, p. 61.)

Imaging

Urgent cranial imaging is needed for this man, whose conscious level is falling. Waiting until the next day could be fatal if he has a space-occupying lesion. CT of the brain will readily exclude space-occupying lesions, such as brain abscess, and gauge whether lumbar puncture is unsafe. CT may show parenchymal features of encephalitis, but MRI is more sensitive. Changes in many cases are non-specific, but temporal lobe involvement suggests herpes simplex encephalitis. Patients often need both imaging modalities.

Other tests

The following may be indicated in some cases:
- EEG: temporal lobe changes strongly suggest herpes simplex encephalitis
- Brain biopsy: now rarely performed for encephalitis since the development of MRI and PCR.

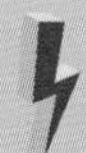

Emerging infections

Outbreaks can occur out of the blue, as happened in New York in 1999, when cases of encephalitis caused by west-Nile-like virus previously undescribed in the USA suddenly appeared [5].

Management

Secure the airway, control seizures and commence empirical therapy as soon as possible.
- Patient with coma: see *Emergency medicine*, Section 1.26
- Patient with meningitis: see Section 1.14, pp. 36–39.

Until a specific diagnosis is confirmed, treat for both meningitis and encephalitis.

Encephalitis

Once you suspect encephalitis, you must consider the likely aetiological agents (see Table 13), particularly the treatable ones. In the UK, the most common identifiable agent in a patient with encephalitis is HSV. Other treatable causes include *Mycoplasma pneumoniae*, VZV and HIV infection. Empirical therapy before an aetiological agent is identified should include parenteral aciclovir 10 mg/kg for 10 days three times daily (reduced in renal failure), together with a macrolide. It is important to start therapy early for herpes simplex [6] because death or severe brain damage is likely once the Glasgow Coma Score has fallen below 8.

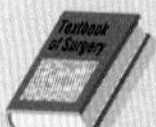

1 Cassidy KA, Whitely RJ. Acute and chronic encephalitis. In: Armstrong D, Cohen J (eds) *Infectious Diseases*. London: Mosby, 1999: Section 2, Chapter 16.
2 Whitley RJ, Kimberlin DW. Viral encephalitis. *Paediatr Rev* 1999; 20: 192–198.
3 Dumpis U, Crook D, Oksi J. Tick-borne encephalitis. *Clin Infect Dis* 1999; 28: 882–890.
4 Gilden DH, Kleinschmidt-DeMasters BK, LaGuardia JJ *et al.* Neurologic complications of the reactivation of varicella-zoster virus. *N Engl J Med* 2000; 342: 635–645.
5 Update: West Nile-like viral encephalitis—New York, 1999. *MMWR* 1999; 48: 890–892.
6 Levitz RE. Herpes simplex encephalitis: a review. *Heart Lung* 1998; 27: 209–212.

1.16 Fever in the neutropenic patient

Case history

A 24-year-old man develops a high fever 3 weeks after bone-marrow transplantation for acute myeloid leukaemia.

Clinical approach

The patient is highly immunosuppressed and neutropenic. He is at high risk of serious sepsis and treatment must not be delayed [1]. There is usually a protocol, based on local antimicrobial sensitivity patterns, guiding urgent therapy

	Neutropenia	Cell-mediated deficiency	Recovery (unless GvHD)
			Hyposplenism
Fungi	Candida + aspergillus	Aspergillus	
Viruses	HSV	CMV	VZV
Bacteria	Gram positive and Gram negative	G+ G–	Pneumococcus
	1st month	2nd, 3rd months	>3 months

Fig. 24 Risk of infection following bone-marrow transplantation. The early phase with chemotherapy-related mucositis and neutropenia is dominated by bacterial and fungal infections. GvHD, graft versus host disease; HSV, herpes simplex virus; CMV, cytomegalovirus; VZV, varicella-zoster virus.

in haematology units (see *Haematology*, Sections 1.6 and 1.7), but this should not prevent a rational diagnostic approach.

History of the presenting problem

This patient will have been monitored very closely and so large amounts of data should already be available. The timescale after the graft is important in guessing the likely pathogens (Figs 24 and 25). In the first month or so neutropenia is the main concern. Thereafter, the main defects are in cell-mediated immunity, and the opportunistic infections in the second and third months are similar to those in solid organ transplants or HIV. After the third month, immune reconstitution is sufficient so that opportunistic infections are less of a problem, although patients remain hyposplenic.

Locating the site

This is often a difficult task in neutropenic patients who fail to 'localize' infections in the same way as the immunocompetent. Commonly, infection enters through a decrease of the normal barrier function of the mucosae, so the portal of entry may not be obvious. Nevertheless, assess symptoms relating to individual systems carefully. Discuss the case with the nurses on the unit who often notice relevant changes in the patient.

Lines as the source

Rigors and fever are occasionally associated with infusion of fluids or drugs. A drug fever is obviously a possibility here, but consider also a line infection. Rarely, the infusion fluids themselves may become contaminated. If this is suspected, retain the fluid and contact microbiology for advice.

Routine surveillance

According to local protocol, surveillance cultures or CMV studies (PCR or antigen detection) may be ongoing. Review all results with the microbiologist and also ask about recent infections in other patients within the unit. If the patient is CMV IgG antibody negative (pretransplantation), has he received exclusively CMV-negative blood products?

Antimicrobial prophylaxis

Antibacterial, antifungal, antiprotozoal and antiviral prophylaxis may be used according to protocol, based on pretransplantation serology and past infections. Review what has been prescribed and administered. Drug reactions may have led to cessation of prophylaxis.

Leucocyte-depleted blood reduces CMV transmission but protection is not complete. Primary CMV disease in the bone-marrow transplant recipient is very severe if not treated aggressively and early.

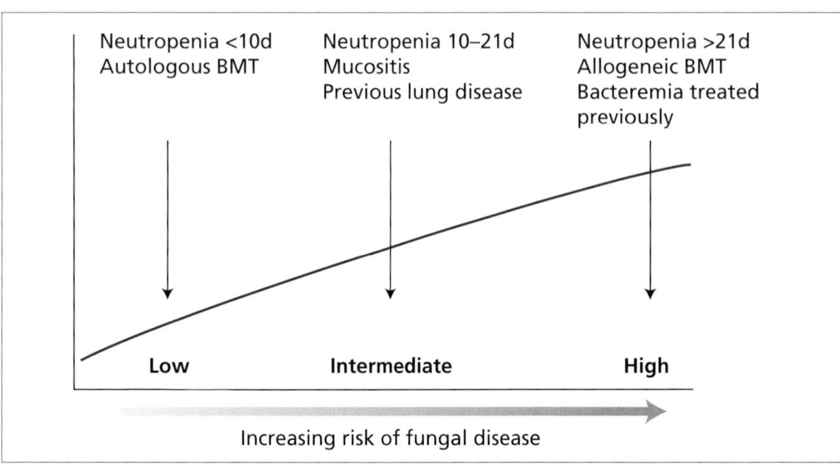

Fig. 25 Fungal infection in bone-marrow transplantation (BMT).

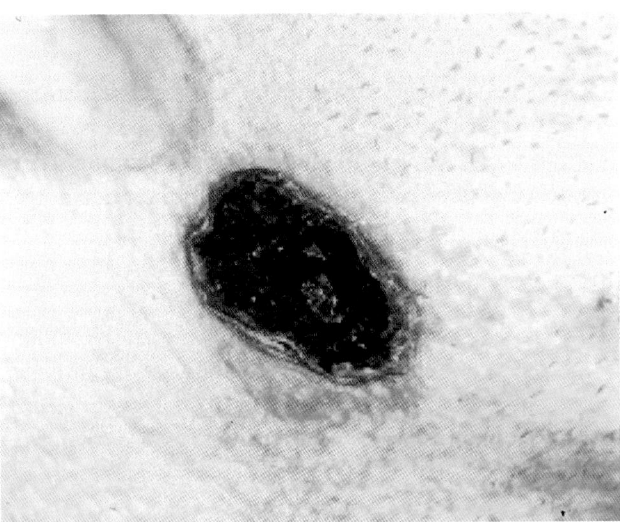

Fig. 26 Ecthyma gangrenosum in a neutropenic patient. Focal areas of necrosis start as dark-red patches and quickly turn black. This lesion occurs only in neutropenia and is almost always the result of metastatic *Pseudomonas aeruginosa*.

Examination

Is the patient cardiovascularly stable? If not, resuscitate. (See Section 1.2, p. 5 and see also *Emergency medicine*, Section 1.2.) A full examination is required, but physical signs may be subtle or absent in neutropenic patients as a result of the lack of an inflammatory response. Pay particular attention to the following:

- Intravenous line site(s)
- Skin: looking for lesions of disseminated bacterial (Fig. 26) or fungal infection, pressure sores or other sites of skin breakdown
- Perianal area: a common site of cellulitis
- Oral cavity: looking for mucositis, candidal and herpetic infection
- Fundoscopy: for evidence of fungal or viral infection.

Approach to investigation and management

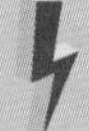

Do not await culture results before treatment. Take cultures and treat immediately according to local protocols.

Investigations

Blood tests

- Routine surveillance of these patients will include FBC, clotting, electrolytes, renal and liver function. Check to see the degree of neutropenia at this stage of treatment.
- Send blood to the lab for detection of CMV by PCR or antigen testing. Candida or aspergillus antigen detection is available in some centres and may be useful. Test for cryptococcal antigen in blood and CSF if central nervous system infection suspected.

Cultures

The following are needed:

- Blood cultures in all cases. Ideally these should be taken peripherally because central line cultures have a poor positive predictive value. A paired line and peripheral culture may be taken if line sepsis is possible.
- Culture of urine in all cases, stool (if diarrhoea is present) and CSF (if there are meningeal or neurological symptoms).
- Respiratory samples: these are essential if there are respiratory symptoms or an abnormal chest radiograph, or if hypoxia is present. Send sputum for bacterial, fungal and mycobacterial culture. Bronchoscopy and lavage may be required to obtain an adequate specimen and to detect respiratory viruses or *Pneumocystis carinii*. Mouth washings or nasopharyngeal aspirate for respiratory virus culture and immunofluorescence can be useful.
- Vesicular lesions should be sampled and sent to virology for electron microscopy PCR or culture for herpes viruses. Other skin lesions may be biopsied and cultured for bacteria and fungi.

Imaging

A chest radiograph should be taken in all cases to exclude obvious disease. CT of the chest is more sensitive in detecting pulmonary infection, particularly the peripheral lesions of aspergillosis (Fig. 27) [2,3]. Ultrasonography, CT and MRI are valuable in localizing focal sites of infection.

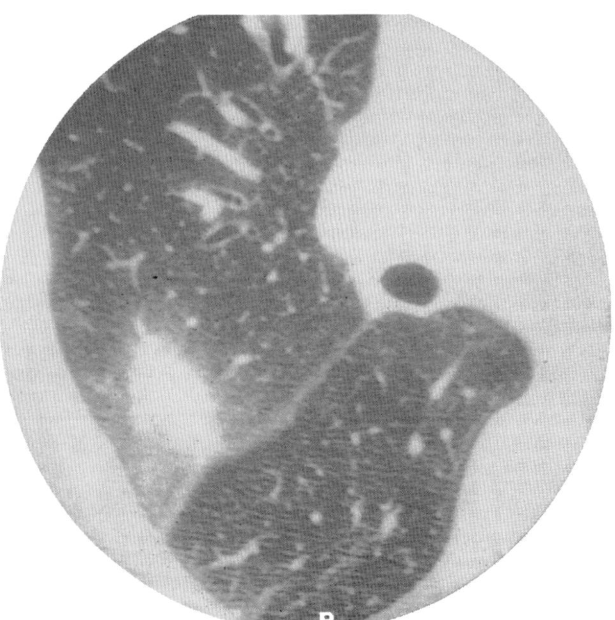

Fig. 27 Pulmonary CT scan showing an area of dense peripheral consolidation caused by invasive aspergillosis. (Courtesy of Dr C Conlon.)

Invasive procedures

Tissue biopsies, guided by imaging techniques, may establish the diagnosis of deep-seated infection, e.g. hepatosplenic candidiasis, but can be difficult in the face of thrombocytopenia or coagulation abnormalities. Have a low threshold for bronchoscopy if respiratory symptoms are present, or upper and lower gastrointestinal endoscopy for appropriate symptoms. Send samples to both microbiology and cytology/histology.

Treatment

Aggressive supportive care will almost certainly be required. (See Section 1.2, p. 5.)

Empirical antimicrobial treatment

This must be instituted immediately in a 'blind' manner to cover the likely pathogens according to protocol (see *Haematology*, Sections 1.6 and 1.7). Most regimens start with antibacterial cover, including *Pseudomonas* spp., and escalate therapy in a sequential manner. If initial antibacterial therapy fails, the likelihood of fungal infection (*Candida* or *Aspergillus* spp.) is increased, and blind antifungal therapy in the form of amphotericin B is usually added at 72–96 h if there is no response [4].

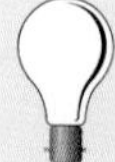

Gram-positive bacterial infections and antimicrobial resistance have been increasing in frequency in the neutropenic population. Consider this when formulating treatment protocols [5].

Although *Candida albicans* is susceptible to fluconazole, other *Candida* spp. may not be. There has been an increase in non-*albicans* candida infection, possibly related to the use of fluconazole prophylaxis. These require antifungal therapy with amphotericin B [6].

Review

Keep reviewing the patient's clinical state and investigations. If necessary, re-image or take further invasive samples.

Line infection

If an intravascular line, e.g. a tunnelled Hickman catheter, is a potential site of infection, it is often possible to treat without having to remove it. However, removal should be considered if the patient remains septic, in suspected endocarditis (rare in neutropenia), when there is venous thrombosis around the line or if the line tunnel becomes infected.

Specific therapy

If a specific pathogen is isolated, adjust the antimicrobial regimen with microbiology advice. There is a great temptation to leave the patient on multiple different antimicrobial agents, which increases the risk of adverse reactions.

Immunomodulation

If neutropenia persists, the outlook from invasive fungal infection, in particular, is poor. Efforts should be directed towards trying to restore bone marrow function as soon as possible. The role of colony-stimulating factors is discussed in *Haematology*, Sections 1.6 and 1.7.

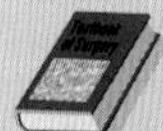

1 Quadri TL, Brown AE. Infectious complications in the critically ill patient with cancer. *Semin Oncol* 2000; 27: 335–346.
2 Warnock DW. Fungal infections in neutropenia: current problems and chemotherapeutic control. *J Antimicrob Chemother* 1998; 41(suppl D): 95–105.
3 Denning DW. Invasive aspergillosis. *Clin Infect Dis* 1998; 26: 781–803.
4 Richardson MD, Kokki MH. Diagnosis and prevention of fungal infection in the immunocompromised patient. *Blood Rev* 1998; 12: 241–254.
5 Zinner SH. Changing epidemiology of infections in patients with neutropenia and cancer: emphasis on gram-positive and resistant bacteria. *Clin Infect Dis* 1999; 29: 490–494.
6 Rex JH, Walsh TJ, Sobel JD *et al.* Practice guidelines for the treatment of candidiasis. Infectious diseases society of America. *Clin Infect Dis* 2000; 30: 662–678.

1.17 Fever after renal transplant

A 64-year-old man presents with a temperature of 39°C 6 weeks after a successful renal transplantation.

Clinical approach

This patient has significant immunosuppression, in particular of cell-mediated immunity (helper T cells, killer T cells and macrophages). (See Sections 2.2, p. 97 and 2.11, p. 134; see also *Immunology and immunosuppression*, Section 8.) The differential diagnosis is wide, requiring careful evaluation and investigations [1]. CMV must be high on the list of probabilities (depending on the CMV status of the donor and recipient), but bacterial infection, e.g. urinary tract infection, must be excluded. Specific therapy once a diagnosis is available is preferable, but if the patient is severely ill treatment must be initiated immediately on a 'covering the possibilities' basis while waiting for the results of investigations.

History of the presenting problem

Immunosuppression

What immunosuppression has the patient received? If he was at high risk of rejection, e.g. because he was highly sensitized, or had suffered graft rejection, he is likely to have received more immunosuppression than would otherwise be the case. Agents such as antithymocyte globulin (ATG) increase the risk of invasive CMV disease.

Site of infection

A detailed history looking for an infective focus is essential (see Section 1.16, p. 41):

• Localizing symptoms? Take respiratory, urinary, gastrointestinal and neurological symptoms particularly seriously.

• Systemic infection? Ask about symptoms of systemic disease.

• Prosthetic material? Many renal patients will have indwelling catheters or the like, e.g. central venous haemodialyis catheters, Tenckhoff catheters for peritoneal dialysis, or arteriovenous connections with Gortex or similar materials.

• Haematuria? This would be rare, but frank haematuria suggests haemorrhagic cystitis or interstitial nephritis caused by polyoma viruses (JC and BK) [2].

Other history

• Hospital-acquired infection? Is there an outbreak on the ward (see Section 2.3, p. 99)?

• Medication? Drug fever is often overlooked and, once blind antibiotic therapy is started, this is difficult to disentangle. What antimicrobial prophylaxis has been taken?

• Travel? Reactivation of tuberculosis is common in renal failure or transplantation [3]. Strongyloides hyperinfection syndrome may occur when immunosuppression is commenced many years after the initial infection (see Section 2.14.2, p. 145).

Relevant past history

What was the cause of renal failure? Is this the patient's first transplant? What happened to previous graft(s)? How much immunosuppression has he received in the past? Is there a history of previous infections, e.g. TB or aspergillosis? What happened around the time of the transplantation? Could this be transfusion-acquired CMV or viral hepatitis?

Examination

Monitor vital signs regularly for evidence of shock or organ dysfunction necessitating urgent intervention (see Section 1.2, p. 5 and *Emergency medicine*, Sections 1.2 and 1.28). Pay attention to the following.

Skin

Examine the operation site for redness, tenderness, exudate or necrosis. Check all lines, fistulas and dialysis catheter sites. Vesicles suggest herpes simplex or herpes zoster (see Section 2.10.2, p. 127). Fungal infection may present with scattered maculopapular lesions (see Section 2.9, p. 120).

Respiratory

Classic chest signs may be masked by immunosuppression. *Pneumocystis carinii* and CMV pneumonitis often present with cough, breathlessness and oxygen desaturation, but with no abnormalities on auscultation (see Section 1.26, p. 65).

Abdomen

Localized signs or ileus may be the result of surgical complications, gut ischaemia or intra-abdominal abscess. Infectious diarrhoea may represent nosocomial infection, especially *Clostridium difficile* in a patient who has received previous antibiotics. Bleeding or diarrhoea may be caused by CMV colitis.

Neurology

Change in mental state, headache or photophobia, or localized neurological signs require urgent investigation. Signs of meningism are often mild/absent in severe immunocompromise.

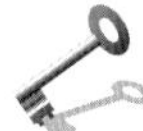

CMV disease in renal transplant recipients

• Primary or secondary (reactivation) is common after solid organ transplantation

• Multisystem infection can involve lung, eye, gut, liver, bone marrow or brain

• Most common 1–3 months after the transplantation

• More common and severe if a CMV-negative patient receives a CMV-positive graft; risk related to the intensity of immunosuppression—particularly high after ATG [4]

• Regular monitoring (blood CMV antigen or PCR detection) allows for pre-emptive therapy.

Approach to investigation and management

Keep in mind the wide differential diagnosis (Figs 28 and 29) and remember that immunocompromised patients may be infected by more than one pathogen.

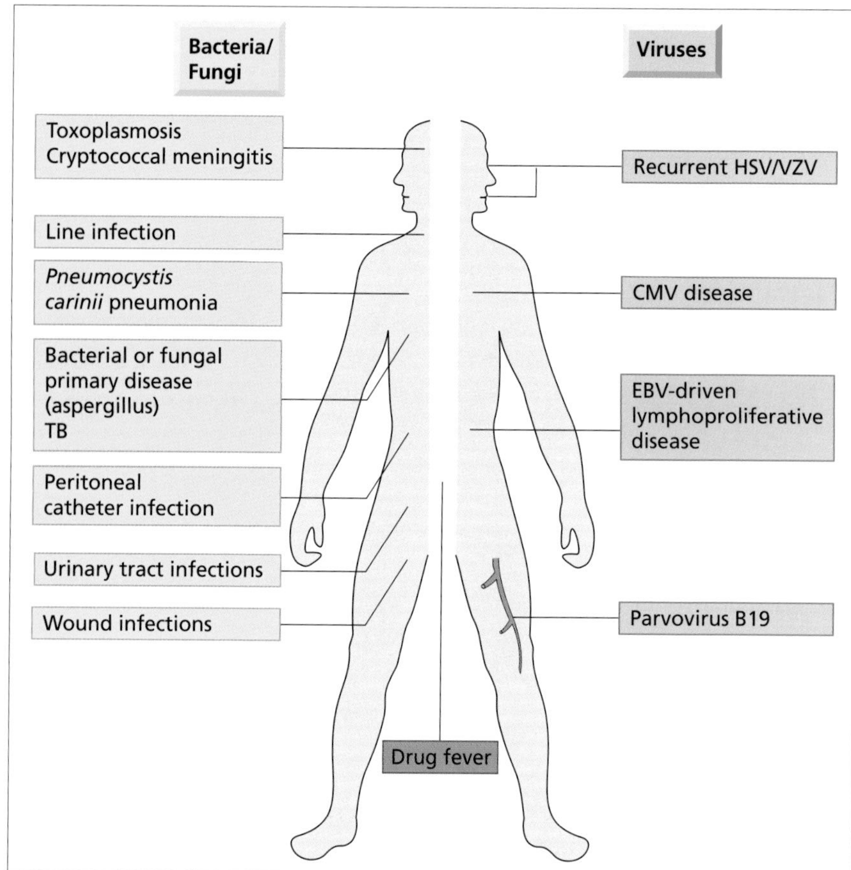

Fig. 28 Potential causes of fever in renal transplantation. CMV, cytomegalovirus; EBV, Epstein–Barr virus; HSV, herpes simplex virus; VZV, varicella-zoster virus.

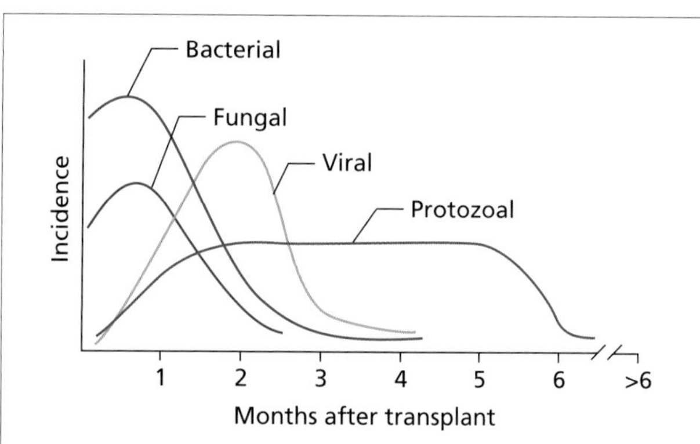

Fig. 29 Timing of infections after transplantation.

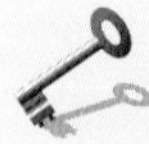

- Examine, culture, image and biopsy until you have obtained a diagnosis
- If the patient looks very ill, give broad-spectrum antibacterial cover immediately.

Investigations

Blood tests

Check the FBC, electrolytes, renal and liver function, glucose, clotting and (possibly) arterial blood gases. Neutropenia will change the clinical approach (see Section 1.16, p. 41). Leucopenia may suggest CMV and anaemia is common in parvovirus B19 infection [5], but these could simply be an effect of drugs, e.g. azathioprine, mycophenolate mofetil.

Cultures

These should be directed by specific symptoms, but should include culture of blood, urine, stool and infected sites. Note the following:

- Blood culture for CMV has been replaced by rapid estimation of CMV viraemia by PCR or antigen detection. Candida or aspergillus antigen tests are not universally available, but may prove useful in the future to aid early diagnosis and therapy.
- Sputum culture has a low yield for bacterial pathogens but may detect TB. Induced sputum and/or bronchial lavage is indicated for the diagnosis of *Pneumocystis carinii* pneumonia (PCP), TB, fungi, CMV and respiratory viruses [6] (see Section 3.1, p. 150).
- Stool culture, *C. difficile* toxin measurement and stain for cryptosporidia if diarrhoea present. If there is a history of foreign travel, request microscopy for ova, cysts and parasites.

Have a low threshold for bronchoscopy if there are respiratory symptoms, desaturation or abnormal imaging. If you delay, bronchoscopy may not be possible as a result of worsening hypoxia.

Imaging

A chest radiograph is mandatory. Other imaging should be as indicated by clinical or laboratory findings. Ultrasonography, CT and MRI are increasingly used to image the chest/abdomen in transplant recipients with pyrexia of unknown origin (see Sections 1.10, p. 26 and 1.11, p. 29) and to direct aspiration/biopsy of suspect lesions. Nuclear medicine imaging, such as indium-111-labelled white cell or gallium-67 scanning, may occasionally localize inflammation in difficult cases.

Histology

This can often establish the diagnosis and is required for the formal diagnosis of invasive fungal or CMV disease; it may detect malignancy. Send samples to both microbiology and cytology/histology.

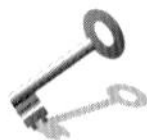

Transplant-associated lymphoproliferative disease [7]

- Increased incidence of EBV-related non-Hodgkin's B-cell lymphoma after transplantation
- Commonly presents with unexplained fever
- Often extranodal and high rate of CNS involvement
- Responds poorly to chemotherapy.

Management

The level of supportive care required will be determined by the severity of haemodynamic or respiratory disturbance (see Section 1.2, p. 5). A full discussion of therapy for individual infections is included in Section 2 of this module (see p. 96), but your first decision in this regard is whether empirical antimicrobial treatment is needed.

- Base this judgement on your clinical findings, exposure history and local policies.
- Review the patient regularly—rapid deterioration can occur.
- If empirical treatment is needed, you cannot cover every possible organism—concentrate your efforts on the most likely and most dangerous causes while continuing with investigations.

Failure of fever to respond to treatment

- Wrong diagnosis
- Drug resistance
- Malabsorption or drug interactions
- A second infection
- Drug reaction
- Malignancy (EBV-related lymphoma).

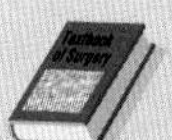

1 Dunn DL, Acton RD. Solid organ transplantation. In: Armstrong D, Cohen J (eds) *Infectious Diseases*. London: Mosby, 1999; Section 4: 3.1–3.16.
2 Boubenider S, Hiesse C, Marchand S. Post-transplantation polyomavirus infections. *J Nephrol* 1999; 12: 24–29.
3 Sayiner A, Ece T, Duman S. Tuberculosis in renal transplant recipients. *Transplantation* 1999; 68: 1268–1271.
4 Nichols WG, Boeckh M. Recent advances in the therapy and prevention of CMV infections. *J Clin Virol* 2000; 16: 25–40.
5 Marchand S, Tchernia G, Hiesse C *et al*. Human parvovirus B19 infection in organ transplant recipients. *Clin Transplant* 1999; 13: 17–24.
6 Wendt CH. Community respiratory viruses: organ transplant recipients. *Am J Med* 1997; 102: 31–36.
7 Dockrell DH, Strickler JG, Paya CV. Epstein–Barr virus-induced T cell lymphoma in solid organ transplant recipients. *Clin Infect Dis* 1998; 26: 180–182.

1.18 Chronic fatigue

Case history

A 29-year-old man is referred by his general practitioner with persistent fatigue.

Clinical approach

Is this chronic fatigue syndrome (CFS) [1–3]? This is essentially a diagnosis of exclusion, although there may be some 'positive' clues, and the first priority must be to rule out significant treatable organic disease. Many patients will include fatigue as one of their symptoms, but in most cases there will be other more specific symptoms and a cause will be apparent. It is probably true to say that any illness can cause fatigue, and lists of conditions that can do so run the risk of simply becoming a catalogue of all known diseases (Tables 14 and 15). However, the first step in evaluating patients with fatigue is a detailed history and examination.

History of the presenting problem

Many acute problems cause fatigue, but this man has persistent symptoms.

Pathological fatigue

Fatigue means different things to different people. The art here is to recognize everyday stress and avoid over-investigation, while not dismissing people with significant fatigue. Ask specific questions about the level of activity and how it has changed:

- Are you still working?
- Take me through what you do in a typical day.
- Is there anything you are prevented from doing?

Table 14 Non-infective causes of fatigue.

Category	Examples	Category	Examples
Haematological	Anaemia, Vitamin B_{12}/folate deficiency Lymphoreticular malignancy	Endocrine	Hypothyroidism Addison's disease Cushing's syndrome Hypopituitarism Diabetes mellitus
Sleep disorders	Sleep apnoea Narcolepsy	Metabolic	Hepatic or renal failure Hyponatraemia, hypokalaemia, hypercalcaemia
Neurological	Multiple sclerosis Myasthenia gravis	Psychological/ psychiatric	Depression/anxiety Substance abuse
Cardiorespiratory	Heart failure Chronic airway disease	Medication	β Blockers, benzodiazepines, neuroleptics Anticonvulsants, corticosteroid withdrawal
Neoplastic	Many cancers	Autoimmune/ inflammatory	SLE, vasculitis, Crohn's disease, sarcoidosis

Table 15 Infective causes of chronic fatigue.

Type of infection	Examples	Type of infection	Examples
Viral	HSV, CMV, EBV Hepatitis B and C HIV Parvovirus B19	Bacterial	Occult abscess Osteomyelitis Chronic sinusitis Infective endocarditis Brucellosis Lyme disease Syphilis Tuberculosis
Fungal	Histoplasmosis and other dimorphic fungi	Parasitic	Toxoplasmosis Tropical parasites

EBV, Epstein–Barr virus; CMV, cytomegalovirus; HSV, herpes simplex virus; HIV, human immunodeficiency virus.

Reason for tiredness

Patients often become worried that tiredness is a sign of serious disease and have not linked it to a change in lifestyle. Ask about occupation, home and social life.

- Is there a new baby?
- Relationship difficulties?
- Is he working two jobs to make ends meet?
- Is he partying all night?
- Medications, recreational drugs and alcohol?

Depression

The symptoms of depression are very similar to CFS and depression may complicate the condition. Find out how well he is sleeping, and about his appetite, life events, stress and mood. (See *Psychiatry*, Section 1.6.)

Serious underlying disease

Ask about weight loss, fever, sweats and any significant localizing symptoms such as cough or early morning joint stiffness. Such patients do not have CFS.

Exposure to infective risk

Take a careful travel history (see Section 1.20, p. 52), sexual history (see Sections 1.31, p. 76 and 1.33, p. 81) and history of hepatitis risk factors. Ask about possible exposure to animals or chemicals.

Relevant past history

Have there been previous episodes of fatigue (some cases of CFS are recurrent) or of infections, e.g. osteomyelitis may relapse after many years? Autoimmune, endocrine and psychiatric disorders could also be relevant.

Examination

Chronic fatigue syndrome has no specific examination findings, although some patients have prominent cervical lymphadenopathy. A careful examination is needed to look for signs associated with the conditions shown in Tables 14 and 15. Pay particular attention to the following:

- Skin, looking for signs of vasculitis or endocarditis
- Joints for arthritis
- Mouth, looking for oral hairy leucoplakia or candidal infection, indicating immunosuppression
- Lymph nodes or masses?
- Hepatosplenomegaly?
- Postural hypotension?

Approach to investigation and management

Your aim is to detect and treat definable causes of fatigue. If none is found, and the diagnosis of CFS is made, the patient needs appropriate supportive management. Explain this at the outset, so that the patient is not angry when you cannot find the 'infection' and give him or her the 'magic' cure.

Fever, sweats or weight loss will accompany most infectious causes of chronic fatigue. Acute infections such as glandular fever have usually resolved by the time the patient comes to clinic. It is therefore quite unusual to make an infectious diagnosis in patients presenting with persistent fatigue.

Blood tests

Specific tests are dictated by clinical suspicion but a typical core screen is as follows.

- FBC and blood film
- Electrolytes, renal and liver function tests, calcium
- CRP or ESR
- Glucose, thyroid function
- Testing for adrenal insufficiency (see *Endocrinology*, Section 3.1).

Cultures and serology

- Routine cultures are not helpful unless there are localizing symptoms or fever
- Serology for CMV, EBV and *Toxoplasma* spp. is worthwhile
- Other serological tests may be indicated, e.g. *Brucella* with a history of travel to southern Europe; Lyme disease after camping trip to an endemic area; hepatitis C if there is a history of past intravenous drug use.

Imaging

Do a chest radiograph in all cases, looking for TB, malignancy and lymphadenopathy. Other imaging should be as directed by clinical suspicion.

Management

If there are any abnormal findings, investigations or documented fever, patients should not be labelled as CFS. Once CFS has been diagnosed, do not send patients away with 'don't worry, there's nothing wrong' ringing in their ears: tell them that:

- you can find no serious progressive disease
- this is good news
- this does not mean that you do not believe them
- CFS is real
- the long-term outlook for most patients is good, with only 10% having significant ongoing disability [4].

Drug therapy

No pharmacological intervention has been proven to work for CFS. Some small studies of antibacterial, antiviral or antifungal agents have been promising, but others show no benefit. Antidepressants are also ineffective in CFS, but may be worth considering if you suspect coexistent depression. If sleep disturbance is prominent, using a sedative antidepressant such as amitriptyline is preferable. Corticosteroids are not beneficial unless adrenal insufficiency is present. A small subgroup of patients with postural hypotension appears to benefit from mineralocorticoids. Many patients take numerous vitamins, minerals and other supplements but the merits of these are unproven.

Non-drug therapy

Non-medication treatments have been proven to work but are not always available [5,6]. Bedrest is detrimental, but a supervised graded exercise programme has been shown to speed rehabilitation. This works best in conjunction with cognitive–behavioural therapy, which is of proven benefit in CFS.

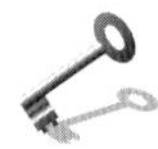

Lifestyle advice to the patient with chronic fatigue

- Limit excessive intake of tea, coffee, alcohol and recreational drugs
- Daily gentle exercise building up over time
- Avoid over-exercise
- Balanced diet
- Lose weight if obese
- Adjust work/social life to energy level.

Management of chronic fatigue syndrome

- Exclude other causes of fatigue
- Tell the patient the diagnosis and prognosis
- Provide support
- Develop rehabilitation plan.

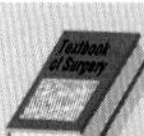

See *Psychiatry*, Section 1.6; *Endocrinology*, Section 1.20; *Rheumatology and clinical immunology*, Section 1.24.

1 Royal College of Physicians. *Chronic Fatigue Syndrome. Report 1996*. London: Royal College of Physicians, 1996.
2 Reid S, Chalder T, Cleare A *et al.* Chronic fatigue syndrome. *BMJ* 2000; 320: 292–296.
3 Schluederberg A, Straus SE, Peterson P *et al.* NIH conference. Chronic fatigue syndrome research. Definition and medical outcome assessment. *Ann Intern Med* 1992; 117: 325–331.
4 Kroenke K, Wood N, Munglesdorg AD *et al.* Chronic fatigue in primary care. Prevalence, patient characteristics, and outcome. *JAMA* 1988; 260: 929–934.
5 Sharpe M, Huwton K, Simkins S *et al.* Cognitive behaviour therapy for the chronic fatigue syndrome: a randomized controlled trial. *BMJ* 1996; 312: 22–26.
6 Fulcher KY, White PD. Randomised controlled trial of graded exercise in patients with the chronic fatigue syndrome. *BMJ* 1997; 314: 1647–1652.

1.19 Varicella in pregnancy

Case history

A 23-year-old pregnant woman is referred with chickenpox.

Clinical approach

The rash is usually characteristic and the diagnosis of chickenpox clear. Although a relatively benign illness in children, severe disease is not uncommon in adults. Life-threatening complications such as pneumonitis are more common in people who smoke, are immunocompromised or are pregnant, when there is also the fetus to consider. These groups therefore need urgent assessment and therapy.

Complications of chickenpox

- Pneumonitis
- Secondary bacterial infection of skin lesions
- Hepatitis
- Post-infectious cerebellar encephalitis is more common in children, occurring in 1 in 6000 cases
- Effect on the fetus.

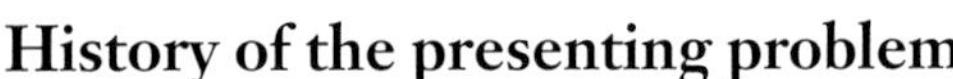

History of the presenting problem

Ask about the following:

- Duration of illness? The earlier treatment is started the better.
- Stage of pregnancy? Risk of fetal abnormalities is highest (about 2.2%) if maternal infection occurs before 20 weeks' gestation [2]. If maternal chickenpox develops within 7 days of delivery, the neonate may develop severe chickenpox up to 3–4 weeks after birth. The highest risk of pneumonitis to the mother is in the third trimester [3].
- Dyspnoea, cough or haemoptysis? Must exclude varicella pneumonitis.
- Smoker? More likely to develop pneumonitis.

Relevant past history

Immune dysfunction increases the risk of severe complications, particularly if there is cell-mediated immune deficiency, e.g. after transplantation, immunosuppressive therapy or HIV infection (see Section 1.17, p. 44).

Examination

General

Examine the skin for vesicles and look for evidence of secondary bacterial infection.

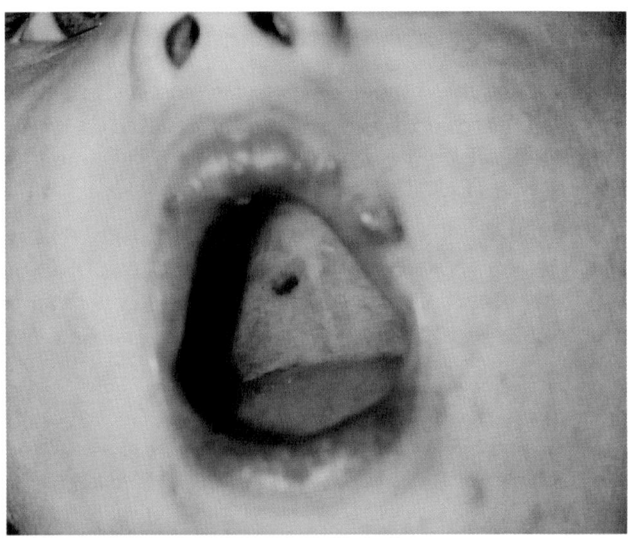

Fig. 30 Child with typical palatal lesion of chickenpox.

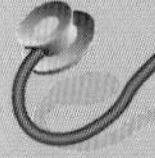

Rash of varicella

Starts as crops of vesicles containing clear fluid on an erythematous base. These evolve into pustules and then scabs. The lesions start on the trunk and spread peripherally. Examine the mouth for lesions (Fig. 30): these may be so severe as to interfere with eating and drinking.

Respiratory assessment

Check for central cyanosis, respiratory rate and focal chest signs. Cough is typically non-productive, or produces clear sputum streaked with blood; purulent sputum suggests secondary bacterial infection.

Approach to investigation and management

Assess for maternal complications, such as pneumonitis, review the potential fetal risk and decide on therapy.

Investigations

Blood tests

- FBC, electrolytes and renal function—hyponatraemia is common in severe varicella
- Liver function tests to detect varicella hepatitis
- Arterial blood gas estimation (if very unwell).

Cultures and serology

- Vesicle fluid for electron microscopy, viral and bacterial culture (see Section 3.1, p. 150)
- Anti-varicella IgM antibodies can be used to confirm the diagnosis
- Blood and sputum cultures because bacterial superinfection is common.

Imaging

A chest radiograph should be performed in any pregnant woman referred to hospital with chickenpox. In pregnancy, the radiation risk of a chest radiograph (minimal with shielding) is far outweighed by the mortality of pneumonitis (Fig. 31).

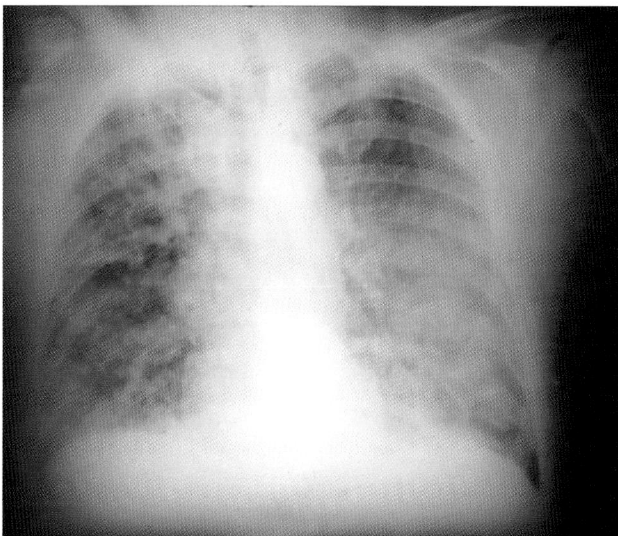

(a)

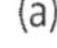

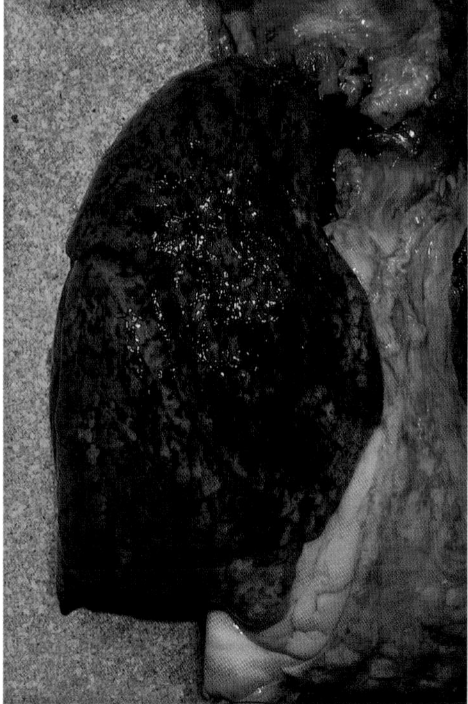

(b)

Fig. 31 (a) Chest radiograph of a 43-year-old smoker presenting 5 days after the onset of the rash with cough and breathlessness. Widespread interstitial shadowing is present throughout the lungs. This may progress to form calcific nodules in survivors. (b) Lung of the same patient *post mortem*. The haemorrhagic lesions of varicella can be seen on the lung surface.

Management

For details of supportive care, see Section 1.2, p. 5; see also *Emergency medicine*, Sections 1.2 and 1.5 [1].

The patient

Adults presenting within 72 h of developing skin lesions should be treated with aciclovir (valaciclovir and famciclovir are suitable alternatives). Transmission is by respiratory droplets and hospitalized isolation in a single room is essential. Intravenous therapy with aciclovir 10 mg/kg three times daily (adjusted depending on renal function) is indicated for severe disease, pneumonitis, hepatitis or acute encephalitis, or in significant immunocompromise [3]. Consider secondary bacterial pneumonia, bacteraemia or cellulitis and treat appropriately.

The fetus

Inform obstetricians because of the possibility of premature labour. There is a small risk of spontaneous abortion or fetal abnormality to 20 weeks' gestation [2]. Aciclovir is not associated with any teratogenic effects. There is a high risk (30%) of disseminated varicella, encephalitis and death if the child is born before maternal immunity to varicella has developed. Neonates born between 5 days before and 3 days after the onset of maternal chickenpox should be treated with hyperimmune antivaricella immunoglobulin (VZIG).

Contacts

Varicella non-immune pregnant women who are exposed to chickenpox should be referred for assessment. If varicella IgG negative, confirming a non-immune status, consider administering VZIG to the mother [4]. VZIG supplies are limited and kept at the Public Health Laboratory Service. VZIG should also be considered for any immunocompromised contacts.

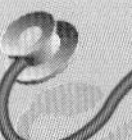

Fetal varicella syndrome

- Occurs in 2.2% of pregnant women infected before 20 weeks' gestation
- Causes microcephaly, cicatricial limb deformities and skin scarring, cataracts and eye defects.

Varicella pneumonitis

Pneumonitis is more likely in people who smoke, pregnant women and immunocompromised patients. Patients may deteriorate very rapidly and their clinical condition, including oxygen saturation, should be monitored.

1 Wilkins EGL, Leen CLS, McKendrick MW, Carrington D. Management of chickenpox in the adult. A review prepared for the UK Advisory Group on Chickenpox on behalf of the British Society for the Study of Infection. *J Infect* 1998; 36(suppl 1): 49–58.
2 Pastuszak AL, Levy M, Schick B *et al*. Outcome after maternal varicella infection in the first 20 weeks of pregnancy. *N Engl J Med* 1994; 330: 901–905.
3 Nathwani D, Maclean A, Conway S, Carrington D. Varicella infections in pregnancy and the newborn. *J Infect* 1998; 36(suppl 1): 59–71.
4 Ogilvie MM. Antiviral prophylaxis and treatment in chickenpox. *J Infect* 1998; 36(suppl 1): 31–38.

1.20 Imported fever

Case history

A 19-year-old student has been feeling hot and cold for the last 3 days and is found to have a temperature of 39°C. Ten days ago he returned from a round-the-world trip.

Clinical approach

Your aim is, as always, to prevent morbidity and mortality from treatable disease, but also to consider transmissible infections of public health importance. Analyses of the final diagnosis in patients with fever after travel to the tropics reveal that about half are the result of tropical disease (Table 16). In assessing an individual patient, formulate two differential diagnoses—first including and then excluding the travel history. Your primary concern is early recognition of malaria: this is the most common single diagnosis and can kill, death being associated with delay in diagnosis.

Table 16 Important infectious causes of fever after travel to the tropics.

Tropical	Common	Malaria (N)
		Acute viral hepatitis* (N)
		Diarrhoeal illness* (N)
		Dengue fever
		Enteric fever* (N)
	Less common	Rickettsial infection
		Amoebic abscess
		Filariasis
		Acute HIV infection*
	Must consider	Viral haemorrhagic fevers* (N)
Cosmopolitan		Respiratory infection
		Urinary tract infection
		Pharyngitis
		Tuberculosis* (N)
		Meningitis* (N)

N, notifiable.
*Transmission of public health significance.

History of the presenting problem

Possibility of malaria

There are no clinical features that are specific for malaria (see Section 2.13.1. p. 141). You must consider this diagnosis immediately in any febrile traveller who may have been exposed within the last 6 months.

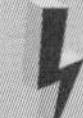

Malaria pitfalls

- Malaria typically presents with abrupt onset of fever accompanied by myalgia and headache. Misleading localizing features occur, such as abdominal pain, diarrhoea, breathlessness or jaundice.
- Brief exposure is sufficient to acquire malaria; the patient may be unaware that he has visited a malarious area or reassured that there was no risk. If in doubt assume potential exposure.
- Malaria chemoprophylaxis does not exclude malaria. It is at best 70–90% effective and compliance is poor.

Travel history

A comprehensive travel history is required to assess exposure to malaria (and other infections) [1,2].

Where, when and what

WHERE?

- Ask for specific countries, regions and descriptions (city, rainforest, etc.).
- Did he stay in a hotel, hostel or tent?

WHEN?

- Exactly when was he in each place? The incubation period limits the differential diagnosis [1].

WHAT?

- Was it holiday or work, such as disaster relief or a zoological expedition?
- Did he have any freshwater contact? Risk of schistosomiasis, amoebiasis or leptospirosis.
- Did he come into close contact with animals? Risk of anthrax.
- Did he eat unpasteurized dairy products or undercooked food? Risk of enteric pathogens and brucellosis.
- Was the water local, bottled, sterilized? Risk of enteric pathogens.
- Did he have sex while abroad?
- Did he do any unusual activities, e.g. caving? Risk of histoplasmosis in America.
- Any illness or treatment while away?

Precautions

Did he take any precautions?
- Pre-travel immunizations
- Malaria prophylaxis and insect bite deterrents
- Safe sex.

What else have you noticed?

A detailed history of symptoms associated with the feverishness is required. Give particular weight to volunteered symptoms, but also perform a systematic enquiry in relation to all organ systems. You will gain little by trying to analyse the fever pattern.

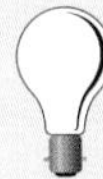

Viral haemorrhagic fevers

Viral haemorrhagic fevers (VHFs) are not a major threat to public health, but some (Lassa, Marburg, Ebola and Congo–Crimean haemorrhagic fever [CCHF]) can be transmitted to nursing, medical and laboratory staff and carry a high case-fatality rate.

VHFs are rare in travellers but difficult to distinguish from other febrile illnesses and you need to maintain vigilance. Case identification depends on recognition of epidemiological risk, i.e. travel to rural, sub-Saharan West Africa (except CCHF, which is distributed sporadically in Africa, the eastern Mediterranean, the Middle East and parts of southern Asia) and contact with known or suspected human cases. The upper limit of the incubation period is 21 days, beyond which these diseases are effectively excluded [3].

Examination

A full examination is required. Your primary survey should ensure that breathing and circulation are adequate, followed by a detailed examination of each system. Your general impression of how ill the patient is will determine whether or not you start immediate empirical treatment. Take particular note of the following:
- Lymphadenopathy
- Jaundice
- Hepatomegaly and/or splenomegaly
- Rash, e.g. look carefully for the eschar of a tick bite or the generalized rash of dengue fever (Fig. 32).

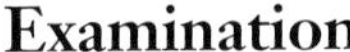

Approach to investigation and management

Investigations

blood tests

Check the FBC, thick and thin malaria films (see Sections 2.13.1, p. 141 and 3.2, p. 151), renal and liver function tests and CRP. Creatine phosphokinase may be elevated in leptospirosis or severe septicaemia. Save serum for serological tests.

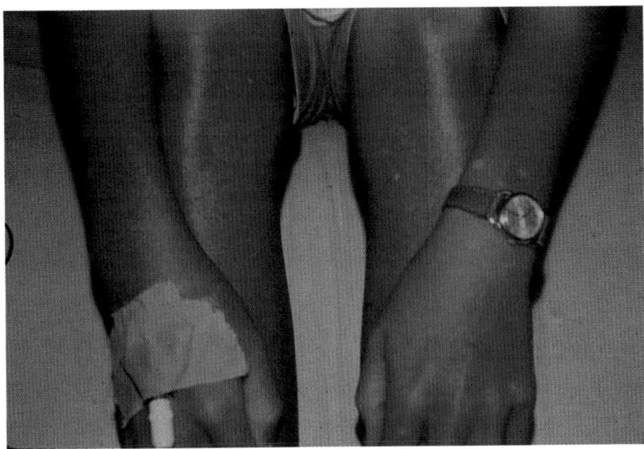

Fig. 32 Evanescent macular rash of dengue fever. The rash resembles scarlet fever or a toxic drug reaction, but may be difficult to see. (Courtesy of T Loke.)

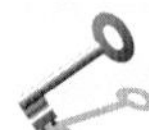

Malaria films

- The timing of the blood sample in relation to the fever is unimportant.
- A single negative malaria film does not exclude the diagnosis. Repeat every 12–24 h in a patient at risk. Malaria is highly unlikely after three negative films, but remains a possibility until the illness resolves or an alternative diagnosis is confirmed.
- Rapid diagnostic tests for malaria can be helpful if available (see Section 2.13.1, p. 141).

Cultures

Take blood, throat swab, MSU, and stool microscopy and culture. Other body sites should be cultured according to the clinical picture.

Imaging

Check a chest radiograph in all cases. Look for consolidation and mediastinal lymphadenopathy. A raised right hemidiaphragm suggests the possibility of an amoebic abscess (Fig. 33). Ultrasonography and/or CT are needed if a liver abscess or other intrathoracic/intra-abdominal collection is suspected.

Management

You must exclude malaria; if malaria films are positive, institute therapy and seek specialist advice in severe malaria (see Section 2.13.1, p. 141). Benign malaria can be treated as an outpatient but all patients with *P. falciparum*

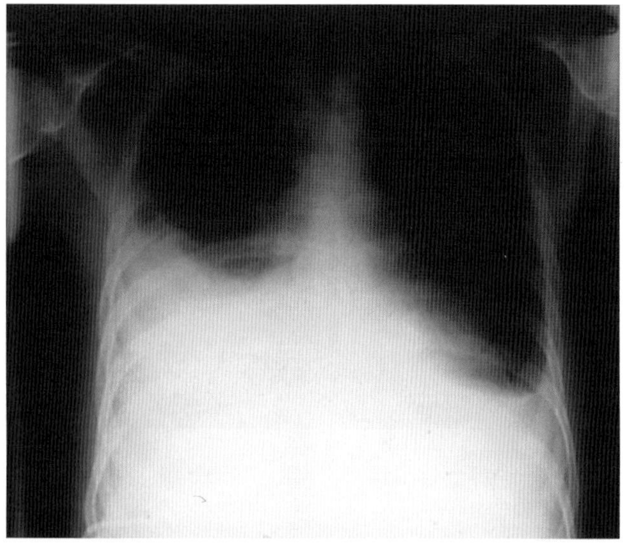

(a)

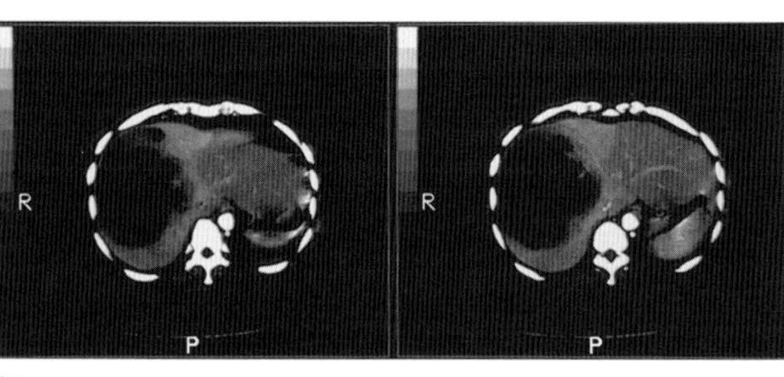

(b)

Fig. 33 (a) Chest radiograph of a patient from India presenting with fever and right upper quadrant pain. (b) CT scan from the same patient revealing a large liver abscess later confirmed as amoebic.

malaria should be admitted. If another specific diagnosis is made, treat appropriately—the challenge is the febrile traveller without a diagnosis!

Fever of unknown cause

IS ADMISSION REQUIRED?

• Your management depends on judgement of the most likely diagnoses and how ill the patient is. Review the history, examination and investigations carefully. If the patient is well enough to be discharged, make arrangements for repeat malaria films, early clinic review, and instruct the patient to return sooner if his condition deteriorates. If in doubt admit for observation.

SHOULD THE PATIENT BE GIVEN EMPIRICAL THERAPY?

• Patients whom you judge to be (or at risk of becoming) seriously unwell should be given 'best guess' empirical antimicrobial therapy once specimens for culture have been obtained. Empirical therapy should be designed to cover the likely diagnoses and those with potentially serious consequences if left untreated (see Section 1.2, p. 5). You rarely need to treat for malaria unless the blood film is positive (see Section 2.13.1, p. 141).

WHAT SORT OF CONTINUED EVALUATION?

• The patient will need regular review until the diagnosis and treatment are clear or the illness resolves. Consider taking advice or referring to a communicable disease or tropical unit if the fever is persistent or the patient deteriorating.

Failure to report notifiable infections is an offence.

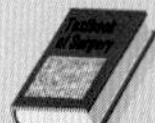

1 Felton JM, Bryceson ADM. Fever in the returning traveller. *Br J Hosp Med* 1996; 55: 705–711.
2 Jacobs MG. Imported fever—a survival guide. *J R Soc Med* 2000; 93: 124–128.
3 Advisory Committee on Dangerous Pathogens. *Management and Control of Viral Haemorrhagic Fevers.* London: The Stationery Office, 1996.

1.21 Eosinophilia

Case history

A 29-year-old soldier has recently returned from a 'jungle assignment'. He has fatigue and is found to have marked eosinophilia.

Clinical approach

Most cases of eosinophilia in patients who have been abroad are caused by infection with multicellular (metazoan) parasites, in particular tissue-invasive helminths [1] (Table 17). Your initial assessment and investigations should be

Table 17 Common parasitic causes of eosinophilia.

Disease	Geographical distribution
Strongyloidiasis	Throughout the tropics and subtropics
Schistosomiasis*	Africa, Arabia, Caribbean, South America, Japan, China, The Philippines
Filariasis	Throughout the tropics and subtropics
Trichinosis	Worldwide
Toxocariasis	Worldwide
Ascariasis	Worldwide

*Combined distribution of multiple species. (See Section 2.14.1, p. 145.)

Table 18 Non-infectious causes of eosinophilia.

Cause	Examples
Allergic reactions	Atopy
	Drug reactions
Solid neoplasms	Carcinoma of lung
	Renal cell carcinoma
	Cervical carcinoma
	Tumours of the large bowel
	Melanoma
Lymphoreticular malignancy	Hodgkin's disease
	B- and T-cell lymphoma
	T-cell leukaemia
	Myelomonocytic leukaemia
Vasculitic diseases	Churg–Strauss disease
	Wegener's granulomatosis
Idiopathic	Hypereosinophilic syndrome

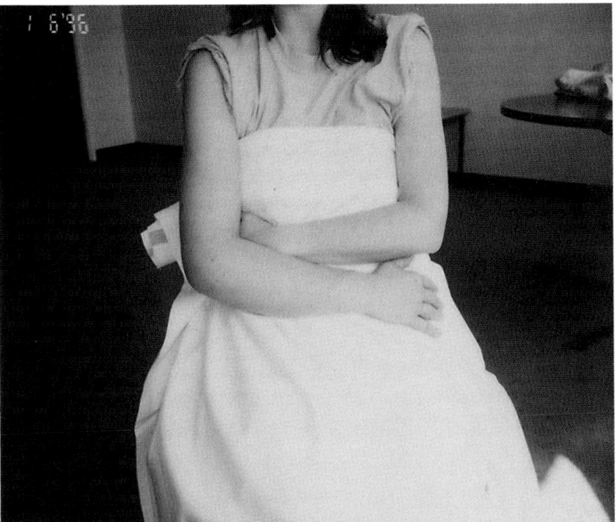

Fig. 34 This young woman presented with fever, swelling of the right arm and tender right axillary lymph nodes after a prolonged trip to sub-Saharan Africa. She had a marked eosinophilia with filariasis confirmed serologically.

directed towards these conditions—eosinophilia is not a feature of the host response to single-celled (protozoal) parasites. A wide range of non-infectious conditions can also cause eosinophilia [2]; the most important are allergic reactions, either atopic or drug related (Table 18). If parasitic and allergic causes are excluded, a search for rarer causes of eosinophilia is required.

History of the presenting problem

Exposure to metazoan parasites

The major risk is travel to areas of endemic parasite infections. Essentially, travel to any tropical or subtropical part of the world is a significant risk. Parasites can remain asymptomatic for years, so you should take a life-time travel and detailed exposure history. This particular patient is likely to have all of these exposures:

- Have you ever travelled to the tropics or subtropics and when?
- Which countries did you visit?
- Did you have any freshwater contact? (schistosomiasis)
- Did you walk barefoot? (strongyloidiasis)
- Have you eaten undercooked meat? (trichinosis)

Clues to particular infections

Most infections with metazoan parasites are asymptomatic, making the exposure history vital. However, the history may contain some specific clues to certain parasites.

- Have you been feeling feverish? (schistosomiasis)
- Have you had any cough or wheeze? (pulmonary eosinophilia, e.g. from *Ascaris*)
- Have you had any diarrhoea?
- Have you noticed any blood in your urine or stool?
- Have you had a rash?
- Have you had muscle aches or pains? (trichinosis)

Allergy

Ask carefully about symptoms of atopy. Take a careful drug history. Drug reactions can occur even after long-term use, so potential culprits are not limited to recent changes in medication.

Relevant past history

Pay particular attention to allergies, medication, previous autoimmune disease and cancer.

Examination

Perform a full examination, but don't be disappointed if there are no external signs of disease. Specific clues to parasites include the following:

- Lymphoedema: suggests filariasis (Fig. 34)
- Rash, e.g. cutaneous larva migrans, dermatitis in onchocerciasis
- Subcutaneous nodules: may be present in onchocerciasis
- Lymphadenopathy
- Urine dipstick for microscopic haematuria—suggests schistosomiasis in this context.

Approach to investigation and management

Investigations

Unless there is a strong clinical suspicion of an alternative diagnosis, the first round of tests is usually directed towards helminthic infection.

Blood tests

Check the FBC and film, eosinophil count, electrolytes, renal and liver function, CRP and ESR. Measure total serum IgE—a normal level weighs against parasitic infections and allergic diseases.

Imaging

Serial chest radiographs may reveal transient infiltrates suggestive of pulmonary eosinophilia [3]. A chest radiograph may also be abnormal in allergic bronchopulmonary aspergillosis and Churg–Strauss disease. Plain radiographs may reveal calcified cysts in cysticercosis or trichiniasis. (See Section 2.14.3, p. 146.)

Parasitological investigations

Specific tests are guided by the exposure history:
- Stool microscopy for ova, cysts and parasites in all cases (see Section 3.1, p. 150). This may need to be repeated several times—expert interpretation is required.
- Blood films are indicated to detect some forms of filariasis, e.g. *Loa loa*. (See Section 2.14.4, p. 147.)
- Skin snips (see Section 3.2, p. 151) can detect onchocerciasis. (See Section 2.14.4, p. 147.)
- Duodenal biopsy or aspirate can detect *Strongyloides stercoralis*. (See Section 2.14.2, p. 145.)
- Serological tests as directed, but note that these may be difficult to interpret with considerable crossreactivity between species.
- Terminal urine sample or rectal biopsy for schistosomiasis (Fig. 35). (See Section 2.14.1, p. 145.)

Other tests

If there has been parasitic exposure, it is unlikely to be necessary to investigate for the diseases listed in Table 18.

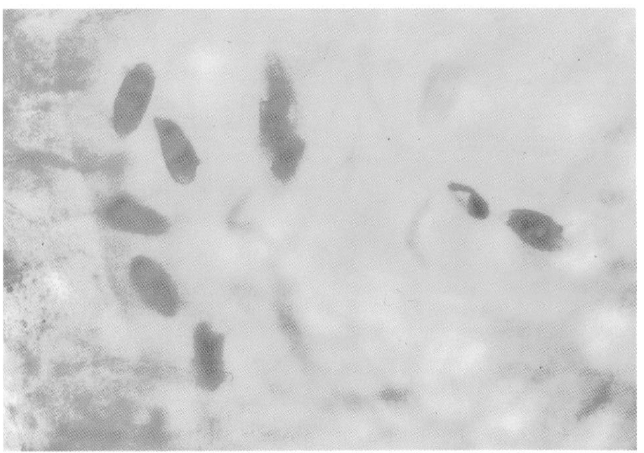

Fig. 35 *Schistosoma mansoni*, identified by the lateral spine, on a rectal biopsy. (See Section 2.14.1, p. 145.)

Management

Appropriate investigation is the cornerstone of management. While this is progressing, stop all drugs that are not absolutely necessary. Treatment is virtually always given only when a firm diagnosis has been established. If the condition defies diagnosis, there is sometimes a role for empirical antihelminthic treatment in consultation with an expert. Treatment of specific infections is covered in Section 2.14, p. 145.

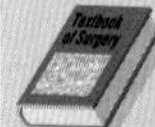

See *Haematology*, Section 2.6.

1 Wolfe MS. Eosinophilia in the returning traveler. *Med Clin North Am* 1999; 83: 1019–1032.
2 Bain BJ. Hypereosinophilia. *Curr Opin Hematol* 2000; 7: 21–25.
3 Ong RK, Doyle RL. Tropical pulmonary eosinophilia. *Chest* 1998; 113: 1673–1679.

1.22 Jaundice and fever after travelling

Case history

A 48-year-old woman presents with fever and jaundice after a trip to the Indian subcontinent to visit her parents.

Clinical approach

The differential diagnosis of jaundice is extensive (see *Gastroenterology and hepatology*, Sections 1.5 and 1.6), but the history of travel and fever makes infection likely (Table 19) [1–3]. A common mistake is to limit your thinking to infectious agents that primarily infect the liver, in particular the hepatitis viruses. Jaundice may be a manifestation of systemic infection that can have severe

Table 19 Important infectious causes of fever and jaundice after travel to the tropics.

Tropical	Common	Acute viral hepatitis A, B and E
		Malaria
	Less common	Leptospirosis
		Typhoid
	Uncommon	Fascioliasis
		Relapsing fever
		Yellow fever
Cosmopolitan		Ascending cholangitis
		EBV, CMV, hepatitis A and B
		Toxoplasmosis

EBV, Epstein–Barr virus; CMV, cytomegalovirus.

consequences if untreated. Spaceoccupying infections within the liver (such as bacterial or amoebic abscess) rarely present with jaundice.

History of the presenting problem

Possibility of malaria

Always consider malaria in a febrile traveller who has been exposed within the last 6 months. (See Section 1.20, p. 52.)

Acute viral hepatitis

In acute viral hepatitis, systemic symptoms occur in the prodromal phase and typically resolve with the onset of jaundice. Fever rarely persists into the icteric phase. This holds true for acute hepatitis A, B and E, which cannot be distinguished reliably from each other clinically. Hepatitis C rarely presents with acute hepatitis.

A detailed history of the progression of the illness is required:

- When were you last completely well?
- When did you notice that you were looking yellow?
- What was the first thing that you noticed was wrong?
- Is your urine darker than usual and when did it change? Dark urine is caused by excretion of conjugated bilirubin in intrahepatic and posthepatic jaundice.
- Are your stools pale? Have you been itchy? Intrahepatic inflammation, such as in acute viral hepatitis, can cause cholestasis with pale stools and pruritus.
- How are you feeling now? Patients with acute viral hepatitis generally feel better once they become jaundiced.

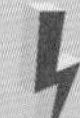

Do not accept the diagnosis of acute viral hepatitis in a patient with jaundice and high fever. Make sure that you consider life-threatening illnesses such as malaria, ascending cholangitis and typhoid.

How infection was caught

Remember that hepatitis A and E are spread via the faecal–oral route and hepatitis B by blood or sex. Also keep the different incubation periods in mind. (See Section 2.10.8, p. 131.)

- Where have you been, when and what did you do? (See Section 1.20, p. 52.)
- Then concentrate on risks for conditions listed in Table 19. Tact and care will be required to elicit this information without causing offence (see *General clinical issues*, Section 2).
- Was the water safe and what did you eat (e.g. shellfish)?
- Have you had unprotected sex in the last 6 months?
- Have you ever injected yourself with drugs?

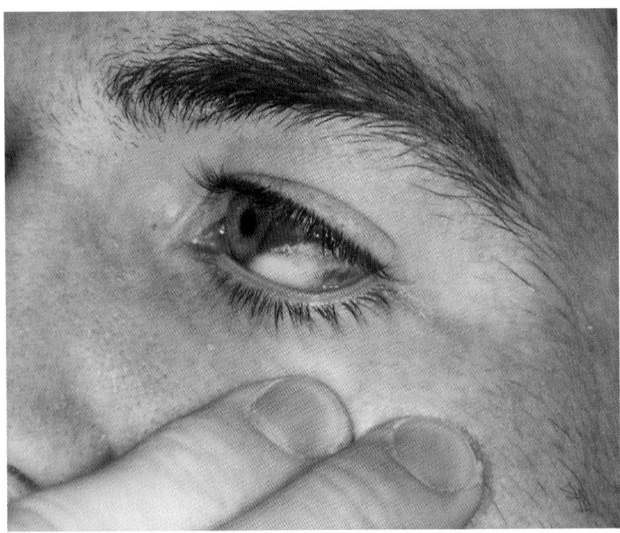

Fig. 36 Subconjunctival haemorrhage.

- Did you have any injections, transfusions or surgical treatment while abroad?
- Did you have a tattoo or any body piercing?
- Have you been immunized against hepatitis? Which type and when? [4]
- Where were you brought up? Individuals who spent their childhood in the tropics are likely to have acquired hepatitis A previously and have lifelong immunity.

Fever and jaundice

Consider the following:

- Leptospirosis: this is common in 'adventure' travellers with freshwater exposure. Fever is usually low grade and the exposure history, along with associated features such as myalgia, meningism or subconjunctival haemorrhages (Fig. 36), suggest the diagnosis. (See Section 2.7.4, p. 116)
- Ascending cholangitis: abdominal pain, jaundice and high fever, often with rigors, raises the possibility of ascending cholangitis. This may result in severe sepsis, which can be rapidly fatal.

Drugs and alcohol

- Ask about prescription and over-the-counter medication. Could the patient have glucose-6-phosphate dehydrogenase (G6PD) deficiency?
- Some recreational drugs, e.g. Ecstasy, can cause acute hepatitis.
- Increased alcohol consumption on holiday may induce alcoholic hepatitis.

Relevant past history

Ask specifically about a previous history of jaundice or biliary disease and risk factors such as alcohol intake. Acute viral hepatitis is much more severe where there is pre-existing liver disease. This woman is 48 years old but, if a younger woman, could she be pregnant? Hepatitis E is generally benign but has a high mortality in pregnancy [5].

Examination

General

Is she well, ill or very ill? Take careful note of the following:
• Fever
• Lymphadenopathy
• Conjunctival haemorrhage in viral haemorrhagic fever or leptospirosis.

Hepatic failure

Check for the following:
• Liver flap
• Confusion
• Spontaneous bruising or bleeding at venepuncture sites. (See *Gastroenterology and hepatology*, Sections 1.7 and 1.16.)

Hepatobiliary system

• Is there really jaundice? Ask the patient to turn her eyes downwards while you retract the upper eyelids, so that you can see the part of the sclerae protected from dust exposure.
• Is the liver enlarged or tender?
• Is there splenomegaly?
• Look for signs of chronic liver disease. (See *Gastroenterology and hepatology*, Sections 1.3 and 1.6.)

Approach to investigation and management

Investigations

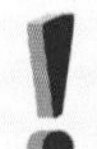

Initial investigations of jaundice

If you were allowed only two tests, which would you choose? The correct answer is:
• Urine dipstick for bilirubin: conjugated bilirubin is water soluble and excreted in urine, so the absence of urine bilirubin in the presence of jaundice implies a prehepatic cause such as haemolysis. If bilirubin is present, the cause of jaundice is intrahepatic or posthepatic.
• Hepatic ultrasonography: intrahepatic or posthepatic causes of jaundice can be distinguished by looking for dilated biliary ducts on ultrasonography.

These simple tests therefore allow you to divide jaundice into prehepatic, intrahepatic and posthepatic types.

Blood tests

Check the following:
• FBC and film for malaria and evidence of haemolysis. (See *Haematology* Section 2.1.7.)
• Renal function: abnormal in leptospirosis, haemolytic uraemic syndrome (see *Nephrology*, Section 2.7.3), or simply a marker of impending acute renal failure or hepatorenal syndrome.
• Clotting and serum albumin to assess hepatic synthetic function.
• Liver function tests: see *Gastroenterology and hepatology*, Section 3.1. In acute viral hepatitis liver transaminases are always significantly elevated. Repeat measurements are useful to follow the course of the illness—typically there will be a shift from a hepatic to a cholestatic pattern as the viral hepatitis begins to resolve. (See Section 2.10.8, p. 131.)
• Monospot/Paul–Bunnell test may allow rapid diagnosis of EBV.

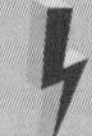

Consider paracetamol overdose in any patient presenting acutely with jaundice.

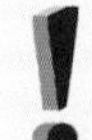

Mild elevation of transaminases is non-specific and can occur in many infections including malaria, typhoid, dengue and bacterial sepsis.

Cultures and serology

Blood cultures should be done in all cases.

Consider serological tests for the following:
• Hepatitis A, B, C and E: see Section 2.10.8, p. 131
• CMV and EBV: see Sections 2.10.3, p. 128 and 2.10.4, p. 129
• Toxoplasmosis: see Section 2.13.4, p. 144
• Leptospirosis: see Section 2.7.4, p. 116.

Always save the serum.

Management

It is essential to recognize life-threatening infections such as cholangitis, bacterial sepsis, malaria, leptospirosis and haemolytic uraemic syndrome, and treat urgently (see Section 1.2, p. 5). In other patients, you can wait for the results of tests and then institute specific management.

Viral hepatitis

There is no antiviral therapy for acute viral hepatitis:
• Is admission needed? In general, patients can be managed at home unless there is evidence of impaired liver synthetic function or hepatic failure. Follow liver function and the prothrombin time closely until liver function is improving.

• What if the patient goes into liver failure? Refer to a specialist unit sooner rather than later: intensive support and possibly transplantation may be needed. (See *Gastroenterology and hepatology*, Section 2.9.)
• Is there a risk of spread? Give advice on hygiene and safe sex to limit spread. Don't forget that hepatitis A can be transmitted though sexual activity. If hepatitis A, household contacts should be offered immunoglobulin and/or hepatitis A vaccine. If hepatitis B, trace, screen for chronic hepatitis B and then immunize sexual contacts.
• For how long should they come to the clinic? Hepatitis A and E need to be followed only until they are clearly improving. Hepatitis B and C need monitoring for chronic disease. (See Section 2.10.8, p. 131.)

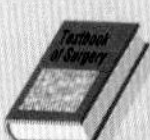

See *Gastroenterology and hepatology*, Sections 1.6, 1.7, 1.16, 2.9 and 2.10.

1 Koff RS. Hepatitis A. *Lancet* 1998; 351: 1643–1649.
2 Aggarwal R, Krawczynski KJ. Hepatitis E. An overview and recent advances in clinical and laboratory research. *Gastroenterol Hepatol* 2000; 15: 9–20.
3 Winn WC Jr. Enterically transmitted hepatitis. Hepatitis A and E viruses. *Clin Lab Med* 1999; 19: 661–673.
4 Loscher T, Keystone JS, Steffen R. Vaccination of travellers against hepatitis A and B. *J Travel Med* 1999; 6: 107–114.
5 Duff P. Hepatitis in pregnancy. *Semin Perinatol* 1998; 22: 277–283.

1.23 A traveller with diarrhoea

Case history

A 35-year-old Australian woman has travelled through south-east Asia, India and Africa before arriving in the UK. On the flight from South Africa to London, she developed abdominal discomfort and diarrhoea.

Clinical approach

This is most probably a case of infectious enterocolitis (Table 20) [1,2]. Try to decide if the infection is non-invasive or invasive, because this will guide therapeutic decisions. A bewildering array of tropical parasites can cause diarrhoea, but few require urgent treatment; consideration of these can be delayed until test results become available and, if diarrhoea persists, efforts to find parasites can be intensified. The only exception is amoebic colitis [3], which needs early treatment. (See *Gastroenterology and hepatology*, Section 2.13.)

Table 20 Causes of infective diarrhoea.

Enterocolitis	Organism	Common examples
Non-invasive	Viruses	Rotavirus, Norwalk, calicivirus, adenovirus, astrovirus, SRSV
	Bacteria	EPEC, ETEC, *Vibrio* spp., *Staph. aureus, Bacillus cereus, Clostridium perfringens*
	Parasites	*Giardia lamblia, Cryptosporidium parvum, Isospora belli, Cyclospora* spp.
Invasive	Bacteria	EHEC, *Shigella* spp., *Salmonella* spp., *Campylobacter jejuni, Clostridium difficile*
	Parasites	*Entamoeba histolytica, Balantidium coli, Schistosoma mansoni/japonicum*
Enteric fever	Bacteria	*Salmonella typhi, S. paratyphi* A and B, *Yersinia* spp.

EHEC, enterohaemorrhagic *E. coli*; EPEC, enteropathogenic *E. coli*; ETEC, enterotoxigenic *E. coli*; SRSV, small, round, structured virus.

Do not fall into the trap of making a cursory assessment. As you approach the patient, do not limit your thinking to infectious enterocolitis. Diarrhoea can be a prominent symptom in severe systemic infections such as bacterial sepsis or toxic shock syndrome (see Section 1.2, p. 5). In travellers, consider malaria or typhoid. Do not forget surgical causes such as appendicitis.

History of the presenting problem

Type of enteric infection

The history will help you decide whether the infection is non-invasive or invasive:
• What is the diarrhoea like? Ask about frequency, volume, consistency, blood and mucus.
• Abdominal pain? Is the pain continuous or colicky? Is it relieved by defaecation?
• Tenesmus?
• Nausea or vomiting?
• Fever/shivers/chills or other systemic symptoms?

Non-invasive diarrhoea

This is caused by viruses, bacterial enterotoxins or protozoa affecting the proximal small bowel. Typically the diarrhoea is watery and associated with nausea and vomiting. Abdominal cramps may be prominent, but the pain is not relieved by defaecation. There is usually minimal or no systemic upset.

Invasive diarrhoea

This is commonly bacterial but consider amoebic colitis. Typically, bowel movements are frequent and may contain mucus or blood (dysentery). Cramping pain is relieved by defaecation and tenesmus is common. Low-grade fever is common, but high fever or rigors suggest blood-stream invasion.

Source of infection

Unless more than one person has been affected, a food history rarely identifies the source of enteric infection. You need to take a travel history. (See Section 1.20, p. 52.)

Systemic infection

Marked systemic symptoms imply invasion from bacterial colitis, infection at another site or generalized infection (e.g. malaria or enteric fever). Take particular note of the following:

- Symptoms of infection outside the gastrointestinal tract
- Symptoms of severe sepsis: see Section 1.2, p. 5
- Menstrual history/tampon use: see Section 1.2, p. 5
- Travel history: see Section 1.20, p. 52.

Relevant past history

The following are particular points to note:

- Underlying illness, particularly immunosuppression
- Antacid drug use: increases the risk of infectious enterocolitis
- Recent antibiotic use: consider antibiotic-associated colitis (see Section 2.5.1, p. 103).

Examination

Is the woman well, ill, very ill or nearly dead? Check the vital signs—temperature, peripheral perfusion, pulse, BP (lying and standing/sitting). Begin resuscitation immediately if required. (See Section 1.2, p. 5; see also *Emergency medicine*, Section 1.2.)

Attention will then obviously focus on the abdomen. Are there are signs of peritonism? This should not occur in uncomplicated infectious enterocolitis. Splenomegaly implies systemic infection such as malaria or typhoid.

Look for focal signs of infection outside the gastrointestinal tract.

Approach to investigation and management

Investigations

Blood tests

- FBC, eosinophil count (see Section 1.21, p. 56), electrolytes, renal and liver function, CRP.
- Malaria films are mandatory if the patient is febrile and has visited a malarious area (see Section 1.20, p. 52).

Cultures and serology

- Blood and stool cultures: if stool is not available, take a rectal swab for culture.
- Stool microscopy for ova, cysts and parasites. Even if the illness does not suggest parasitic infection, gastrointestinal infection with multiple pathogens is common as a result of a shared route of transmission.
- Hot stool? Microscopic examination of a fresh stool specimen is useful if amoebic dysentery is suspected. Neutrophils within the specimen imply invasive or inflammatory diarrhoea, but may be absent in amoebic colitis because they are destroyed by the amoebae.
- Check amoebic serology in dysentery, but note that this may be negative early in disease.

Imaging

Plain abdominal film is rarely helpful unless marked tenderness suggests the possibility of toxic megacolon (Fig. 37).

Management

General

Fluid replacement is the mainstay of management. Use the oral route if possible. Intravenous replacement is needed if the patient is shocked or vomiting. Antidiarrhoeal agents should be avoided if there are signs of invasive disease.

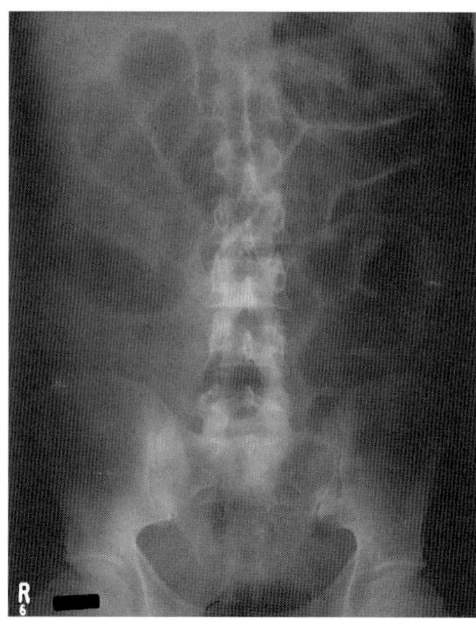

Fig. 37 Toxic megacolon in a case of *Clostridium difficile* colitis.

Antibiotic therapy

Most cases of diarrhoea do not require specific antimicrobial therapy and will settle with rehydration and time [4]. In uncomplicated salmonella infection, antibiotics are of no benefit and prolong stool carriage [5]. When therapy is indicated sensitivity data may help, but empirical therapy is required while awaiting culture results. Indications for this are the following:

- Marked systemic symptoms, particularly severe sepsis or shock, extraintestinal manifestations or a very marked inflammatory response. Ciprofloxacin is widely used but note increasing ciprofloxacin resistance.
- Moderate-to-severe bloody diarrhoea: ciprofloxacin for presumed bacterial dysentery; add metronidazole if at risk of amoebic dysentery.
- Very profuse non-inflammatory diarrhoea, which suggests cholera—consider tetracycline.

Specific antibiotics are indicated for the following:

- Positive blood cultures
- Typhoid/paratyphoid
- Parasitic infections (including amoebiasis).

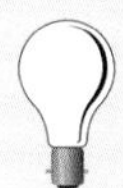

Immunocompromised host

- Increased range of pathogens, e.g. CMV enterocolitis
- Increased disease severity with invasive pathogens
- Antimicrobial therapy more likely to be required
- Increased incidence of salmonella bacteraemia
- Prolonged infection/carriage may occur, e.g. cryptosporidia

Public health

Note the following:

- Nurse in side room if admitted
- Give advice on hygiene if patient is discharged
- Food poisoning, suspected or proven, and typhoid are notifiable
- Salmonella infections require repeat stool cultures to detect chronic carriage, particularly if the patient is a food handler.

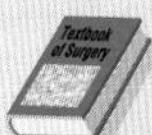

See *Gastroenterology and hepatology*, Section 1.1.

1 Cook GC. Diarrhoeal disease: a world-wide problem. *J R Soc Med* 1998; 91: 192–194.

2 DuPont HL. Diarrhoeal disease: current concepts and future challenges. Antimicrobial therapy and prophylaxis. *Trans R Soc Trop Med Hyg* 1993; 87(suppl 3): 31–34.

3 Li E, Stanley SL Jr. Protozoa. Amebiasis. *Gastroenterol Clin North Am* 1996; 25: 471–492.

4 Caeiro JP, DuPont HL. Management of travellers' diarrhoea. *Drugs* 1998; 56: 73–81.

5 Sirinavin S, Garner P. Antibiotics for treating salmonella gut infections. *Cochrane Database Syst Rev* 2000; (2): CD001167.

1.24 Malaise, mouth ulcers and fever

You are asked to review a 54-year-old gay man complaining of malaise, rash, mouth ulcers and pyrexia.

Clinical approach

Is this primary HIV infection (seroconversion illness) [1,2]? The differential diagnosis (Table 21) is wide and you must assess the HIV risk, exclude other conditions and consider antiretroviral therapy.

History of the presenting problem

A seroconversion illness occurs in 50–75% of patients acquiring HIV, but is often mild. Primary HIV infection has an incubation period of 2–4 weeks (range 1–6) and typically resolves within 14 days.

Exposure risk

- A full sexual history is needed—what sexual exposure has occurred both recently and in the past, how many partners and what type of sex? There is no 100% safe sex: unprotected receptive anal sex carries the highest risk, but oral sex still confers a risk.
- Does the man use recreational drugs? Drugs and alcohol increase high-risk behaviour. Intravenous drug use may directly transmit HIV.
- Is there a travel history? Sex abroad may carry a higher risk.

Symptoms

Symptoms associated with HIV seroconversion are shown in Table 22. Similar symptoms are seen in many other

Table 21 Differential diagnosis of malaise, rash, mouth ulcers and fever in a gay man.

Cause	Example
Viral	Primary HIV infection
	Mononucleosis (CMV, EBV, toxoplasmosis)
	Primary herpes simplex
	Enteroviruses
	Rubella and parvovirus infection
Bacterial	Secondary syphilis
	Disseminated gonorrhoea
	β-Haemolytic streptococcus
	Meningococcal infection
Non-infective	Crohn's disease
	Behçet's syndrome
	Leukaemia

CMV, cytomegalovirus; EBV, Epstein–Barr virus.

Table 22 Presenting symptoms in primary HIV.

System	Comments
General	Fever, sweats, malaise, myalgia, arthralgia
Mouth	Sore throat, mouth ulcers
Gastrointestinal	Odynophagia resulting from oesophageal ulcers (Fig. 38)
	Nausea, vomiting, diarrhoea, rectal ulcers
Skin	Rashes (Fig. 39)
Genitourinary	Ulceration
Neurological	Headache, photophobia, confusion, neuropathic pain

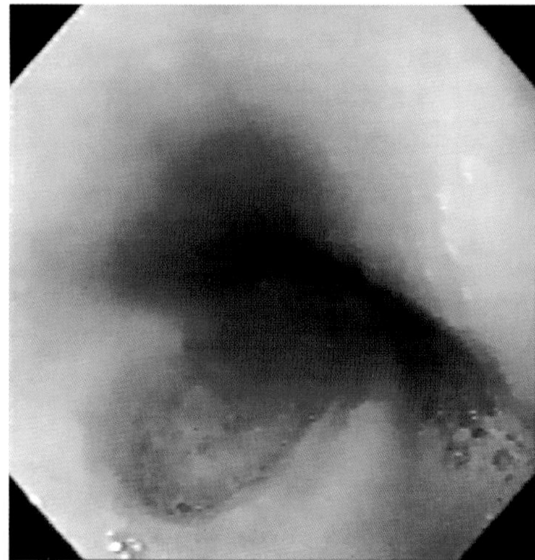

Fig. 38 Oesophageal ulcer during HIV seroconversion.

conditions and it is linking these with the exposure risk that will lead to a correct diagnosis (Fig. 38).

Examination

A full physical examination is required, noting the following in particular:

• Pyrexia is invariable in primary HIV.
• Mouth ulcers are common in HIV seroconversion, but by contrast to EBV disease tonsillar enlargement is rare.
• Rashes are frequent and most often macular (Fig. 39), although nodular and vesicular forms may be seen. Alopecia and desquamation may follow the rash.
• Lymphadenopathy: typically generalized, smooth, non-tender nodes appear in 70% of cases in the second week.
• Hepatosplenomegaly may be present.

Approach to investigation and management

Investigations

Blood tests

• FBC, electrolytes, renal and liver function tests, and inflammatory markers. Reactive lymphocytes are common. Thrombocytopenia may occur but anaemia is unusual. Liver enzymes are often raised but jaundice is rare. Elevated CRP and ESR are seen, and also creatine phosphokinase.

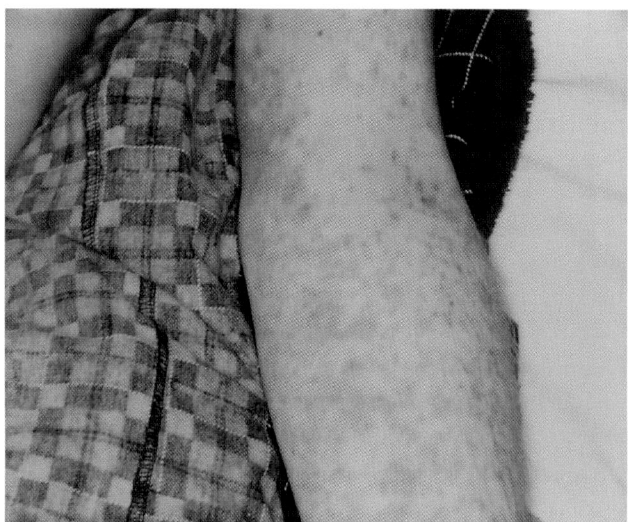

Fig. 39 Macular rash of HIV seroconversion.

• Differential lymphocyte count: in the second week of the illness CD8 cells increase and CD4 cells fall (see Section 2.11, p. 134). Occasionally CD4 cells can fall below 200/μL and opportunistic infections have been described. The ratio of CD4/CD8 cells is measured for prognostic reasons and is not a surrogate HIV test.

Serology and cultures

HIV DETECTION

• Anti-HIV antibodies appear 2–6 weeks after the onset of symptoms. HIV P24 antigen appears within 2–3 days of the onset of illness and PCR can detect HIV plasma RNA from 1 to 2 days before the onset of symptoms.

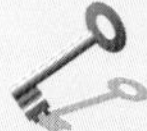

HIV testing

• In the mentally competent this must always be performed with consent.
• Testing without consent is only acceptable if the patient is *not* competent *and* the test is in their best interests.
• Pre- and post-test counselling should be available.

OTHER INFECTIONS

• Send blood cultures and throat swab for bacterial culture
• Viral culture from stool and throat for enteroviruses; viral throat swab for herpes simplex
• Syphilis serology will always be positive if there is secondary disease
• Positive Paul–Bunnell test suggests EBV, but false positives may occur
• Send specific serology for CMV, EBV and toxoplasmosis.

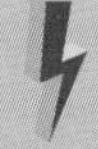

Primary HIV mimics other illnesses. HIV risk should be assessed in all cases of unexplained fever, fever plus rash, meningoencephalitis, hepatitis and oesophageal/rectal ulceration.

Serological diagnosis of HIV infection

- Enzyme-linked immunosorbent assay (ELISA) tests are used to screen for anti-HIV-1 and HIV-2 antibodies
- Approximately 1% equivocal or false-positive rate
- Confirm positive tests by further ELISA or western blot
- Window period from exposure to seroconversion of up to 3 months

Management

Other infections, particularly secondary syphilis, must be excluded. When primary HIV is confirmed consideration must be given to antiretroviral therapy (ART). There is a compelling theoretical argument to commence treatment immediately while the virus is still genetically homogenous and before extensive spread has occurred [3].

This must be weighed against committing patients with early disease to long-term, potentially toxic therapy (see Section 1.28, p. 70). In one study, zidovudine monotherapy for 6 months after seroconversion appeared to slow disease progression [4] and small studies with combination ART are encouraging.

Long-term clinical studies are awaited to define the role of ART in primary HIV infection. If ART is not started, treatment is essentially symptomatic and the patient should be monitored closely. Patients who appear high risk for rapid progression can then be targeted for early ART [5,6].

Factors associated with rapid HIV progression

- Age over 40 at seroconversion
- Severe or prolonged seroconversion illness
- CD4 fall to <200/μL during seroconversion
- Failure of CD4 to rise >500/μL after seroconversion
- High HIV viral load after seroconversion

1 Carr A, Cooper D. Primary HIV infection. In: Sande MA, Volberding PA (eds) *The Medical Management of AIDS* (5th edn). Philadelphia: WB Saunders, 1997: 89–106.
2 Cooper DA, Gold J, Maclean P *et al.* Acute AIDS retrovirus infection. Definition of a clinical illness associated with seroconversion. *Lancet* 1985; i: 537–540.
3 Jolles S, Kinloch-de Loes S, Johnson MA *et al.* Primary HIV-1 infection: a new medical emergency? *BMJ* 1996; 312: 1243–1244.
4 Kinloch-de Loes S, Hirschel BJ, Hoen B *et al.* A controlled trial of zidovudine in primary human immunodeficiency virus infection. *N Engl J Med* 1995; 333: 408–413.
5 Pedersen C, Katzenstein T, Nielsen C, Lundgren JD, Gerstoft J. Prognostic value of serum HIV-RNA levels at virologic steady state after seroconversion: relation to CD4 cell count and clinical course of primary infection. *J Acquir Immune Deficiency Syndr Hum Retrovirol* 1997; 16: 93.
6 Veugelers PJ, Kaldor JM, Strathdee SA *et al.* Incidence and prognostic significance of symptomatic primary human immunodeficiency virus type 1 infection in homosexual men. *J Infect Dis* 1997; 176: 112–117.

1.25 Needlestick exposure

Case history

A 32-year-old surgical registrar calls having had a needlestick injury while she was operating on an HIV-positive patient

Clinical approach

You must act quickly if postexposure prophylaxis (PEP) is to be effective. Assess the level of risk, decide on a therapeutic plan and counsel/support the member of staff.

History of the presenting problem

The risk of HIV transmission will depend on the HIV inoculum, which is the product of the concentration of virus in the blood and the volume transmitted.

The injury

- When did the incident occur? PEP must be given as soon as possible.
- What was the gauge of the needle? Was it hollow or solid?
- Had the needle come into direct contact with the patient's blood?
- How deep was the injury and did she make it bleed afterwards?

The HIV positive 'donor'

- Is the HIV viral load known? The higher the load, the more likely there is to be transmission.
- What is the stage of the HIV disease? Viral load tends to be highest at the time of seroconversion and in advanced AIDS.
- Is the patient on ART: if so, what drugs and are they working?
- ART history? You may need to consider drug resistance when choosing the PEP.
- Is the patient's syphilis and hepatitis status known?

Unknown source of any blood inoculum

Often the source is unknown, such as with injury from a needle from a sharps bin, or when the patient has not been tested for transmissible viruses. Knowledge of the local epidemiology can assist decision-making.

Personal history

This is delicate and should be discussed in a confidential setting. Ask the surgeon about other risk factors for acquiring HIV as part of pretest counselling. You should discuss sexual partners who may be at risk should the surgeon seroconvert to HIV.

Infections transmissible by needlestick

- HIV, hepatitis B and hepatitis C
- Malaria, South American trypanosomiasis
- Syphilis
- Ebola and Lassa fever.

Examination

Look at the actual wound because this can help assess risk.

Approach to investigation and management

The event should be reported immediately and an incident form completed. Expert evaluation of the need for PEP should occur quickly and with preserved confidentiality. Needlestick injuries are stressful even if there is no risk of HIV—counselling and support should be made available as required.

Investigations

Testing the source of any blood inoculum

If the source is known but the infection status is unclear, you can request that the patient is tested for transmissible infections. This must be done with consent. A senior member of staff should approach him or her and not the surgeon who suffered the needlestick.

Testing the healthcare worker

Check immunity to hepatitis B. Check baseline HIV and hepatitis C status at the healthcare worker's request and store serum for retrospective testing if necessary.

Management

Postexposure prophylaxis for HIV

The risk of HIV seroconversion after a high-risk needlestick is 0.32% (95% confidence interval of 0.18–0.46) [1]. Risk can be assessed as higher or lower using the questions outlined above. HIV risk from blood splashing on to intact skin is minimal and mucous membrane exposure is estimated at 0.03%. A retrospective case–control study indicated that PEP with zidovudine monotherapy was associated with a 79% fall in transmission [2].

Come to a joint decision on PEP with the healthcare worker after discussing the HIV risk, medications and side effects. Current guidelines for HIV PEP are shown in Table 23 [3]. A 28-day course is recommended, but less than 50% complete the course and follow-up. Different medication may be needed if drug-resistant HIV is suspected.

Table 23 Department of Health recommendations for postexposure prophylaxis in the UK.

Regimen	Comment
Zidovudine (AZT) 300 mg + lamivudine 150 mg twice daily	Minimum standard. Can be taken as Combivir one tablet twice daily Anaemia, nausea and headache may occur
Zidovudine (AZT) 300 mg + lamivudine 150 mg twice daily + nelfinavir 750 mg three times daily	Recommended regimen for maximal efficacy Diarrhoea from nelfinavir
Zidovudine (AZT) 300 mg + lamivudine 150 mg twice daily + indinavir 800 mg three times daily	Alternative protease inhibitor-based regimen Renal toxicity from indinavir; must drink 3 L/day

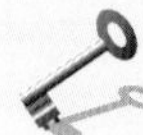

Risk of blood-borne viruses

Risk of acquiring blood-borne viruses from a needlestick injury:

- HIV 0.32%
- Hepatitis C 3–5%
- Hepatitis B 'e' antigen positive: 30–50% in non-immune

Factors increasing HIV risk

Factors increasing risk of HIV transmission by needlestick:

- Source patient with advanced disease
- Deep injury
- Visible blood on the needle/scalpel
- Needle used to enter a blood vessel

Postexposure prophylaxis for other infections

If the healthcare worker is non-immune, hepatitis B can be prevented with hyperimmune globulin and immunization. There is no recommended PEP for hepatitis C, although early experience with interferon is promising.

Counselling and follow up

If PEP for HIV is started, an FBC and liver function should be checked at 2 and 4 weeks. PEP may delay rather than prevent seroconversion and HIV antibody (and hepatitis C if relevant) should be checked at 6 and 26 weeks after the event. Any febrile illness in this period should be reported and investigated as possible HIV seroconversion (see Section 1.24, p. 61). Safe sex should be recommended until these tests are clear and women warned not to become pregnant [4,5].

Continuing to work

The surgeon is allowed to continue to operate during the period of surveillance.

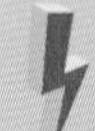

Failure of HIV PEP has occurred and there is no proven prophylaxis after hepatitis C exposure. Avoiding blood exposure is the best way to minimize risk.

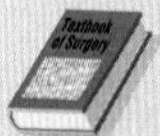

1 Gerberding JL. Management of occupational exposure to blood-borne viruses. *N Engl J Med* 1995; 332: 444–451.
2 Case–control study of HIV seroconversion in health-care workers after percutaneous exposure to HIV-infected blood—France, United Kingdom, and United States, January 1988–August 1994. *MMWR* 1995; 44: 929–933.
3 Chief Medical Officers' Expert Advisory Group. *HIV Post-Exposure Prophylaxis*. Guidance from the UK Chief Medical Officers' Expert Advisory Group on AIDS, July 2000. London: Department of Health. Available at: www.doh.gov.uk/eaga/index.htm.
4 *Serious Communicable Diseases*. General Medical Council, October 1997. Available on www.gmc-uk.org.
5 Department of Health. *AIDS/HIV Infected Health Care Workers. Guidance on the Management of Infected Health Care Workers*. London: Department of Health. Available at: www.doh.gov.uk/aids.htm.

1.26 Breathlessness in an HIV-positive patient

Case history

An HIV-positive patient presents with a dry, non-productive cough and breathlessness.

Clinical approach

There are many causes of breathlessness in HIV-positive patients (Table 24). A key priority is to determine whether or not this is *Pneumocystis carinii* pneumonia (PCP) [1–3].

Table 24 Breathlessness in HIV infection.

Category	CD4 count	More common conditions
Pulmonary infection	Any	Bacterial pneumonia Tuberculosis
	<200	*Pneumocystis carinii* pneumonia (PCP) Viral: RSV, CMV (uncommon) Fungal: *Cryptococcus*, *Histoplasma* spp.
Malignancy	Very low	Kaposi's sarcoma
	Any	Lymphoma
Anaemia	Not relevant	HIV related Caused by infection or malignancy Drug induced
Pulmonary: non-infective	Not relevant	Pneumothorax: may complicate PCP Primary pulmonary hypertension Thromboembolic disease Non-infective pulmonary effusion Lymphoid interstitial pneumonitis (LIP) Interstitial lung disease
Cardiac	Not relevant	HIV-related cardiomyopathy Pericardial effusion
Metabolic	Not relevant	Bacterial sepsis Drug-induced lactic acidosis Renal failure

CMV, cytomegalovirus; RSV, respiratory syncytial virus.

History of the presenting problem

Degree of immunosuppression

This relates well to the risk of infection (see Section 2.11, p. 138):

- Does he have AIDS? This implies severe immunodeficiency.
- Does he know his most recent CD4 cell count and HIV viral load?

Symptoms

You will need to assess the degree of breathlessness. The following may help in the differential diagnosis:

- How long has he been breathless? PCP is generally indolent or subacute.
- Are you coughing anything up? PCP is usually non-productive and purulent sputum suggests bacterial infection. If there is haemoptysis, tuberculosis must be excluded.
- Has there been chest pain? PCP is generally painless.
- Fever and sweats? If these have been totally absent, consider non-infective causes. Abrupt onset of high fever suggests bacterial infection.

Medication history

- Is he on anti-HIV therapy, what are the drugs and have they been working? Most clinics will have these data to hand.
- Has he been prescribed, and is he taking, prophylactic therapy for PCP?

Exposure to pathogens

Ask about travel (TB, histoplasmosis), birds (cryptococci, *Chlamydia*), hospital admissions (resistant bacteria, TB) and specific contacts with TB. Has there been a local influenza or mycoplasma outbreak?

Relevant past history

Has he had any HIV-related infections? (See Section 1.28, p. 70.)

AIDS-defining infections

AIDS describes the occurrence of serious opportunistic infections or certain malignancies in HIV-positive individuals. More common indicator conditions in the UK include the following [4,5]:

- Infections: oesophageal candidiasis, PCP, toxoplasmosis, tuberculosis, invasive atypical mycobacteria, cryptosporidiosis, CMV
- Malignancy: Kaposi's sarcoma, invasive cervical carcinoma, lymphoma
- Others: HIV-wasting syndrome, HIV dementia.

Examination

Is the patient well, ill, very ill or nearly dead? Immediately assess the airway, breathing and circulation.

- Can the patient speak?
- Is he using accessory muscles?
- Is he cyanosed?
- Is there a pneumothorax?
- Are there focal lung signs? Often there are few chest signs in PCP, although there may be fine or coarse crackles. Focal consolidation suggests bacterial pneumonia.
- Does he look exhausted?
- Check pulse oximetry.

Have a low threshold for asking for help from the ICU if the patient has, or is developing, respiratory failure. (See *Emergency medicine*, Section 1.5.)

Fundoscopy may show focal lesions from extrapulmonary PCP or signs of CMV retinitis (see Section 1.27, p. 68). Look for signs of the other conditions listed in Table 24, including bacterial sepsis, heart failure and anaemia.

Approach to investigation and management

The baseline CD4 cell count is critical. If significantly above 200 cells/μL, PCP and viral and fungal pneumonia are unlikely.

Investigations

Blood tests

- FBC, electrolytes, glucose, renal and liver function tests to exclude anaemia and hepatic or renal failure.
- CD4 cell count unless a recent clinic result is available. This may fall in any acute illness.
- Arterial blood gas: pulse oximetry is a good guide to hypoxia, but an arterial blood gas breathing room air is needed to assess respiratory failure and exclude acidosis. If acidotic, measure blood lactate levels (see below).
- Exercise oximetry: in early PCP, arterial oxygen saturation is normal at rest but will fall on exercise.
- Lactate dehydrogenase (LDH) is typically raised in PCP.

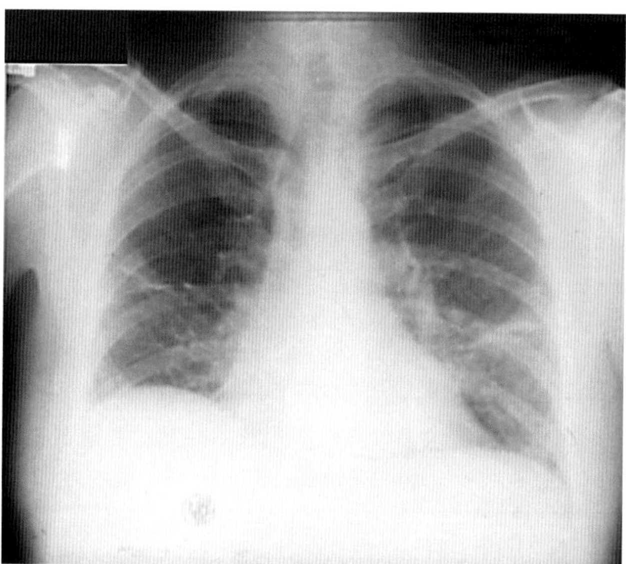

Fig. 40 Chest radiograph of a patient with severe *Pneumocystis carinii* pneumonia.

Imaging

- Chest radiograph typically reveals a fine interstitial and/or nodular infiltrate in PCP with relative sparing of the bases and apices (Fig. 40): 5–10% have a normal chest radiograph at presentation. Occasionally, PCP may present with focal infiltrates or thin-walled cavities (pneumatoceles), but cavitation is more suggestive of tuberculous, bacterial or fungal (histoplasmosis) aetiology.
- High-resolution CT reveals a 'ground-glass' pattern of alveolar consolidation in PCP.

Pulmonary function

In PCP the key abnormality is impaired diffusing capacity (KCO) (see *Respiratory medicine*, Section 3.6). Lung volumes may be reduced with a restrictive pattern.

Microbiology

Imaging is not diagnostic and you should strive to obtain a microbiological diagnosis. Alveolar specimens are needed to diagnose PCP, whereas other pathogens may be identified in ordinary sputum. Inducing sputum with nebulized saline produces specimens suitable for PCP, TB and bacterial studies (see Section 3.1, p. 150). If induced sputum is negative, proceed to bronchoalveolar lavage. Lung biopsy (transbronchial, CT-guided or thoracoscopic) may rarely be needed to establish the diagnosis.

Breathlessness in an HIV patient with a normal chest radiograph

- PCP is suggested by exercise desaturation.
- Lactic acidosis is an increasingly recognized and serious complication of anti-HIV therapy. The patient will usually have abdominal pain, abnormal liver function and hepatic steatosis.
- Bacterial sepsis.
- Cardiac failure or thromboembolism.

Do not delay bronchoscopy in immunocompromised patients with unexplained respiratory symptoms. Pneumonia may progress rapidly and the patient become too hypoxic to bronchoscope safely.

Management

Respiratory support

Respiratory support up to and including artificial ventilation may be required depending on the severity of breathing difficulty (see *Respiratory medicine*, Section 2.12). Monitor pulse oximetry. Give supplemental oxygen as needed. Consider non-invasive ventilation if hypoxia is not corrected (see *Respiratory medicine*, Section 2.12). Consider the need for assisted ventilation early and notify intensive care if this is likely—the indications for mechanical ventilation are the same as for any respiratory condition, and the man's HIV status should not prevent transfer to intensive care if appropriate to the clinical situation.

Antimicrobial therapy

Empirical therapy for bacterial infection and PCP (if low CD4) is needed for those who are very ill. Treatment options for the therapy of PCP are given in Table 25 [6]. In moderate-to-severe hypoxia, adjunctive corticosteroids (oral prednisolone 40–60 mg/day or equivalent) significantly reduce morbidity and mortality [7]. After acute therapy prophylaxis should be continued and primary prophylaxis instituted in all patients with CD4 <200/μL or a diagnosis of AIDS. Prophylaxis can be discontinued if the CD4 cell count stabilizes above 200/μL on ART [8].

Table 25 Options for the therapy of *Pneumocystis carinii* pneumonia (PCP).

Scenario	When to use	Medication
Acute disease	First line	High-dose co-trimoxazole (5 mg/kg trimethoprim component four times daily) Oral sufficient in mild illness; increased adverse reactions in HIV
	Second line	Dapsone + trimethoprim (check G6PD) Clindamycin + primaquine (check G6PD) Pentamidine 4 mg/kg per day i.v. (nebulized insufficient) Atovaquone
Prophylaxis	First line	Co-trimoxazole 960 mg three times a week or 480 mg/day
	Second line	Dapsone 100 mg/day alone Dapsone 100 mg + pyrimethamine 25 mg three times a week Pentamidine 300 mg via nebulizer every 2–4 weeks Atovaquone 750 mg once daily

G6PD, glucose-6-phosphate dehydrogenase.

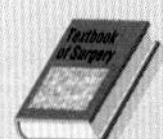

1 Stansell JD *et al. Pneumocystis carinii* pneumonia. In: Sande MA, Volberding PA (eds) *The Medical Management of AIDS* (5th edn). Philadelphia: WB Saunders, 1997; 275–300.
2 Breen RJM, Johnson M. Respiratory infections in patients with HIV. *J R Coll Physicians Lond* 1999; 33: 430–433.
3 Thomas CF Jr *et al.* Pneumocystis pneumonia: clinical presentation and diagnosis in patients with and without acquired immune deficiency syndrome. *Semin Respir Infect* 1998; 13: 289–295.
4 www.aidsmap.com—contains excellent up-to-date advice on management of all aspects of HIV.
5 www.hopkins-aids.edu—contains excellent up-to-date advice on management of all aspects of HIV.
6 Bozzette SA, Finkelstein DA, Feinberg J *et al.* A randomized trial of three antipneumocystis agents in patients with advanced human immuno-deficiency virus infection. NIAID AIDS Clinical Trials Group. *N Engl J Med* 1995; 332: 693–699.
7 Bozzette SA, Sattler FR, Chiu J *et al.* A controlled trial of early adjunctive treatment with corticosteroids for *Pneumocystis carinii* pneumonia in the acquired immunodeficiency syndrome. *N Engl J Med* 1990; 323: 1451–1457.
8 Schneider MM, Borleffs JC, Stolk RP *et al.* Discontinuation of prophylaxis for *Pneumocystis carinii* pneumonia in HIV-1-infected patients treated with highly active antiretroviral therapy. *Lancet* 1999; 353: 201–203.

1.27 HIV+ and blurred vision

Case history

A patient with AIDS phones the HIV unit complaining of altered vision in one eye.

Clinical approach

This is an emergency and the patient must be assessed promptly. Rapid visual loss can occur directly from opportunistic infection (Table 26) or as a result of retinal detachment. Cytomegalovirus is responsible for 80–90% of retinal infection in patients with AIDS [1].

Table 26 Ocular complications in HIV.

Site	Causes/comments
Conjunctiva	Bacterial conjunctivitis Kaposi's sarcoma
Cornea	Keratitis from HSV or VZV
Anterior chamber, uveitis	HIV, CMV if recently started on ART, TB, syphilis, drug reactions
Posterior chamber and retina	HIV retinopathy (Fig. 41) CMV retinitis (Fig. 42) PORN, caused by VZV/HSV (Fig. 43) *Candida* spp. rare unless neutropenic Retinal detachment after infection
Choroidoretinitis	Toxoplasmosis, TB, syphilis

PORN, progressive outer retinal necrosis [2]; HSV, herpes simplex virus; VZV, varicella-zoster virus; CMV, cytomegalovirus; ART, antiretroviral therapy; TB, tuberculosis.

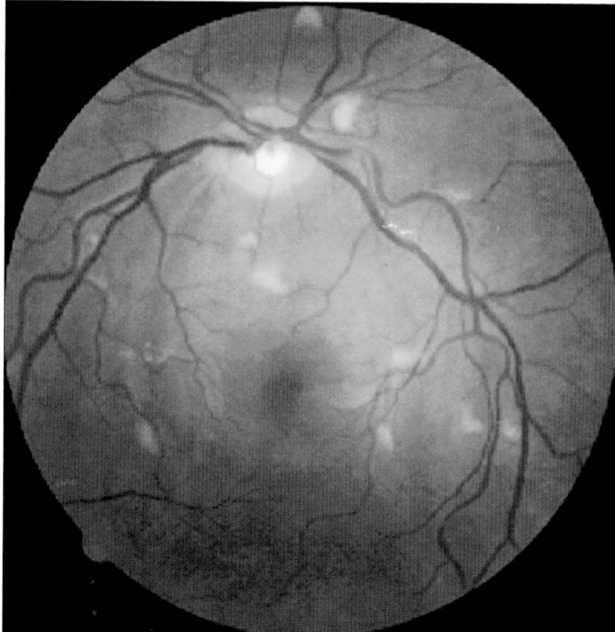

Fig. 41 Changes of HIV retinopathy. There are numerous 'cotton-wool' spots on the retina. These are generally asymptomatic and disappear when antiretroviral therapy is commenced.

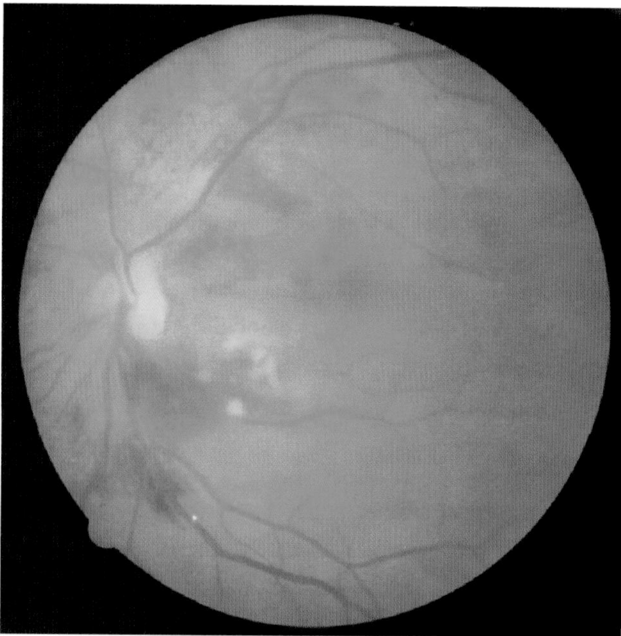

Fig. 42 Cytomegalovirus retinitis. Typical mixture of haemorrhage and exudate often referred to as a 'pizza pie' appearance.

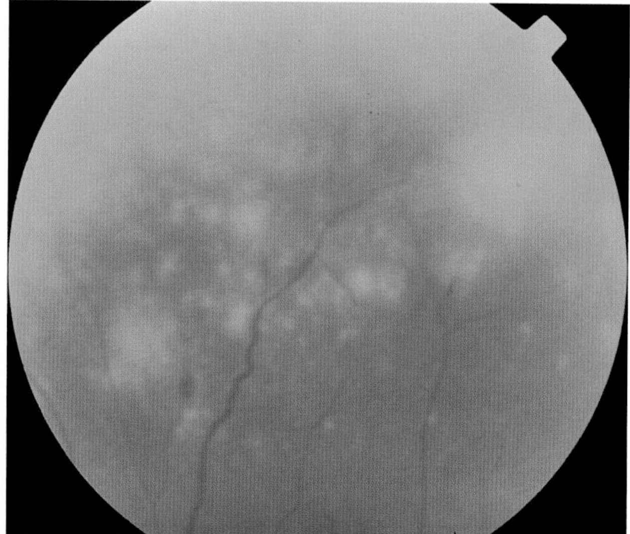

Fig. 43 Progressive outer retinal necrosis (PORN): pale necrotic retina with an advancing edge. This is most commonly the result of varicella-zoster virus; untreated it rapidly leads to blindness. PORN requires a combination of high-dose systemic and intraocular therapy. (Courtesy of Professor S Lightman.)

History of the presenting problem

Assess the immune function using a similar initial approach to that described in Section 1.26, p. 65. CMV retinitis is rarely seen with a CD4 count >75 cells/μL.

Ocular symptoms

What has happened?
- Does it affect one or both eyes? Most retinal infections will start in one eye and a problem affecting vision in both eyes may have an extraocular cause.
- How much is the vision affected? Can he still read?
- Is there pain and is the eye bloodshot? A painful red eye is unusual in retinal infections in AIDS unless the patient has recently been started on ART [3].
- Are there 'holes' in his vision, flashing lights or floaters? These features suggest retinal disease.
- Was it like a 'curtain' coming down? If so, refer urgently to exclude retinal detachment.

Other features

Ask about the following:
- Symptoms that give clues about other sites of infection.
- CD4 count—the patient will usually know this.
- What medication is being taken? Ethambutol may cause visual loss, and rifabutin and fluconazole can interact leading to pseudojaundice and uveitis.

Relevant past history

Note in particular the following:
- Previous ocular disease: inflammatory disease can lead to cataract and retinal disease to detachment.
- Previous infections in the eye or elsewhere, e.g. CMV, TB, toxoplasmosis and syphilis. CMV in particular may reactivate if the CD4 counts falls when HIV therapy is failing.

Examination

Perform a full general examination, looking for signs of infection elsewhere.

Ocular examination

Look at *Ophthalmology*, Section 3.1, for a description of how to examine the eye.

Check the following carefully (Figs 41–43):
- Conjunctiva: looking for inflammation, ulcers, pus or Kaposi's sarcoma.
- Red eye: if so, refer for slit-lamp examination.
- Visual acuity: if there is a sudden documented change, urgent ophthalmological review is needed.
- Pupillary reflexes and visual fields: a field defect in one eye suggests retinal disease; consider intracerebral pathology if there is a homonymous defect.
- Fundoscopy: look for debris/abscess in the anterior and posterior chambers, but these are best seen with a slit lamp. Look at as much of the retina as possible, dilating the pupils to get a good view. Pay particular attention to the area around the macula and the edge of the optic disc—disease in this area, known as zone 1, is sight threatening and needs immediate attention.

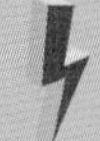

HIV and a visual problem

If in doubt seek an expert ophthalmological opinion. Retinal infection or detachment can rapidly lead to permanent visual loss unless managed correctly.

Approach to investigation and management

The aim must be to exclude sight-threatening disease as rapidly as possible. Most infections can be recognized clinically. The opinion of an HIV-experienced ophthalmologist is invaluable.

Investigations

Blood tests

Check the FBC (neutropenia is a risk factor for fungal infection) and CD4 cell count, unless a recent clinic result is available (CMV retinitis is unlikely with a count >75/μL).

Infection screen

Serology can assess the risk of latent infection for toxoplasmosis, CMV and syphilis, but it cannot establish a definitive diagnosis. CMV may be cultured from blood, but PCR or antigen detection is more sensitive [4]. However, patients can have CMV retinitis without detectable CMV in the blood, when the diagnosis is made on the basis of the characteristic clinical picture. Vitreal or retinal samples can be sent, where indicated, for microscopy, culture and PCR. Examination of the CSF is occasionally helpful.

Imaging

Cranial CT/MRI is appropriate if optic nerve or cortical involvement is suspected.

Management

This depends entirely on the cause (see Sections 2.10, p. 124 and 2.11, p. 134). Management of serious infection should involve an ophthalmologist. Many drugs penetrate the eye poorly so that a combination of systemic and intraocular therapy is often needed for viral or fungal retinitis [5]. Antimicrobial therapy cannot eradicate some infections such as CMV and toxoplasmosis, necessitating continuous suppressive therapy [6]. Prolonged remission requires restoration of immune function with effective ART.

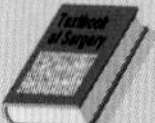

See *Ophthalmology*, Sections 1.4, 1.5 and 3.1.

1 Cunningham ET Jr, Margolis TP. Ocular manifestations of HIV infection. *N Engl J Med* 1998; 339: 236–244.
2 Batisse D, Eliaszewicz M, Zazoun L *et al.* Acute retinal necrosis in the course of AIDS: study of 26 cases. *AIDS* 1996; 10: 55–60.
3 Whitcup SM. Cytomegalovirus retinitis in the era of highly active antiretroviral therapy. *JAMA* 2000; 283: 653–657.
4 Dodt KK, Jacobsen PH, Hofmann B *et al.* Development of cytomegalovirus (CMV) disease may be predicted in HIV-infected patients by CMV polymerase chain reaction and the antigenemia test. *AIDS* 1997; 11: F21–28.
5 Katlama C. Management of CMV retinitis in HIV infected patients. *Genitourin Med* 1997; 73: 169–173.
6 USPHS/IDSA 1999 guidelines for the prevention of opportunistic infections in persons infected with human immunodeficiency virus. *Clin Infect Dis* 2000; 30(suppl 1): S29–65.

1.28 Starting anti-HIV therapy

Case history

A 33-year-old woman has recently been diagnosed as HIV positive.

Clinical approach

This is a complex situation and time is needed. You need to consider several issues [1]:

- Counselling and support
- Staging of HIV disease
- Consideration of ART
- Risk of opportunistic infections.

History of the presenting problem

Tested for HIV

Why was she tested for HIV? Has she had a high-risk exposure? Is she unwell? If she is unwell, this implies more advanced disease. Find out what she understands about HIV and how it is transmitted.

Risk factors

What are her risk factors for HIV and other sexually transmitted diseases? This is important, but may cause distress, so be sensitive (see *General clinical issues*, Section 2). Ask about intravenous drug use and medical therapy abroad.

Current symptoms

Fatigue, muscle aches, joint pains, night sweats, dry skin, diarrhoea and poor concentration may all be HIV related. Marked weight loss, pyrexia or focal symptoms such as cough or headache should not be attributed to HIV alone.

Social history

Find out about her occupation, living conditions, current sexual partner and children. Is there anyone else at risk of HIV, i.e. sexual partner (see Section 1.30, p. 74), does she have children or could she be pregnant? Ask about lifestyle, medications, recreational drug use, alcohol, smoking and diet. These are all important when planning ART.

Relevant past history

Past infections

Many infections can cause chronic disease or reactivate in patients with HIV. Ask about hepatitis or jaundice, labial and genital herpes, syphilis and other STDs, TB, shingles and thrush. Minor infections such as thrush, gingivitis, skin or nail fungal infection, respiratory infection or shingles suggest moderate immunodeficiency. AIDS-defining infections indicate severe immunodeficiency. (See Section 1.26, p. 65.)

Travel history

Take a detailed and life-long history to detect potential exposure to pathogens not endemic to the UK, e.g. leishmaniasis or histoplasmosis.

Examination

Look for evidence of advanced HIV disease and signs of infection or malignancy. Features to look for include the following:

- Mouth: oral hairy leucoplakia (Fig. 44), oral candida, gingivitis (Fig. 45), Kaposi's sarcoma (hard palate)
- Skin: seborrhoeic dermatitis, Kaposi's sarcoma (Fig. 46)
- Nails: chronic infections
- Lymphadenopathy: typical HIV-related lymphadenopathy is of nodes that are generalized, 1–2 cm in size, smooth, mobile and non-tender; an isolated mass of nodes, or focal abnormalities in chest, abdomen or central nervous system are unlikely to be the result of HIV alone
- Full genital examination is essential (see Sections 1.31, p. 76 and 1.33, p. 81).

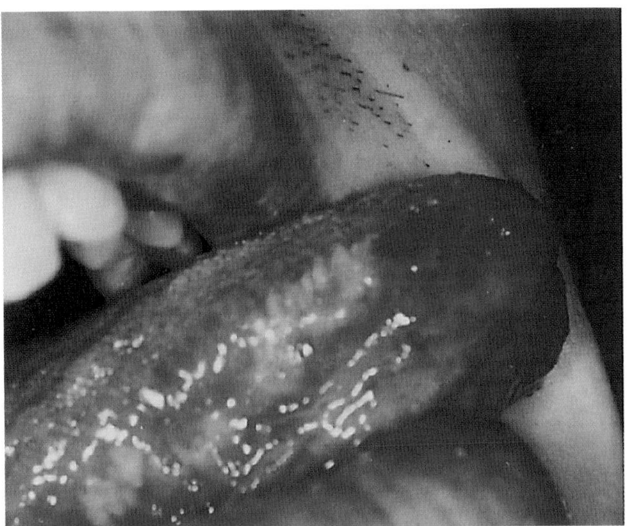

Fig. 44 Oral hairy leucoplakia.

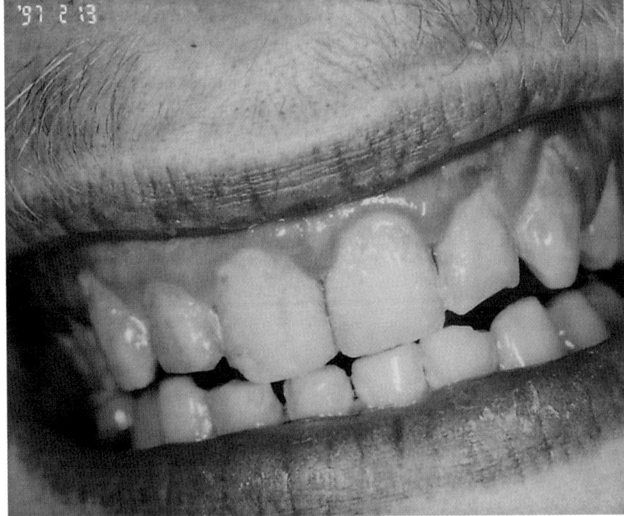

Fig. 45 Gingivitis complicating HIV infection.

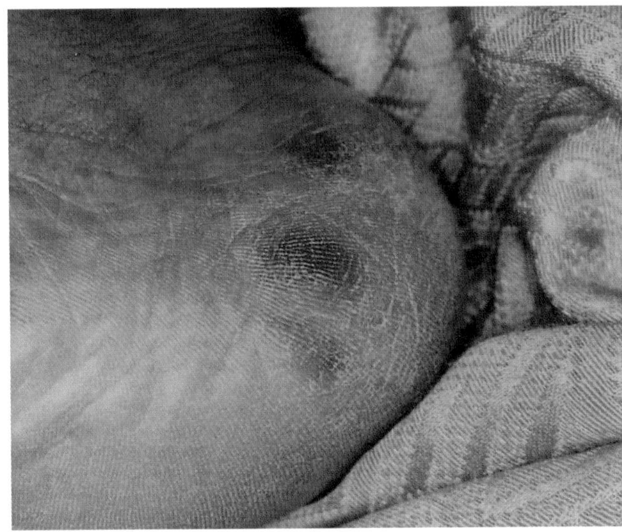

Fig. 46 Lesions of Kaposi's sarcoma on the foot.

Approach to investigation and management

The aim is to stage her HIV disease, screen for infection and prepare the patient for ART [2,3].

Investigations

Baseline blood tests

Check the FBC, electrolytes, renal and liver function tests, calcium, amylase, fasting glucose and lipids. Baseline tests are essential because HIV or opportunistic infections can affect any body system and antiretroviral medication has many side effects. (See Section 2.11, p. 134.)

Screen for infection

Assess for current infection and the risk of reactivation of latent infections. If she is ill, further investigations will be required based on the clinical picture:

• Serology for toxoplasmosis, syphilis, hepatitis B and C and CMV IgG

• Perform a full genitourinary screen, including a cervical smear (see Section 1.33, p. 81)

• Chest radiograph.

Stage HIV

You need to consider the clinical picture, immune function and HIV activity:

• Clinical staging: detailed clinical staging is useful for research studies, but in clinical practice patients can be divided into three groups—asymptomatic, symptomatic non-AIDS and AIDS.

• Immune function: CD4/CD8 cells are measured by flow cytometry and expressed in absolute numbers and as a percentage of total lymphocyte count. During disease progression CD4 cells decline (CD4/CD8 ratio <1) and the CD4 level is a reasonably accurate guide to the risk of opportunistic infection (see Section 2.11, p. 134). CD4 counts are, however, a poor predictor of HIV progression.

• HIV measurement: HIV viral load, assayed with PCR technology, is a quantitative measure of viraemia and reflects HIV replication. Results are expressed as HIV particles/mL and are predictive of disease progression. Viral load is also the cornerstone of therapeutic monitoring.

Management

Support and counselling

Learning that you are HIV positive is very frightening and can affect every aspect of life. Refer to appropriate support staff or outside agencies. Many patients have fears surrounding HIV or ART and, unless these are dealt with successfully, therapy is less likely to be successful. Education about HIV and ART is vital and ongoing over many clinic visits. Safe sex and general health issues should be covered.

Infection prevention

Screen and immunize for hepatitis B. Gay men should also be offered hepatitis A vaccine, and consider pneumococcal and influenza vaccines for all patients. Give PCP prophylaxis if CD4 <200/μL (see Section 1.26, p. 65). Investigate and treat any problems found at screening, e.g. cervical neoplasia or syphilis. Give lifestyle and travel advice where appropriate.

Starting antiretroviral therapy

Key issues are when to start, what to use, how to start and how to monitor [2,3].

WHEN TO START

There are no clear trial data regarding the best time to start therapy. The decision should be individualized, based on the patient, CD4 count and viral load. Theoretical arguments favour early treatment but this may expose patients to toxic therapy for years before clinical benefit is seen [4]. In the UK, most physicians broadly follow the British HIV Association (BHIVA) guidelines [5]. These aim to commence treatment before severe immune damage has occurred, generally with a CD4 count of 300–400/μL. Patients with serious opportunistic infections or a CD4 <200/μL should all be offered therapy. Consider acute therapy during seroconversion. (See Section 1.24, p. 61.)

HIV in pregnancy

- Untreated vertical transmission rate is 16% in Europe
- Risk of transmission is related to maternal HIV viral load
- Zidovudine (AZT) monotherapy for the last 6 weeks of pregnancy, intravenous during labour and orally for the baby, can reduce the rate of transmission to 8%
- Combination antiretroviral therapy may reduce the rate to <2%
- Elective caesarean section reduces transmission by approximately 50%
- HIV may be transmitted by breast milk.

WHAT TO START WITH

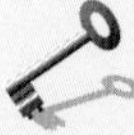

Antiretroviral drug classes

- Nucleoside reverse transcriptase inhibitors (NRTIs)
- Non-nucleoside reverse transcriptase inhibitors (NNRTIs)
- Protease inhibitors (PIs).

Drugs are divided into three classes (see Section 2.11, p. 134). A combination of at least three drugs is required to achieve sufficient HIV suppression, but whether four or five drugs are more effective is not known. PI-based regimens were the first really successful therapy, leading to an 80% fall in AIDS-related deaths [6,7], but PIs are quite toxic and many recommend avoiding them for first-line therapy. BHIVA guidelines suggest that two NRTI + NNRTI or three NRTI drugs are used first line in patients with moderate immunodeficiency.

HOW TO START

Not at the first visit! Poor compliance is strongly linked to failure and success of the first regimen is much more likely when the patient understands and is committed to therapy. The rationale behind therapy, the exact regimen and how it can be managed with diet, lifestyle and side effects must all be discussed. Support from nurses, dietitians, pharmacists, counsellors and psychologists increases the chance of success.

WHAT TO MONITOR

Safety monitoring is mandatory with blood tests at 2 and 4 weeks to check the FBC, renal and hepatic function. Longer-term safety issues include elevated cholesterol/triglycerides. CD4 counts and viral load should be checked at 4–6 weeks with an expected 2–3 $\log_{10}$ fall in viral load. When stabilized on treatment safety tests, CD4 counts and viral load are monitored every 2–3 months, with a treatment aim of keeping the viral load as low as possible, preferably undetectable by the most sensitive available test. Therapeutic drug monitoring is becoming available for NNRTIs and PIs. Side effects should be looked for and compliance assessed and discussed at each visit.

Some HIV medications have potentially fatal side effects, including lactic acidosis (NRTIs), hepatitis (most classes), pancreatitis (didanosine) and allergy (NNRTIs and abacavir). Patients must be warned and followed closely.

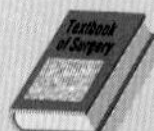

1 Gazzard B, ed. Chelsea and Westminster Hospital AIDS Care Handbook. London: Mediscript, 1999.
2 Clumeck N. Choosing the best initial therapy for HIV-1 infection. *N Engl J Med* 1999; 341: 1925–1926.
3 Gallant JE. Strategies for long-term success in the treatment of HIV infection. *JAMA* 2000; 283: 1329–1334.
4 Harrington M, Carpenter CC. Hit HIV-1 hard, but only when necessary. *Lancet* 2000; 355: 2147–2152.
5 British HIV Association (BHIVA) www.aidsmap.com—contains information on current and future therapy plus the most recent version of the BHIVA treatment guidelines.
6 Katzenstein DA, Hammer SM, Hughes MD *et al.* The relation of virologic and immunological markers to clinical outcomes after nucleoside therapy in HIV-infected adults with 200–500 CD4 cells per cubic millimeter. *N Engl J Med* 1996; 335: 1091–1098.
7 Hammer SM, Squires KE, Hughes MD *et al.* A controlled trial of two nucleoside analogues plus indinavir in persons with human immunodeficiency virus infection and CD4 cell counts of 200 per cubic millimeter or less. *N Engl J Med* 1997; 337: 725–733.

1.29 Failure of anti-HIV therapy

Case history

A 24-year-old HIV-positive patient has been taking anti-HIV medication for the past year and you now find that the HIV viral load is rising.

Clinical approach

This indicates failure of viral control and will inevitably lead to clinical failure [1]. You need to consider why treatment is failing:

- Development of antiretroviral drug resistance
- Pharmacological failure: drug interactions
- Poor compliance
- Malabsorption of drugs
- Coexistent illness.

History of the presenting problem

Antiretroviral therapy record

What and when

When was treatment started, what combinations were used, how good was compliance and what were the side effects? In the past patients may have received one or two drug therapies that failed fully to suppress HIV, and which predispose to later resistance and failure. How many previous regimens have been tried? Heavily drug-experienced patients are less likely to respond to a new regimen.

Stage of disease

At what stage of disease was he originally treated and how did he respond? A very high viral load (>100 000 copies/mL) or a very low CD4 count is associated with a poorer long-term response to therapy.

Response to previous therapy

When treatment is started, the viral load should fall by 2–3 $\log_{10}$ within the first 6 weeks. A slower rate of fall or failure to reach an undetectable level predicts subsequent failure.

Drug interactions that can lead to toxicity or therapeutic failure are common. Warn patients to check all new over-the-counter drugs and alternative therapies with their HIV pharmacist [2].

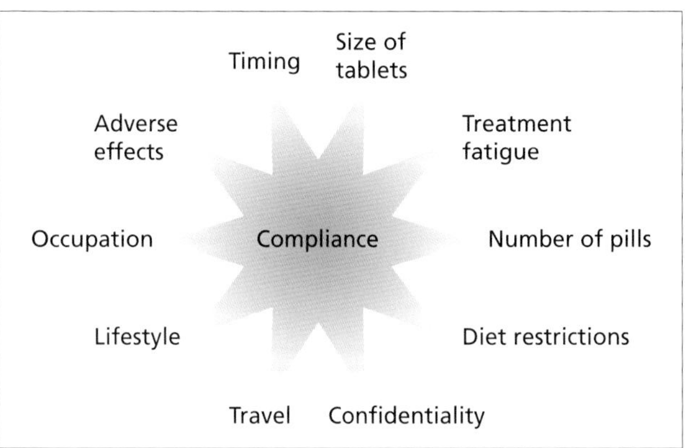

Fig. 47 Factors underlying poor compliance.

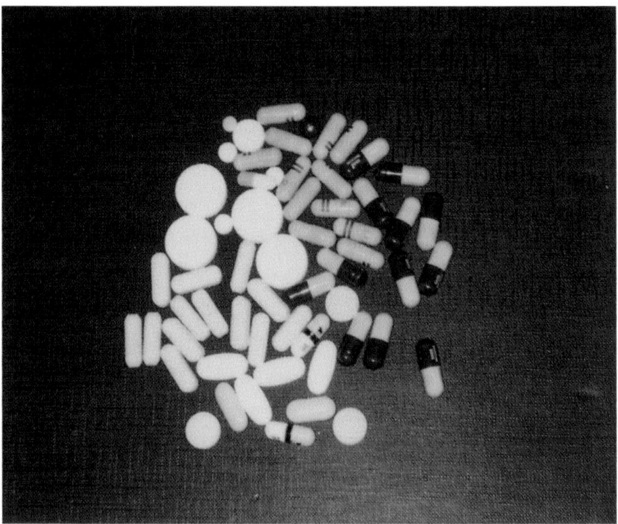

Fig. 48 Daily pill burden in a patient with advanced AIDS and invasive cytomegalovirus disease.

Compliance, lifestyle and side effects

Poor compliance is a major predictor of treatment failure [3]. Reasons underlying poor compliance are complex (Fig. 47). Patients may have to take very large numbers of tablets (Fig. 48)—some have to be taken with food and others on an empty stomach, and there are numerous side effects (see Section 2.11, p. 138).

Compliance is difficult to assess objectively:

- Have you missed any drug doses in the last day/week/month?
- Are you late with doses?
- Do you find it difficult to remember to take your medicines?
- How does the medication fit in with your work, lifestyle, diet, etc.?
- What side effects have you had and how are you coping with them?

Pharmacy and nursing staff often have a good idea of compliance, which can be monitored by counting pills and with recording devices.

General history

Take a full general history, looking for evidence of underlying infection or malignancy because this can directly increase the viral load. Ask about symptoms of malabsorption, history of bowel and pancreatic disease.

Examination

This is of limited value in this situation, except for looking for signs of infection or malignancy such as a new mass of lymph nodes.

Approach to investigation and management

Investigations

Routine blood tests

Check the FBC, electrolytes, renal and liver function tests, and inflammatory markers, looking for evidence of opportunistic infection and drug side effects.

Repeat CD4 and HIV viral load

Confirm the original results. Viral load can increase transiently with minor infections and you do not want to alter therapy on the basis of a single result. If the CD4 count is falling, changing therapy is more urgent. Do not forget to initiate PCP prophylaxis if CD4 <200/μL.

HIV resistance testing

This is available in some centres. There are problems with methodology and interpretation but the results may improve the choice of therapy. Genotypic testing detects drug-resistance mutations in the viral genome; phenotypic tests (not routinely available) look directly at drug inhibition of viral replication.

Therapeutic drug monitoring

This is available at some centres for PI and NNRTI agents. It can give a guide to non-compliance and pharmacological failure.

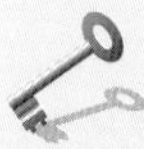

Factors associated with HIV drug resistance

- Pretreatment: very high HIV viral load or very low CD4 count
- Slow/incomplete viral load response to therapy
- Previous exposure to HIV drugs
- Compliance <95%

Management

Discuss the possible reasons for increasing viral load with the patient. If he understands these, it makes the success of further therapy more likely. Depending on previous therapy, new options available, CD4 count and the clinical picture, you may decide to monitor closely or switch therapy [4,5]. Ideally you should aim to change all (at least two) drugs in the failing regimen, and one of the new drugs should be from a class of HIV drugs that he has not previously been exposed to. Consider clinical trials of newer agents. The new regimen needs careful consideration and choice is based on the following:

- Antiretroviral history
- Risk of drug interactions
- Resistance testing (if available)
- Side effects
- Pill burden and patient preference.

Safety monitoring and multidisciplinary support are essential following the switch (see Section 1.28, p. 70).

Transmission of multidrug-resistant HIV does occur. Up to 20% of patients currently acquiring HIV may have a degree of drug resistance.

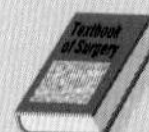

1 d'Arminio Monforte A, Testa L, Adorni F *et al.* Clinical outcome and predictive factors of failure of highly active antiretroviral therapy in antiretroviral-experienced patients in advanced stages of HIV-1 infection. *AIDS* 1998; 12: 1631–1637.
2 Burman WJ, Gallicano K, Peloquin. Therapeutic implications of drug interactions in the treatment of human immunodeficiency virus-related tuberculosis. *Clin Infect Dis* 1999; 28: 419–429.
3 Carpenter CC, Cooper DA, Fischl MA *et al.* Antiretroviral therapy in adults: updated recommendations of the International AIDS Society-USA. *JAMA* 2000; 283: 381–390.
4 Moyle GJ, Gazzard BG, Cooper DA, Gatell J. Antiretroviral therapy for HIV infection. A knowledge-based approach to drug selection and use. *Drugs* 1998; 55: 383–404.
5 www.aidsmap.com—contains up-to-date information on new therapeutic options and developments in resistance testing.

1.30 Don't tell my wife

Case history

A man tests positive for HIV but asks you not to tell his wife.

Clinical approach

You are faced with an ethical dilemma. The HIV-positive man is your patient to whom you have a duty of care. So do you respect his confidentiality or do you have an equal or greater duty to protect his partner? Your initial approach here must be to continue to communicate with him and try to help him come to the decision to inform his wife. This is not easy and is best handled by those with experience of the problem.

Being told you are HIV positive is devastating and very much like a grief reaction. Be sensitive and take time.

History of the presenting problem

You need more information to plan your approach. He has just tested positive for HIV and a common reaction is to want no one else to know. At the first visit you must make it clear that he is your main priority and that your aim is to help him to understand HIV and what options will be open to him. Reassure him about confidentiality. Integral to this discussion will be an explanation of how HIV is transmitted. This affords an opportunity to discuss those whom he might be putting at risk.

Determining who is at risk

If he is not sexually active with his wife, there will not be an immediate concern about her contracting HIV from him. She will still need to know that she may have been at risk in the past. If high-risk sexual activity is taking place, you must ensure that he has been told clearly about the risk he is placing his wife in, and document that conversation in the medical notes. Do not assume that his wife is his only sexual partner—there may be others, past or present, also at risk. Could anyone be pregnant by him? If they are, and they do not know their risk, an opportunity to prevent transmission to the child may be lost. (See Section 1.28, p. 70.)

Determining his reasons

After establishing who is at risk, discuss directly the need to inform his sexual partners for their own health. If he is still reluctant, try to find out the reasons behind this. He is likely to be frightened that she may leave him or he may have difficulty confronting issues around his sexuality. Understanding his reasons may allow you to provide specific help and support to enable him to tell her.

If he still says no

Do not feel that you have to deal with this alone or try to do it in one session. It is better to work with the patient over several sessions than to try to pressurize him into an instant decision. Use HIV specialist nurses, health advisers and psychologists who have much experience in this area.

Approach to management

How he should tell his wife

There is no easy answer to this question, but fear of how to tell is often the limiting step. Offer him as much support as possible. Offer to give her the information yourself—sometimes people would prefer a doctor or nurse to do this.

Testing her secretly

Sometimes patients ask you to test their partners under the pretext of testing for something else. This must be refused because consent for HIV testing is always required in mentally competent adults [1].

Continued refusal

Tell him directly, and record in the notes, that you have a duty to protect people whom he knowingly puts at risk. The General Medical Council's (GMC's) guidelines on Serious Communicable Diseases [2] support this approach, but state that you must first exhaust all efforts to persuade him to tell his partner. If he continues to decline, you should inform him of your actions and approach his wife directly or through her general practitioner. She needs to be told that she may be at risk of HIV, while trying to preserve the husband's confidentiality. However, it is difficult, if not impossible, to maintain such confidentiality in practice in this unfortunate situation. Wait to be asked specific questions, and record in the notes that information was released only in response to direct questioning.

His wife comes to see you

It is not uncommon for this to happen and it is a breach of confidentiality, and gross misconduct, to discuss his medical problems without specific consent. If, however, the wife requests HIV testing for herself, there is no reason why this cannot be performed after appropriate counselling and discussion.

Ethical issues

Be very careful before taking action that may infringe confidentiality. You must be prepared and able to justify your actions at a later stage.

The patient dies

Your dilemma continues! The GMC's guidelines state that the duty of confidentiality extends after death, but you still have a duty to protect his wife. In this case, the patient's wife should be informed that she may be at risk, and offered counselling and testing. Practically it will be very difficult to avoid disclosing his status, but do not volunteer the information.

They refuse testing of a child

This has recently been tested in the courts, with the ruling going against the parents and in favour of having the child tested. For this to happen is a disaster. In that case, the family immediately left the country, removing themselves and the child from medical care. Becoming confrontational may therefore be counterproductive, and it is best to try very hard to work with the family concerned.

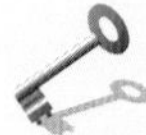

Confidentiality and HIV

- You can divulge an HIV-positive person's status only with explicit consent
- When another individual is at risk, you may make him or her aware of that risk only after all other avenues have been exhausted
- The duty of confidentiality continues even after death.

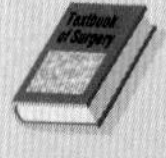

1 Nyrhinen T, Leino-Kilpi H. Ethics in the laboratory examination of patients. *J Med Ethics* 2000; 26: 54–60.
2 General Medical Council. *Serious Communicable Diseases.* London: General Medical Council, October 1997. Available on www.gmc-uk.org.

1.31 A spot on the penis

Case history

A 34-year-old man complains of a lesion on his penis.

Clinical approach

Is this an STD? If so, your aim is not only to diagnose and treat the patient, but also to reduce the level of the STD in the community. Thus, you must assess exposure and potential risk of transmission to others, and educate about safe sex. The advice of an appropriate genitourinary medicine physician will be required.

History of the presenting problem

The differential diagnosis of penile lesions is quite wide, including infectious and non-infectious conditions (Table 27).

The lesion

If the information does not emerge spontaneously, ask about the following:

- How long has the lesion been present? Warts tend to be present for weeks/months before the patient presents; the chancre of primary syphilis lasts for 3–6 weeks.
- Is there more than one lesion? Genital herpes often has multiple lesions, although single lesions can occur in recurrences.
- Is it painful? Herpes and chancroid usually are, but primary syphilis is not.
- How has it changed? A lesion that does not heal could be malignant.
- Did you injure yourself? Shallow ulcers are often the result of minor trauma.

Genitourinary symptoms

Ask about local symptoms suggestive of other STDs, e.g. urethral discharge (see Section 1.32, p. 79).

General health

Ask about associated symptoms suggestive of systemic involvement, such as fever, weight loss or rash.

Exposure

A detailed sexual history is required, which should cover the following risk factors for STDs:

- Have you recently changed your sexual partner?
- Do you have more than one sexual partner at the moment?
- When was the last protected/unprotected sexual intercourse?
- What type of sexual activity took place? Remember that STDs are not confined to the genitalia and oral or rectal lesions may be present.
- What contraception was used?
- Who was it with? Casual encounters or contact with sex workers carry a higher risk.
- Do you get paid for sex? Commercial sex workers are at high risk.
- Who else could be at risk now or in the past?
- Do you use drugs or alcohol during sex? Loss of control increases risk.
- Did you have sex abroad? People are often more sexually adventurous on holiday and may take fewer precautions. Ask about 'red light' districts. Some STDs, notably chancroid and lymphogranuloma venereum, are not endemic to the UK.
- Past sexual history? Broadly speaking, the risk increases with the number of sexual partners.
- HIV risk factors? Any patient with an STD has, by definition, been at risk of HIV. Specific risks should also be explored, which include men having sex with men, intravenous drug use and sexual exposure in countries with a high HIV prevalence.

Table 27 Differential diagnosis of penile lesions.

Condition		Features
Common infections	Herpes simplex	HSV-2 or HSV-1 Cluster of vesicles on penis, progress to shallow painful ulcers Progressive ulceration in immunocompromised individuals
	Warts: human papilloma virus	Condylomata accuminata (Fig. 49), typically raised papillary lesions May extend into the urethra Flat verrucous forms also seen
	Molluscum contagiosum	1–3 mm papule with central umbilicus.
Uncommon but increasing	Primary syphilis	Chancre (Fig. 50), usually single but kissing lesions where mucosal surfaces are opposed Papular and then ulcerates with a painless smooth raised edge and an indurated but clean base Regional lymphadenopathy Heals in 3–6 weeks
Uncommon	Secondary syphilis	Condylomata lata Moist papules in skin creases around genitals, groin and anus
	Chancroid	Painless papule rapidly progresses to painful 1–2 cm ulcer with raised, irregular edges and a necrotic base
	Granuloma inguinale	Painless ulceration with beefy red base and tissue destruction
	Lymphogranuloma venereum	Caused by particular serovars of *Chlamydia trachomatis* Primary lesion small and painless, healing without scarring Most characteristic secondary lesion is buboes Very rare in the UK
	Non-infectious causes	Pearly patches, lichen planus, bowenoid papulosis, Kaposi's sarcoma.
	Carcinoma of the penis	Consider in any non-healing lesion Typically irregular ulcer with a necrotic base and tissue destruction

HSV, herpes simplex virus.

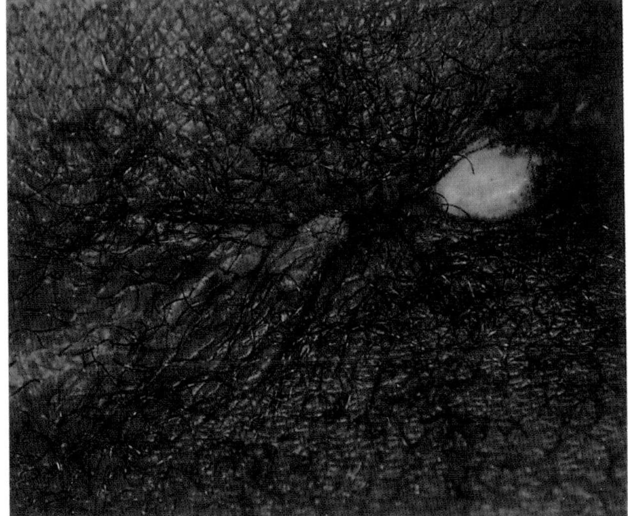

Fig. 49 Perianal condylomata accuminata caused by human papilloma virus.

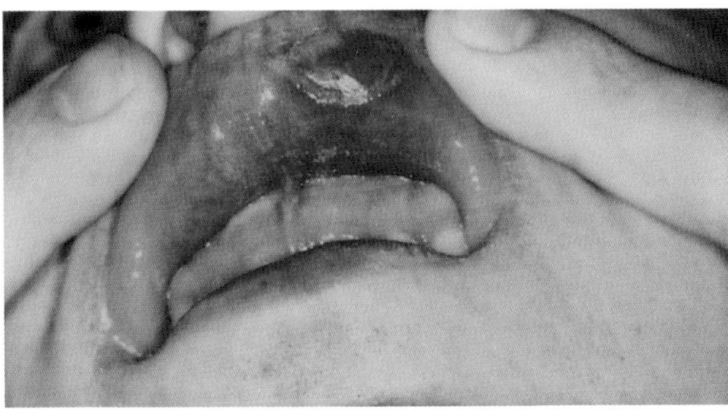

Fig. 50 Chancre of primary syphilis appears at the site of inoculation and can be anywhere. After the genitalia and perianal region, the mouth is the most common site.

Relevant past history

Ask about previous STDs and where/how they were treated. Recurrent infections such as oral candidal infection suggest immunodeficiency. (See Section 1.24, p. 61.)

When taking a sexual history, reassure the patient about confidentiality, explain why an accurate history is important and ensure that you have adequate privacy. (See *General clinical issues*, Section 2.)

Examination

The features of penile lesions are given in Table 27.
• Examine the entire penis, not forgetting to retract the foreskin.
• Look for urethral discharge.
• Examine the scrotum and testicles—tenderness suggests epididymo-orchitis. (See Section 1.32, p. 81.)
• Palpate inguinal lymph nodes.
• Inspect the perianal region and perform a digital rectal examination—a tender, boggy prostate suggests prostatitis. Proctoscopy is indicated if there is a history of unprotected anal intercourse or rectal symptoms, or if perianal warts are present.
• Inspect the mouth for pharyngitis (gonorrhoea), signs of secondary syphilis (see Sections 1.35, p. 86 and 2.7.1, p. 114) or evid- ence of underlying HIV such as oral hairy leucoplakia (see Section 1.28, p. 70).

Approach to investigation and management

Although many lesions can be recognized clinically, microbiological confirmation of diagnosis is required.

Investigations

Blood tests

Routine haematology and biochemistry are rarely helpful. Check glucose in candidal balanitis or recurrent UTI. Serology can be used to confirm syphilis (see Section 1.35, p. 86) it can also be of use in the uncommon condition of lymphogranuloma venereum, and may be useful in detection of past or recent exposure to herpes, although this is controversial.

Samples from the lesion

Check the following:
• Scrape the ulcer base for microscopy and culture—samples from the chancre of primary syphilis reveal spirochaetes on dark-ground microscopy, multinucleate giant cells suggest herpes and specific immunofluorescence can be used to detect HSV-1 or -2.
• Send swabs for viral (herpes) and bacterial (chancroid) culture.
• Biopsy may be required if the lesion is progressive and no diagnosis is forthcoming.

Other tests

A male genitourinary screen is required for anyone presenting with a sore on the penis.

Male genitourinary screen

• Urethral swab: Gram stain, culture for gonorrhoea. DNA-based tests for *Chlamydia trachomatis* (chlamydial infection)
• Rectal swab: culture for *Neisseria gonorrhoeae* (gonorrhoea)
• Throat swab: culture for gonorrhoea
• Swab any lesions: bacterial and viral culture
• Syphilis serology: if exposed to syphilis and serology is negative, repeat in one month [1]
• Hepatitis and HIV testing should be offered.

Management

Treat the condition, trace contacts and educate.

Antimicrobial therapy

Treat specific diagnoses:
• Syphilis: long-acting penicillin remains the treatment of choice [2–4] (Table 28).
• Chancroid: seek advice, a single dose of 1 g azithromycin is currently effective [5].
• Lymphogranuloma: doxycycline 100 mg twice daily for 3 weeks [6].
• Herpes simplex: aciclovir 200 mg five times a day for 5 days is indicated in primary infection. Better dosing schedules are possible with famciclovir and valaciclovir, but these drugs are more expensive. Consider prophylactic aciclovir 400 mg twice daily if there are frequent recurrences [7].
• Condylomata accuminata: variety of topical therapies such as podophyllin or liquid nitrogen.

Table 28 Therapy of syphilis.

Stage	Drug	Duration
Early (<2 years)	Benzathine benzylpenicillin 2.4 MIU i.m.	Single dose
	Procaine penicillin 0.6 MIU i.m. daily*	10–14 days
	Doxycycline 100 mg twice daily	10–14 days
	Erythromycin 500 mg four times daily	10–14 days
Late (>2 years, including cardiovascular)	Benzathine benzylpenicillin 2.4 MIU i.m.	Weekly × 3
	Procaine penicillin 0.6 MIU i.m. daily*	17–21 days
	Doxycycline 100 mg twice daily	21 days
Neurosyphilis	Benzylpenicillin 4 MIU i.v. four times daily	10 days

*Procaine penicillin is available in the UK as a mixture with benzylpenicillin.

Contacts

Contact tracing must be handled with sensitivity. STDs are not notifiable. Reassure the patient about confidentiality, and refer to a health adviser who will organize contact tracing where appropriate.

Contact tracing in syphilis

- Anonymously trace and offer therapy to all sexual contacts
- Trace contacts in the time before disease onset: primary syphilis 3 months, secondary 6 months and latent >1 year
- Offer testing to all partners of patients with late syphilis.

Sexual health

Education is critical in attempting to reduce the risk of reinfection and improve long-term sexual health. Explain why this infection has occurred and how he can protect himself. Be explicit: there is no point unless both you and the client understand what is being said. Most clinics have a variety of health promotion leaflets, but these do not replace face-to-face education. Education in condom use and free condoms can be provided.

Test of cure

Follow-up is essential to ensure successful management of syphilis, gonorrhoea and chlamydial infection.

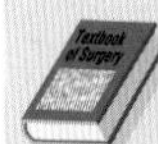

http://www.mssvd.org.uk. This website contains an induction pack for GUM trainees and regularly updated clinical guidelines on the diagnosis and treatment of sexually transmitted diseases.

1 Egglestone S, Turner A. Serological diagnosis of syphilis: PHLS Syphilis Serology Working Group. *Commun Dis Public Health* 2000; 3:158–162
2 Kinghorn GR. Syphilis. In: Armstrong D, Cohen J (eds) *Infectious Diseases*. London: Mosby, 1999: 64.
3 Clinical Effectiveness Group (Association of Genitourinary Medicine and the Medical Society for the Study of Venereal Diseases). National guideline for the management of early syphilis. *Sex Transm Infect* 1999; 75(suppl 1): S29–33.
4 Clinical Effectiveness Group (Association of Genitourinary Medicine and the Medical Society for the Study of Venereal Diseases). National guideline for the management of late syphilis. *Sex Transm Infect* 1999; 75(suppl 1): S34–47.
5 Clinical Effectiveness Group (Association of Genitourinary Medicine and the Medical Society for the Study of Venereal Diseases). National guideline for the management of chancroid. *Sex Transm Infect* 1999; 75(suppl 1): S43–45.
6 Clinical Effectiveness Group (Association of Genitourinary Medicine and the Medical Society for the Study of Venereal Diseases). National guideline for the management of lymphogranuloma venereum. *Sex Transm Infect* 1999; 75(suppl 1): S40–42.
7 Clinical Effectiveness Group (Association of Genitourinary Medicine and the Medical Society for the Study of Venereal Diseases). National guideline for the management of genital herpes. *Sex Transm Infect* 1999; 75(suppl 1): S24–28.

1.32 Penile discharge

Case history

A 37-year-old man presents with a urethral discharge.

Clinical approach

Establish whether a urethral discharge is present and whether it is the result of an STD [1]. There are many causes of urethritis (Table 29). Your aim is not only to diagnose and treat your patient, but also to reduce the level of the STD in the community.

History of the presenting problem

The discharge

- How long after sexual exposure did it start? Gonococcal urethritis has an incubation period of 24–72 h; non-gonococcal urethritis is more indolent.
- How much discharge and what colour? Gonococcal discharge is purulent; non-gonococcal is usually thin and colourless.
- Dysuria or haematuria? Dysuria is frequent in urethritis, but haematuria is uncommon and requires investigation for urinary tract disease. Dysuria in the absence of urethral discharge is more likely to be caused by a UTI.
- Pain on defaecation or sitting down? Pain in the perineum or tip of the penis during defaecation suggests prostatitis.
- Is there pain in the testicles? If present look for epididymo-orchitis.
- Systemic symptoms? Fever, rigors and loin pain suggest a bacterial UTI.
- Fever, a sparse pustular rash and arthralgia are seen in disseminated gonorrhoea. Reiter's syndrome may follow urethritis and present with conjunctivitis, arthritis, keratoderma blenorrhagica and circinate balanitis.
- Full sexual and partner history. (See Section 1.31, p. 76.)

Table 29 Causes of urethritis.

Common causes	*Neisseria gonorrhoeae*
	Chlamydia trachomatis
	Mycoplasma spp.
Uncommon causes	Human papilloma virus*
	Herpes simplex virus
	Candida albicans
Non-infectious	Trauma
	Chemical irritants
	Carcinoma
	Stevens–Johnson syndrome

*Human papilloma virus is a very common infection, but an uncommon cause of urethritis.

Relevant past history

Ask about previous STDs and where/how treated. Recurrent infections such as oral candidal infection suggest immunodeficiency. (See Section 1.28, p. 70.)

Examination

A full genital and general examination should be performed as described in Section 1.31 (p. 78).

Urethral discharge

This is washed out by urination, so it is best if the patient has not urinated for 2 hours beforehand. Inspect the penile meatus looking for spontaneous discharge or crusting. Staining of the undergarments may also be present. Note the volume and colour of the discharge, and immediately transfer some to a swab and spread on a clean microscope slide. If no discharge is visible, proceed to take a urethral swab.

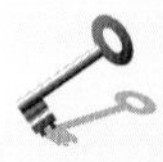

Epididymo-orchitis

- Pain and tenderness in testicle/epididymis
- May complicate chlamydial and non-gonococcal urethritis
- Less common complication of gonorrhoea
- Chronic epididymo-orchitis in TB and brucellosis
- Prolonged antimicrobial therapy required
- Any persistent mass—consider testicular carcinoma.

Approach to investigation and management

Investigations

Do a full male genitourinary infection screen, as described in Section 1.31 (p. 78). The key to diagnosis and management is the urethral swab, which must be taken correctly.

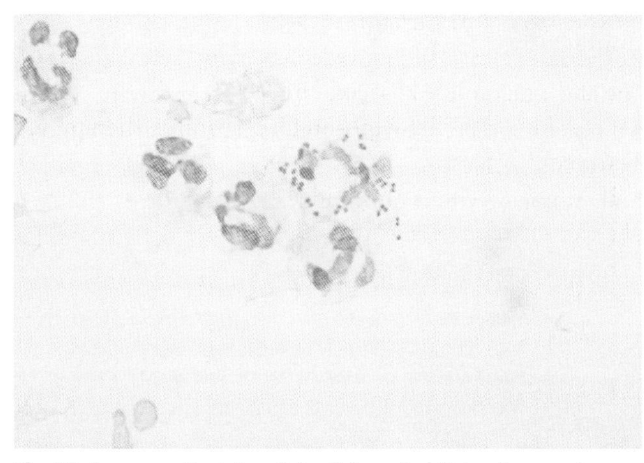

Fig. 51 Gram-negative intracellular diplococci of *Neisseria gonorrhoeae.*

Currently Gram stain (Fig. 51) and culture are the gold standard for the diagnosis of gonorrhoea. DNA amplification-based techniques are replacing immunoassay and culture in the diagnosis of chlamydial infection.

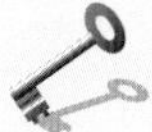

Taking a male urethral swab

1. The man should not have urinated for 2 h
2. Insert a swab 2–4 cm into the urethra and rotate for 5 s
3. Roll the swab on a glass slide for Gram staining
4. Plate on to chocolate agar
5. Use a second specific swab for *Chlamydia trachomatis* (chlamydia) samples.

Management

Management based on the swab results is shown in the algorithm in Fig. 52. For the specific antimicrobial therapy of the following:

- Gonorrhoea: see Section 2.5.2, p. 104 [2]
- Chlamydia: see Section 2.8.4, p. 119 [3]

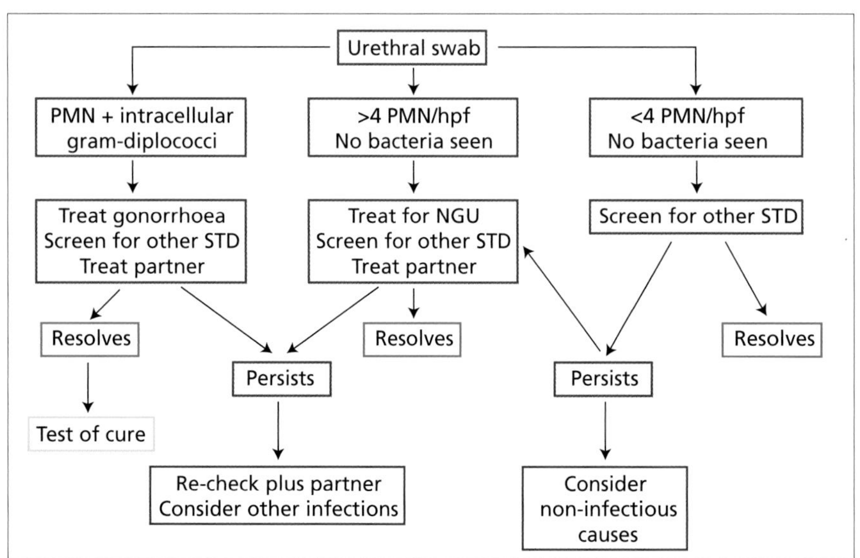

Fig. 52 Algorithm showing the management of urethritis in males. PMN, polymorphonuclear cells; NGU, non-gonococcal urethritis; STD, sexually transmitted disease.

• Non-gonococcal urethritis (NGU) is generally treated with doxycycline 100 mg twice daily for 10 days as first line and a macrolide as second line [4]
• Prostatitis or epididymo-orchitis requires therapy for 4–6 weeks [5]
• If *N. gonorrhoea* has been identified, repeat swabs (test of cure) should be taken after therapy [6].

For contact tracing and education, see Section 1.31, p. 79.

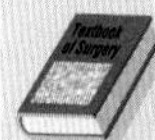

See *Rheumatology and clinical immunology*, Sections 1.18 and 2.3.4.

http://www.mssvd.org.uk. This website contains an induction pack for GUM trainees and regularly updated clinical guidelines on the diagnosis and treatment of sexually transmitted diseases.

1 Erbelding EJ Quinn TC. Urethritis treatment. *Dermatol Clin* 1998; 16: 735–738.
2 Clinical Effectiveness Group (Association of Genitourinary Medicine and the Medical Society for the Study of Venereal Diseases). National guidelines for the management of gonorrhoea in adults. *Sex Transm Infect* 1999; 75(suppl 1): S13–15.
3 Clinical Effectiveness Group (Association of Genitourinary Medicine and the Medical Society for the Study of Venereal Diseases). National guideline for the management of Chlamydia trachomatis genital tract infection. *Sex Transm Infect* 1999; 75(suppl 1): S4–8.
4 Clinical Effectiveness Group (Association of Genitourinary Medicine and the Medical Society for the Study of Venereal Diseases). National guideline for the management of non-gonococcal urethritis. *Sex Transm Infect* 1999; 75(suppl 1): S9–12.
5 Clinical Effectiveness Group (Association of Genitourinary Medicine and the Medical Society for the Study of Venereal Diseases). National guideline for the management of epididymo-orchitis. *Sex Transm Infect* 1999; 75(suppl 1): S51–53.
6 Carne CA. Epidemiological treatment and tests of cure in gonococcal infection: evidence for value. *Genitourin Med* 1997; 73: 12–15.

1.33 Woman with a genital sore

Case history

A 32-year-old woman complains of a painful spot 'down below'.

Clinical approach

Is this an STD? The area is painful. Could this be genital HSV (Fig. 53)? Your aim is not only to diagnose and treat your patient, but also to reduce the level of the STD in the community. Thus, you must assess exposure and potential risk of transmission to others, and educate about safe sex and contraception. The advice of an appropriate genitourinary medicine physician should be obtained.

History of the presenting problem

The sore spot

Enquire about the following if the details do not emerge:
• How long has the painful spot been present?
• What was it like at the start?
• How did she become aware of the problem?
• Is there one or more area that is sore?
• Is this the first episode?
• Is there a history of trauma?

The chancre of primary syphilis is usually painless, but can become painful if superinfected. Genital herpes starts as a cluster of small vesicles filled with clear fluid, but these soon progress to painful shallow ulcers. Recurrent episodes are strongly suggestive of herpes.

Associated symptoms

Ask about the following:
• Vaginal discharge? Also ask about change in vaginal odour and vulval symptoms [1].
• Dyspareunia? Is sexual intercourse painful and if so, is the pain superficial or deep?
• Dysuria? This may indicate urethritis or a UTI, but is also common with genital herpes in women. Severe primary HSV may be associated with urinary retention.
• Abdominal pain, back and leg pain?
• Systemic symptoms? Fever, headache and arthralgia are often present in genital herpes and constitutional symptoms may start 24 h before the genital lesions develop. Some patients with primary HSV may develop aseptic meningitis.
• Menstrual cycle? When did her last period start? Has there been any blood loss, intermenstrual bleeding or alteration in her cycle?

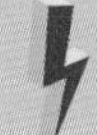

The woman presenting with a probable STD—could she be pregnant?

Exposure

Take a detailed sexual history as described in Section 1.31, p. 76.

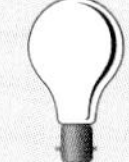

Consider the possibility of a sexual assault and gently explore this where appropriate.

Table 30 Features of vulval lesions.

	Condition	Features
Common	Warts: human papilloma virus	Condylomata accuminata (Fig. 53), typically raised papillary lesions Flat verrucous forms also seen
	Molluscum contagiosum	1–3 mm papule with central umbilicus
	Herpes simplex	Cluster of vesicles at any site including perianal region, progressing to superficial ulcers Severe or progressive ulceration in immunocompromised (Fig. 53)
	Bartholin's cyst	Swelling at base of labia May become infected where inflamed and may drain pus
	Non-infectious causes	Trauma, lichen planus, leucoplakia, Bowen's disease
Uncommon but increasing	Primary syphilis	Chancre at site of inoculation Usually single but kissing lesions where mucosal surfaces are opposed Initially papular then ulcerates Non-tender, smooth raised edge, indurated but clean base, regional lymphadenopathy Heals in 3–6 weeks
Rare in the UK	Secondary syphilis	Condylomata lata Moist papules in skin creases around genitals, groin and anus
	Chancroid	Painless papule rapidly progresses to painful 1–2 cm ulcer with raised, irregular edges and a necrotic base
	Granuloma inguinale	Progressive ulceration with tissue destruction Painless with a beefy red base.
	Carcinoma of the vulva	Consider in any non-healing lesion Rare in young women Often preceded by leucoplakia

Relevant past history

Enquire about previous STDs, including hepatitis, and how and where she was treated. Recurrent minor infections such as shingles may signify underlying immunodeficiency. Ask about previous UTIs (see Section 1.12, p. 31) and past obstetric history. When was her last cervical smear and what was the result?

Sexually transmitted diseases and HIV infection

- Coexistent STD increases the risk of HIV transmission
- HIV prevalence is higher in STD clinic attendees
- STD may have atypical presentation in HIV, e.g. increased reactivation of HSV, rapid progression of syphilis.

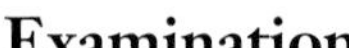

Fig. 53 Extensive anogenital herpes simplex virus and warts in a patient with advanced HIV-related immunodeficiency.

Examination

Genital

Ensure that a properly trained person performs a thorough examination in the presence of a chaperone:

- Inspect the sore area to locate any discrete lesions (Table 30)
- Check for inguinal nodes
- A speculum examination is mandatory because vaginal lesions may be hidden; look at the cervix for irregularity and mucosal abnormalities; check for discharge from the urethra and cervix
- A bimanual vaginal examination may detect uterine, fallopian or ovarian abnormalities
- Have all of the equipment to take screening swabs available to avoid unnecessary repeat vaginal examinations.

General

Look for evidence of immunosuppression (see Section 1.28, p. 70) because HIV co-infection increases the risk of other STDs [2], including disseminated gonorrhoea and secondary syphilis (see Section 1.35, p. 86).

Approach to investigation and management

Investigations

Appropriate samples should be taken from the index lesion. If vesicles are present, vesicle fluid can be sent for culture for HSV. Electron microscopy on vesicle fluid can give a rapid diagnosis, but is impractical in routine situations. Screen for other STDs.

Female genitourinary screen

- High vaginal swab: wet preparation can detect *Trichomonas* spp., bacterial vaginosis and *Candida* spp.
- Urethral swab: Gram stain, culture for gonorrhoea. DNA-based tests for *Chlamydia* spp.
- Endocervical swab: Gram stain low sensitivity; culture for gonorrhoea; chlamydia screen
- Rectal swab: culture for gonorrhoea
- MSU: bacterial culture
- Throat swab: culture for gonorrhoea
- Swab lesions: bacterial and viral culture
- Serology: for syphilis and consider hepatitis B/C, HIV and HSV.

Management

The following are principles underlying management:
- Treat specific infections [3,4].
- Test of cure where applicable.
- Partner notification and contact tracing where appropriate. Screening and therapy of partners are essential to prevent reinfection, but remember that partner notification and tracing may be very difficult in situations where the woman feels at risk of abuse.
- Educate: see Section 1.31, p. 79 [5].
- Discuss contraceptive options and refer for family planning advice if appropriate.
- Make sure that follow-up for cervical smear result has been arranged.

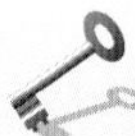

Areas to cover in health promotion

- General education about the routes of transmission, symptoms and consequences of STDs
- Safe sex: discuss risks of different sexual activity, use of male and female condoms
- HIV risk awareness
- Cervical cancer and cervical screening programme
- Family planning advice.

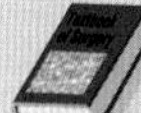

http://www.mssvd.org.uk. This website contains an induction pack for GUM trainees and regularly updated clinical guidelines on the diagnosis and treatment of sexually transmitted diseases.

1 Emmert D. Sexually transmitted diseases in women. Gonorrhea and syphilis. *Postgrad Med* 2000; 107: 181–184, 189–190, 193–197.
2 Capps L. Sexually transmitted infections in women infected with the human immunodeficiency virus. *Sex Transm Dis* 1998; 25: 443–447.
3 Update on drugs for herpes zoster and genital herpes. *Drug Ther Bull* 1998; 36: 77–79.
4 Clinical Effectiveness Group (Association of Genitourinary Medicine and the Medical Society for the Study of Venereal Diseases). National guideline for the management of genital herpes. *Sex Transm Infect* 1999; 75(suppl 1): S24–28.
5 Darrow WW. Health education and promotion for STD prevention: lessons for the next millennium. *Genitourin Med* 1997; 73: 88–94.

1.34 Abdominal pain and vaginal discharge

Case history

A 20-year-old woman presents with fever, lower abdominal pain and vaginal discharge.

Clinical approach

Is this pelvic inflammatory disease (PID) [1]? You must first exclude life-threatening surgical conditions and then decide on the relationship of the vaginal discharge to her abdominal pain.

History of the presenting problem

The most likely diagnosis from the brief details given above is PID, but could the pain be the result of anything else? Ask about the following if the details are not forthcoming:
- What is the site, severity and radiation of the pain? Does it fit the pattern of any well-recognized cause of abdominal pain, e.g. appendicitis? (See *Emergency medicine*, Section 1.13.)
- Has there been diarrhoea, alteration in bowel habit or rectal bleeding? These would suggest an intestinal cause of abdominal pain, with vaginal discharge not directly related to the pain in this context.
- Have there been symptoms to suggest a urinary tract infection, e.g. frequency, dysuria, strong urinary smell, fever? Has she had a urinary infection before?
- When was her last period? Is there any risk of pregnancy? If yes, exclude an ectopic pregnancy urgently.
- Has there been bleeding after sex or between periods?

Table 31 Vaginal discharge.

Cause	Examples	Features
Physiological		Thin watery, non-offensive discharge May vary with menstrual cycle
Vaginitis	Bacterial vaginosis	Malodorous discharge, clue cells on wet prep, risk of preterm labour
	Candidiasis	Moderate white discharge, pruritis
	Trichomonas spp.	Profuse, purulent offensive discharge, pruritis and dyspareunia
Cervicitis	*Neisseria gonorrhoeae*	Often asymptomatic and detected at examination for other genital symptoms May produce a purulent discharge
	Chlamydia trachomatis	
	Herpes simplex	
Urethritis	Same as for cervicitis	Associated dysuria
Non-infectious	Foreign body, allergy	Pruritis, discharge may be profuse and offensive

Vaginal bleeding can occur in spontaneous abortion or ectopic pregnancy and, in an older woman, it may signify underlying malignancy. Irregular bleeding may also be a symptom of endometritis that accompanies PID.

And focusing on the vaginal discharge:

- What is the discharge like? Quantity, consistency, colour and odour (Table 31). Creamy white discharge suggests candidal infection, malodorous discharge may occur with PID or *Trichomonas* spp., and a fishy smell is characteristic of bacterial vaginosis.
- Have there been other genital symptoms? Vaginal itching and dyspareunia occur with vaginitis.
- What about contraceptive use? Ask specifically about intrauterine contraceptive devices (IUCDs) that may be associated with PID. Ask whether she uses tampons and if there is a possibility of a retained tampon—which can predispose to toxic shock syndrome. (See Section 1.2, p. 5.)
- Take a full sexual history (see Section 1.31, p. 76). PID occurs in sexually active women, especially those <20 years, and is increased in relation to the number of sexual partners and the frequency of sexual intercourse.

What if this patient reports a sexual assault?

- Believe her and take immediate action
- This requires privacy, care and sensitivity
- Refer to the appropriate authorities only with her consent
- Do not examine or take samples until you have received expert advice from a genitourinary specialist
- Consider postexposure prophylaxis against STD, including HIV and emergency contraception
- Refer to a specialist rape counselling service.

Issues with 'children'

When dealing with those <16 years (or <18 years in care), consider the following:

- Confidentiality: GMC guidance (see *General clinical issues*, Section 3)
- Children's Act
- Child protection issues.

The issues can be complex in individual cases. If in doubt about medicolegal aspects, consult senior clinicians and/or contact the Medical Protection Society (MPS)/Medical Defence Union (MDU) and GMC before breaching confidentiality.

Relevant past history

Ask about obstetric history, previous treatment or investigations for infertility, endometriosis, menstrual problems and previous episodes of abdominal pain.

Examination

Is the woman well, ill, very ill or nearly dead?

- Check vital signs: temperature, pulse, BP and respiratory rate.
- Is there any evidence of bleeding or sepsis?
- If necessary, obtain intravenous access immediately and begin resuscitation while completing the history and examination. (See *Emergency medicine*, Sections 1.2 and 1.11.)

Then continue with the following:

- General examination: look in particular for evidence of immunodeficiency (see Section 1.24, p. 61). Arthritis or rash suggests Reiter's syndrome or disseminated gonococcal infection.
- Abdominal examination: check for masses, local or generalized peritonitis. Right upper quadrant tenderness may be present in the Curtis–Fitz-Hugh syndrome.
- Genital examination. Vaginal speculum examination to look for fluid in the vaginal vault, check for urethral and cervical discharge. Bimanual vaginal examination is also essential—feel for swelling or tenderness of the adnexae; pain on cervical excitation is typical of PID.
- Rectal examination.

Approach to investigation and management

Investigations

Blood tests

Check the FBC, electrolytes, renal and liver function, and inflammatory markers (ESR/CRP). Check blood gases if severely unwell. Other tests, e.g. amylase, may be indicated depending on the clinical context. Look for anaemia, neutrophilia and an inflammatory response. Abnormal liver function may occur in the Curtis–Fitz-Hugh syndrome or sepsis. Severe sepsis is suggested by thrombocytopenia, renal impairment or acidosis.

Cultures

Take the following:

• Blood cultures may detect gonorrhoea in disseminated disease

• MSU if urinary dipstick abnormal

• Perform urethral and endocervical swabs as well as a full genitourinary screen (see Section 1.33, p. 82).

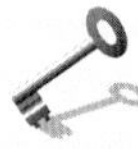

Detection of *Chlamydia* sp.

• Frequently asymptomatic

• Screen all STD clinic attendees

• Culture is difficult and insensitive

• Immunoassays superseded by DNA-based tests

• Screening now possible on urine samples or self-taken vaginal swab [2,3].

Imaging

The following may be needed:

• Abdominal radiograph if renal stones or bowel disease suspected.

• Abdominal ultrasonography may show tubal swelling in PID and detect ectopic pregnancy or tubo-ovarian abscess.

• CT for suspected pelvic abscess (Fig. 54).

Other tests

• Pregnancy test in all potentially fertile women.

• Laparoscopy is the definitive method to diagnose PID and can be used to drain an abscess: consider when there is diagnostic uncertainty or the patient is failing to respond to therapy.

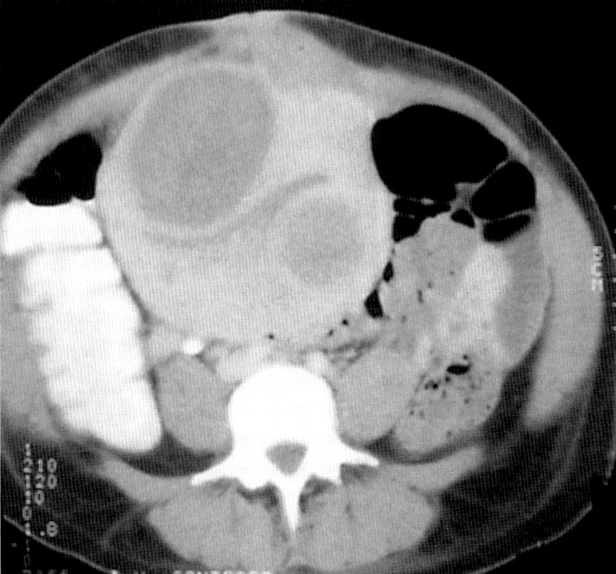

Fig. 54 Pelvic CT scan showing deep-seated abscess formation as a result of *Mycoplasma hominis* infection after premature labour.

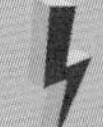

Do not perform a cervical smear when there is obvious cervical infection because inflammatory cells make interpretation difficult.

Management

Surgical cause

If the woman has an acute abdomen or ectopic pregnancy, she requires immediate admission and urgent surgical referral.

Pelvic inflammatory disease

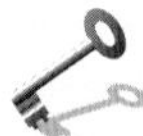

Microbiology of pelvic inflammatory disease

• *Chlamydia trachomatis*

• *Neisseria gonorrhoeae*

• Genital mycoplasmas

• *E. coli* and other enteric bacteria

• Streptococci and anaerobes

If the patient is systemically well, consider outpatient therapy with oral antibiotics (see Sections 2.5.2, p. 105 and 2.8.4, p. 119). If severe pain, high fever, signs of severe sepsis or pregnant, admit for intravenous therapy [4]. Commence empirical therapy based on the likely microbiology and local antibiotic policy. The causative organism is not known at the onset of therapy and, if empirical therapy is failing, you must reconsider the underlying diagnosis and investigate for other causes or abscess formation. Consider genitourinary TB in chronic cases. Infertility as a result of fallopian tube scarring is a potential consequence of PID and should be discussed with the patient [5].

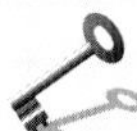

Disseminated gonorrhoea

• Generally follows asymptomatic local gonococcal infection

• Skin: sparse (<30) pustular, papular or petechial lesions

• Joints: tenosynovitis or asymmetrical polyarthritis

• Blood/joint fluid culture: positive in 50%

• Genital/pharyngeal cultures: may be positive.

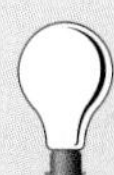

Genitourinary TB

• Males: epididymo-orchitis

• Females: endometritis

• Both males and females may have bladder, ureter or renal disease.

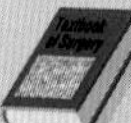

http://www.mssvd.org.uk. This website contains an induction pack for GUM trainees and regularly updated clinical guidelines on the diagnosis and treatment of sexually transmitted diseases.

1 Paavonen J. Pelvic inflammatory disease. From diagnosis to prevention. *Dermatol Clin* 1998; 16: 747–756.

2 Clinical Effectiveness Group (Association of Genitourinary Medicine and the Medical Society for the Study of Venereal Diseases). National guideline for the management of pelvic infection and perihepatitis. *Sex Transm Infect* 1999; 75(suppl 1): S54–56.

3 Clinical Effectiveness Group (Association of Genitourinary Medicine and the Medical Society for the Study of Venereal Diseases). National guideline for the management of *Chlamydia trachomatis* genital tract infection. *Sex Transm Infect* 1999; 75(suppl 1): S4–8.

4 Howell MR, Quinn TC, Braithwaite W *et al.* Screening women for *Chlamydia trachomatis* in family planning clinics: the cost-effectiveness of DNA amplification assays. *Sex Transm Dis* 1998; 25: 108–117.

5 Westrom L, Joesoef R, Reynolds G *et al.* Pelvic inflammatory disease and fertility. *Sex Transm Dis* 1992; 19: 1895–1891.

1.35 Syphilis in pregnancy

Case history

You are asked to see a 29-year-old pregnant woman who has positive syphilis serology at antenatal screening.

Clinical approach

The aim is to establish whether the fetus is at risk of syphilis or other infections and intervene to reduce fetal harm (Table 32) [1–3].

History of the presenting problem

Serological results

Find out exactly what the results are before seeing the patient [1] (Table 33). If in doubt, repeat the test to confirm the result. Telling the woman that she has syphilis only to discover that it is a biological false-positive result must be avoided. If the results suggest syphilis ask the following:

- Have you ever been treated for syphilis and when?
- Why did they treat you? Did you have disease or simply exposure?
- What treatment did you have and for how long?
- Where was the treatment given? If possible, you want to confirm that adequate treatment was indeed given.
- Where have you lived? There might be a possibility of other treponemal infections such as yaws.

Table 32 Sexually transmitted infections and the unborn child.

Infection	Consequence
Syphilis	Congenital disease
Bacterial vaginosis	Premature labour
HIV	Vertical transmission
Gonorrhoea	Ophthalmia neonatorum
Chlamydial infection	Ophthalmia neonatorum, pneumonia
Human papilloma virus	Laryngeal/tracheal papillomas
Herpes simplex	Disseminated infection in neonate

Table 33 Commonly encountered patterns of syphilis serology.

Test results	Interpretation
VDRL or RPR positive TPHA or FTA negative	Biological false positive, e.g. pregnancy, connective tissue disease, HIV
VDRL or RPR positive TPHA or FTA positive	Treponemal infection at some stage If VDRL titre is high the infection with syphilis is recent In latent syphilis the VDRL will be of low titre
VDRL or RPR negative TPHA or FTA positive	Either latent untreated syphilis, fully treated syphilis or a related treponemal infection Can have TPHA false positive, but this is uncommon

VDRL, venereal disease research laboratory; RPR, rapid plasma regain; TPHA, *Treponema pallidum* haemagglutinin assay; FTA, fluorescent treponemal antigen.

Antenatal history

What gestation is she? Has there been an illness consistent with primary or secondary syphilis? This is important because the risk of congenital syphilis is much higher during early infection.

Sexual history

Assess the risk of HIV co-infection and other STDs. (See Section 1.33, p. 81.)

Examination

Full genital and general examination for signs of syphilis (Fig. 55), other STDs and HIV is required. (See Sections 1.28, p. 70 and 1.33, p. 82.)

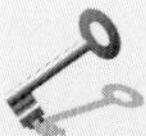

Features of secondary syphilis

- Signs start 6–8 weeks after infection
- Fever, headache, musculoskeletal pains
- Rash: macular, becoming papular on trunk, palms and soles
- Alopecia: moth-eaten
- Oral: mucous patches, snail-track ulcers
- Anogenital: condylomata lata
- Generalized lymphadenopathy

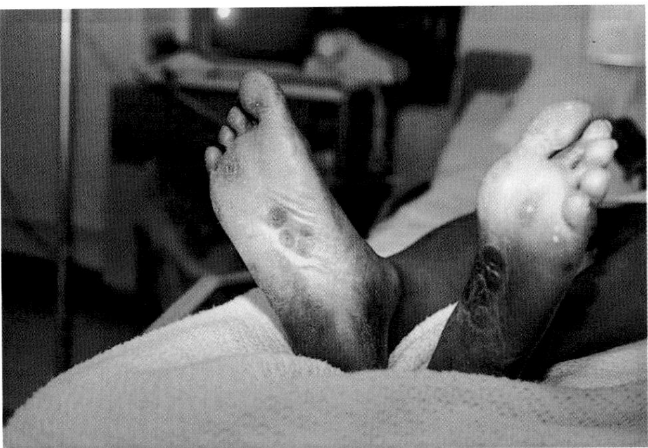

Fig. 55 Soles of a patient who had no antenatal care presenting to A&E in labour, showing characteristic lesions of secondary syphilis.

Approach to investigation and management

Investigations

Serology

Check the following:

• Syphilis serology (see Table 33) is divided into non-treponemal (rapid plasma reagin [RPR], Veneral Disease Reference Laboratory [VDRL]) and treponemal tests (TPHA [*Treponema pallidum* haemagglutination assay], fluorescent treponemal antibody [FTA]) [4]. The non-treponemal tests detect antiphospholipid antibodies: they are non-specific, but their titre relates to disease activity. Treponemal tests are more specific but remain positive life-long, even after effective therapy. A combination of both tests is therefore required for accurate diagnosis and monitoring of the therapeutic response.

• Other serology: counsel and offer hepatitis B and HIV testing.

Cultures

Do a female genitourinary infection screen (see Section 1.33, p. 82) because syphilis means that she should be considered at risk of other STDs.

Management

If the serology suggests active syphilis, therapy is essential to treat the mother and minimize the risk/severity of congenital disease. Parenteral penicillin is the only proven therapy for syphilis in a pregnant woman, and desensitization should be considered in those allergic to penicillin. If the VDRL titre is very low/negative and there is a past history of treated syphilis, check that full therapy was completed, but err on the side of re-treatment if in doubt [5,6].

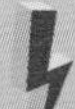

Jarisch–Herxheimer reaction

• Acute reaction to antitreponemal therapy mediated by inflammatory cytokines

• Occurs within 24 h of therapy and is most common with the first treatment dose

• Fever, myalgia, headache and hypotension

• Can (rarely) be fatal

• In pregnancy, it may trigger labour.

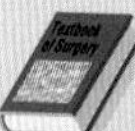

1 Guerina N. Management strategies for infectious diseases in pregnancy. *Semin Perinatol* 1994; 18: 305–320.

2 Emmert D. Sexually transmitted diseases in women. Gonorrhea and syphilis. *Postgrad Med* 2000; 107: 181–184, 189–190.

3 S Eggleston, A Turner. *Serological Diagnosis of Syphilis.* PHLS Syphilis Serology Working Group. London: PHLS, 1999. Available from www.phls.co.uk.

4 Smith C Jr. The management of herpes simplex virus infection in pregnancy. *Br J Obstet Gynaecol* 1998; 105: 255–260.

5 Kinghorn GR. Syphilis. In: Armstrong D, Cohen J (eds) *Infectious Diseases.* London: Mosby, 1999: 64.

6 Clinical Effectiveness Group (Association of Genitourinary Medicine and the Medical Society for the Study of Venereal Diseases). National guideline for the management of early syphilis. *Sex Transm Infect* 1999; 75(suppl 1): S29–33.

1.36 Positive blood cultures

Case history

The microbiologist calls you to report that a patient, who has been sent home from A&E, has a positive blood culture.

Clinical approach

Your priority must be to ensure that a patient with a significant bacteraemia is traced and treated. The information you need at this point is the following:

• When/where/how was the blood culture taken?

• Why was it taken?

• What is growing?

History of the presenting problem

When, where and how

Ask the microbiologist which team sent the culture (you may need to call them), how many cultures were sent and when. One positive bottle from several cultures taken a week ago is less likely to be significant than something growing in all bottles taken yesterday. Was the blood taken peripherally or from a central venous line? Central lines may be colonized with bacteria and line cultures have a poor positive predictive value. (See Section 1.11, p. 29.)

Why the culture was taken

You have to pull the notes:

- What did the patient present with?
- What was there in the history or examination to suggest infection?
- Were other investigations sent?
- Was a diagnosis made?
- Was treatment given?

What is growing

This is the key element of the case. The organism may be significant, suggest a specific diagnosis or focus of infection, or merely be a contaminant [1,2]. (See Section 3.2, p. 151.)

Relevant past history

Is there any predisposing cause for bacteraemia or infection such as an abnormal heart valve, recent surgery or immunocompromise?

Examination

Look at the notes for evidence of a documented fever, signs of sepsis or focal infection. If the patient is recalled, then assess him or her fully. (See Section 1.1, p. 3.)

Approach to investigation and management

The safe approach is to consider that all positive blood culture results are significant until proved otherwise, although some organisms may be skin contaminants. Recall the patient for clinical review if your reading of the notes and microbiology results suggests that there is a risk of a significant infection.

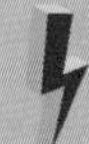

Be safe! If in doubt contact the patient or his or her GP.

Investigations

Blood tests

Review all investigations sent at the time of the original culture, particularly the FBC, liver function and inflammatory markers. If the patient is recalled, repeat testing as appropriate. (See Sections 1.1, p. 3 and 1.2, p. 5.)

Interpretation of blood cultures

The probability that a culture is a true positive depends on several factors [1,2] including the following.

PRETEST PROBABILITY

Is the clinical course consistent with infection with the organisms grown? For example, a single viridans streptococcus in four bottles in a patient suspected of having endocarditis is likely to be real, but the same culture result in a fit healthy young woman with no stigmata of infection is not.

NUMBER OF SAMPLES POSITIVE

A minimum of two sets of blood cultures should always be sent, with three or four sets recommended to exclude a bacteraemia (see Section 3.2, p. 151) [3,4]. More than one culture positive with the same organism is very suggestive of genuine infection.

ORGANISM ISOLATED

Pathogens, e.g. *N. meningitidis* and *Staph. aureus*, are almost always causing significant disease whenever they are grown in blood cultures (Table 34).

PURE VERSUS MIXED CULTURE

Multiple organisms suggest contamination unless the clinical picture is compatible, e.g. intra-abdominal sepsis and mixed faecal-type organisms.

Management

Day 1

Blood culture systems are automated to allow continuous monitoring (Fig. 56). On the first day, the microbiologist will be able to tell you only a Gram stain result, but he or she may have some idea of what the organism is from its morphology (Table 35). The need for empirical antibiotics is decided on the basis of the clinical picture and these preliminary results. For example, if Gram-positive cocci in clumps have been seen in this patient, and there is evidence of infection, repeat cultures and commencement of empirical therapy for *Staph. aureus* with flucloxacillin would be appropriate. By contrast, if there was no

Table 34 Significance of common blood culture isolates.

Organism	Percentage significant (probability of causing disease)
Staphylococcus aureus	90–95
Escherichia coli	99
Candida spp.	90–100
Coagulase-negative staphylococci	5–15
Propionibacterium spp.	1–2

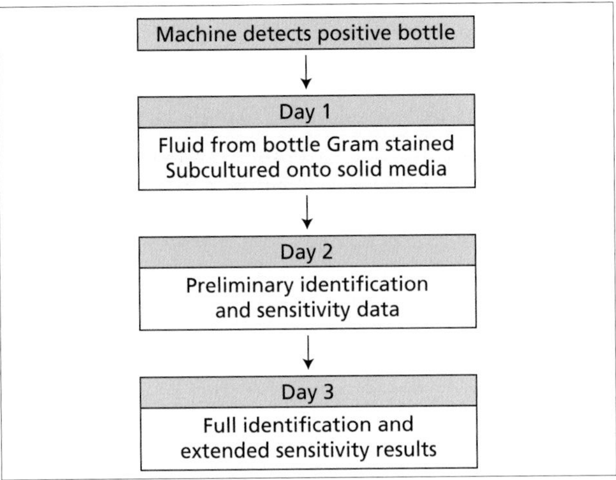

Fig. 56 Blood culture bottles are constantly monitored in an automated machine. When evidence of bacterial growth is detected, the bottle will flag up as positive. The laboratory technicians will remove the culture and process it further.

Table 35 Blood culture isolates.

Gram stain	Morphology	Likely organism
Gram-positive	Cocci in clumps	*Staphylococcus* spp.
	Cocci in pairs	Pneumococci
		Enterococci
	Cocci in chains	*Streptococcus* spp.
	Rods	*Corynebacterium* spp.
		Bacillus spp.
		Listeria monocytogenes
		Clostridia spp.
Gram-negative	Cocci in pairs	*Neisseria* spp.
	Coccobacilli	*Haemophilus* spp.
		Brucella spp.
	Rods	Coliforms and Enterobacteriaceae
		Pseudomonas spp.

evidence of infection, it would be sensible to repeat cultures and observe.

Day 2

At this stage the laboratory should have more information on what is growing and will be in a better position to evaluate its significance. Initial sensitivity data will allow adjustment in antibiotics. For example, the staphylococcus suspected on day 1 may be confirmed as *Staph. aureus* but found to be methicillin-resistant *Staph. aureus* (MRSA) and flucloxacillin switched to vancomycin.

Day 3 onwards

Full identification and susceptibilities should be available. Some organisms are slow growers or prove difficult to identify, and so complete results may take even longer than the 3 days. Review therapy with the microbiologist, particularly if the patient is not improving.

Diagnosis does not stop at the point of a significant blood culture result. It is not enough simply to treat this patient for *Staph. aureus* bacteraemia. Where was the source of infection? Is there a deep-seated focus? Some organisms, including *Staph. aureus*, may seed to distant sites and cause endocarditis, osteomyelitis or deep abscesses. The knowledge of the source and/or evidence of metastatic spread may alter the length of therapy and further management.

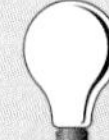

Organisms as markers

Some organisms are markers for underlying/unsuspected disease and should prompt further investigation:

- Non-typhoidal salmonella bacteraemia: consider immunosuppression, HIV
- *Strep. bovis*: consider gastrointestinal malignancy
- Recurrent meningococcaemia: consider complement deficiency.

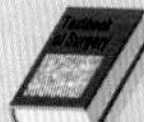

1 Weinstein MP, Reller B, Murphy JR, Lichtenstein KA. The clinical significance of positive blood cultures: A comprehensive analysis of 500 episodes of bacteremia and fungemia in adults. *Rev Infect Dis* 1983; 5: 54–70.
2 Aronson MD, Bor DH. Diagnosis and treatment. Diagnostic decision—blood cultures. *Ann Intern Med* 1987; 106: 246–253.
3 Brown DF, Warren RE. Effect of sample volume on yield of positive blood cultures from adult patients with haematological malignancy. *J Clin Pathol* 1990; 43: 777–779.
4 Durack DT, Lukes AS, Bright DK. New criteria for the diagnosis of infective endocarditis: utilization of specific echocardiographic findings. *Am J Med* 1994; 96: 200–209.

1.37 Therapeutic drug monitoring—antibiotics

Case history

The on-call microbiology technician calls to report that a patient has a 'toxic' gentamicin level.

Clinical approach

First ensure that the sample has been taken correctly and then interpret the result in the light of the clinical situation. Remember that therapeutic monitoring (Table 36) is important to ensure both efficacy and safety of treatment. Decisions on further dosing will require knowledge of the present level, but also of the patient's renal function, previous levels in association with the renal function at that time and the disease process being treated.

Table 36 Antimicrobial agents requiring therapeutic monitoring.

Agent	Monitoring and risk group	Expected levels (mg/L)	Reassay interval (days)
Aminoglycosides: gentamicin, netilmicin two and three times daily dosing	All patients on second to fourth dose Close monitoring if changing renal function	Most infections: trough <2; peak >5 Infective endocarditis: trough <1; peak 2–3	3–5
Aminoglycosides: gentamicin, netilmicin once daily dosing (7 mg/kg)		Follow nomogram (Fig. 57)	6–8
Aminoglycosides: amikacin		Trough <10; peak >20	3–5
Glycopeptides: vancomycin	All patients on >2 days therapy; assay at second to fourth dose	Trough 5–15	6–8
Teicoplanin	Severe infections, e.g. osteomyelitis only or long courses	Trough >10–20 but <60	
Chloramphenicol	In neonates	10–25	5–7
Cycloserine	All patients after 4th–6th dose	Trough 10–20 peak (at 2 h post dose) 20–35	10–30
Flucytosine	All patients	Trough 30–50; peak 70–80	4–8

Therapeutic drug monitoring is important when:
- the drug has a narrow therapeutic–toxic range
- there is a large variability in pharmacokinetics between patients
- the therapeutic effect of the drug is not easily assessed
- there is a direct relationship between concentration and pharmacological effect
- a patient has altered and/or variable renal/hepatic function and the route of drug elimination is via that organ
- the expected or desired therapeutic effect is not observed.

History of the presenting problem

To interpret antibiotic levels correctly you need to know the following:
- Dose and route of administration.
- When the sample was taken in relation to the antibiotic dose. The 'toxic' gentamicin level reported may actually be a perfectly acceptable peak level after a once-daily bolus dose.
- How the sample was taken? If taken through the same line as the antibiotic was given, this may give a falsely high value.
- Organism and site of infection. This will allow you to judge what levels are needed, e.g. target gentamicin levels are lower when treating endocarditis (see Table 36).
- Other medication.
- Renal/hepatic function.

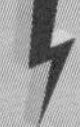

The advice you get is only as good as the information on the request card.

Relevant past history

Renal or ear disease are important because these predispose to toxicity from gentamicin

Gentamicin should be used with caution in renal failure. Take specific advice on dose and monitoring from microbiology or pharmacy.

Approach to investigation and management

Investigations

Consider repeat measurement of the following:
- Renal function: if recent result is not available
- Gentamicin levels: if there is any doubt regarding the validity of the result, take further samples at the appropriate timing for repeat levels.

Management

If a level is toxic for the time it was taken, the dose will have to be modified. It is safest to stop the drug, reassay and reintroduce it only when trough levels are within the acceptable

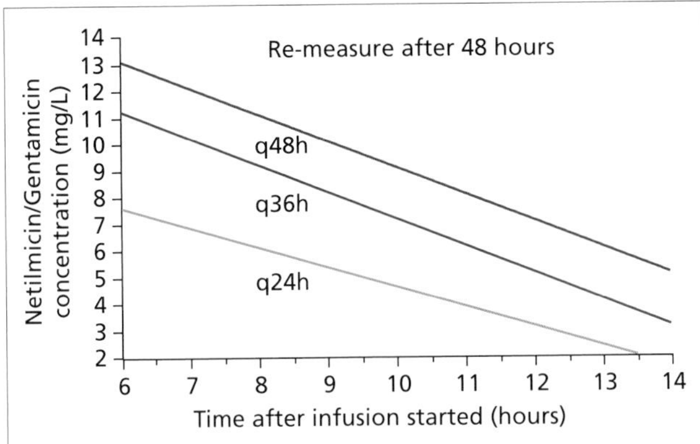

Fig. 57 Nomogram for monitoring once-daily aminoglycoside dosage interval based on 7 mg/kg dose. The dosing should be based on the actual body weight, unless the patient is morbidly obese and then: Obese dosing weight = ideal body weight + (0.4 × [actual weight − ideal weight]). (From Freeman 1997 [1].)

range. If toxicity has occurred, it is likely that the drug will need to be restarted with an altered dosing schedule, about which the microbiology department should be able to advise.

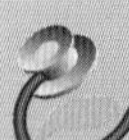

Gentamicin dosing for once-daily use

Understanding of pharmacokinetics has provided the basis for considering once-daily aminoglycoside dosing. Many comparative trials and three meta-analysis studies have been published [1]. These showed equivalent, or a trend towards better, cure rates and significantly less nephrotoxicity with a once-daily dose. This is not validated in endocarditis or pregnancy.

1 Single dose of gentamicin by bolus infusion
2 Take level 6–14 h after start
3 Subsequent dosing by nomogram (Fig. 57).

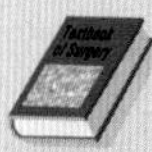

See *Clinical pharmacology*, Sections 2, 3 and 5

1 Freeman CD, Nicolau DP, Belliueau PP *et al.* Once-daily dosing of aminoglycosides: review and recommendations for clinical practice. *J Antimicrob Chemother* 1997; 39: 677–686.

1.38 Contact with meningitis

Case history

You are phoned at home by one of your colleagues who is concerned because he has treated a patient who has probable meningococcal meningitis.

Clinical approach

Meningococcal disease always creates a lot of interest and anxiety, mainly from the general public but also among healthcare workers. You should clarify what your colleague's main concerns are. It is likely that he is worried about the risk to himself and the need for prophylaxis. He needs reassurance and education. The risks to him are extremely low.

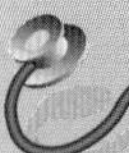

Carriage of meningococci

Humans are the only natural host for meningococci [1]. At any one time, about 10% of the population will be carrying the organism in their nasopharynx, the mean duration of carriage being estimated from community studies as about 9 months. Little is known about the factors that influence progression to invasive disease or maintenance of a carrier state. However, analysis of bacterial population structure and genetics shows that there are certain hypervirulent strains of meningococci that are associated with invasive disease.

History of the presenting problem

Establish the facts

• Did the patient have proven/suspected meningococcal disease? Often staff panic on hearing the term 'meningitis' and the patient may well have a cause other than meningococcal.
• What was the involvement with the patient? Staff prophylaxis is rarely needed but often leads to a chain reaction. One person is treated; they tell everyone else and, within a short time, people who did not even see the patient are on the phone.
• Was mouth-to-mouth resuscitation given? If not, then staff prophylaxis is not required.

Inform the PHLS

The Public Health Laboratory Services (PHLS) [2], usually the Consultant in Communicable Disease Control (CCDC) in England and Wales or the Director of Public Health/Consultant in Public Health in Scotland, should be notified without delay (by telephone) about any suspected case of meningococcal disease. This serves several purposes:
• Point of contact for questions, advice and education for healthcare professionals and the public
• Administration of chemoprophylaxis and immunization
• Management of outbreaks.

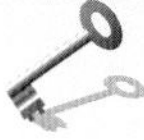

Risk to household contacts

People who live in the same household as a case are at higher risk of developing disease than other members of the community. The attack rate in the month after the index case has occurred is increased by about 500–1200 times (a risk of around 1% per household). This probably reflects the epidemiology of strain carriage, but also the genetic susceptibility of household members.

Approach to investigation and management

Quickly establish whether there is a risk and a need for prophylaxis. At the same time, make sure that the index case has been appropriately managed (see Sections 1.2, p. 7 and 1.14, p. 38) and that the household contacts have been dealt with.

Investigations

No investigations are needed for the staff member.

Confirm index case

It is very important to confirm the diagnosis. This may be by culture from throat swabs, blood or CSF, or based on detection by PCR from blood or CSF.

Management

Staff members

Prophylaxis is indicated only for those involved in mouth-to-mouth resuscitation. If prophylaxis is not indicated, do not give it. Do not acquiesce simply because he or she is a colleague, or because he or she puts pressure on you—if you do, you will very quickly have many staff members queuing up for inappropriate therapy.

Chemoprophylaxis and choice of antibiotic

Chemoprophylaxis is an attempt to reduce risk by eliminating carriage from the network of contacts, thereby reducing the risk of invasive disease in other susceptible family members [3]. Many antibiotics that are useful in treating meningococcal disease are ineffective in eradicating carriage, so do not forget to treat the index case with chemoprophylaxis. The following are effective agents (adult doses shown):

- Rifampicin p.o. 600 mg twice daily for 2 days
- Ceftriaxone i.m. 250 mg single dose
- Ciprofloxacin p.o. 500 mg single dose (not licensed).

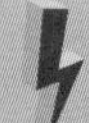

Chemoprophylaxis of meningococcal disease

Side effects should be explained, including the reduction in the efficacy of the oral contraceptive pill with rifampicin.

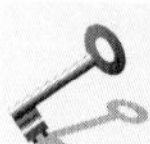

Notification and prophylaxis of meningococcal disease

- The Public Health services should be notified of all clinically or laboratory diagnosed cases of meningococcal disease
- Chemoprophylaxis is recommended for close household contacts or other intimate (kissing) contacts as soon as possible after the diagnosis of the index case
- Health-care workers need prophylaxis only if they have performed mouth-to-mouth resuscitation
- Steps should be taken to confirm the diagnosis
- Immunize household contacts of meningococcal serogroup C or A.

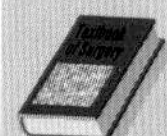

1 PHLS Meningococcal Infections Working Group and Public Health Medicine Environmental Group. Control of meningococcal disease: guidance for consultants in communicable disease control. *Communicable Disease Report* 1995; 5: R189–195.
2 Public Health Laboratory Service. Available at: www.phls.co.uk—contains reports and advice on immunization for meningococcal and other communicable diseases.
3 Stuart JM, Cartwright KA, Robinson PM *et al.* Does eradication of meningococcal carriage in household contacts prevent secondary cases of meningococcal disease? *BMJ* 1989; 298: 569–570.

1.39 Pulmonary tuberculosis—follow-up failure

Case history

An alcoholic patient presents with smear-positive pulmonary TB. He is started on antituberculous chemotherapy but fails to attend to follow up.

Clinical approach

Tuberculosis is caused by *Mycobacterium tuberculosis* complex (see Section 2.6.1, p. 110). In the UK, about 75% of cases involve the lung and the infection is usually acquired by inhalation of infected droplets. The sputum smear status reflects the ability to visualize organisms on direct microscopy. Smear positivity correlates with a higher burden of bacilli in the sputum ($\geq 10^5$–10^7 organisms/mL) and higher infectivity [1]. Thus, this patient is a high risk to his family and the community.

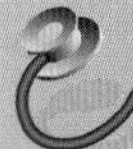

Tuberculosis in the UK

All forms of TB are notifiable to the PHLS [2]. Notification provides data to monitor epidemiological trends and triggers contact tracing. Worldwide there has been a resurgence of TB, including drug resistance and in the UK there has been an increase in notifications since the early mid-1990s. UK policy [3] aims to minimize morbidity and transmission of infection by early diagnosis, effective treatment and infection control measures. Homeless people have been highlighted by the Interdepartmental Working group on TB, established in 1994, as a particular group of concern.

History of the presenting problem

Why has he not attended clinic? Possibilities include the following:

- He has moved away
- He is in a psychiatric institution or prison
- He is homeless
- He is drunk all the time
- He is scared of hospitals.

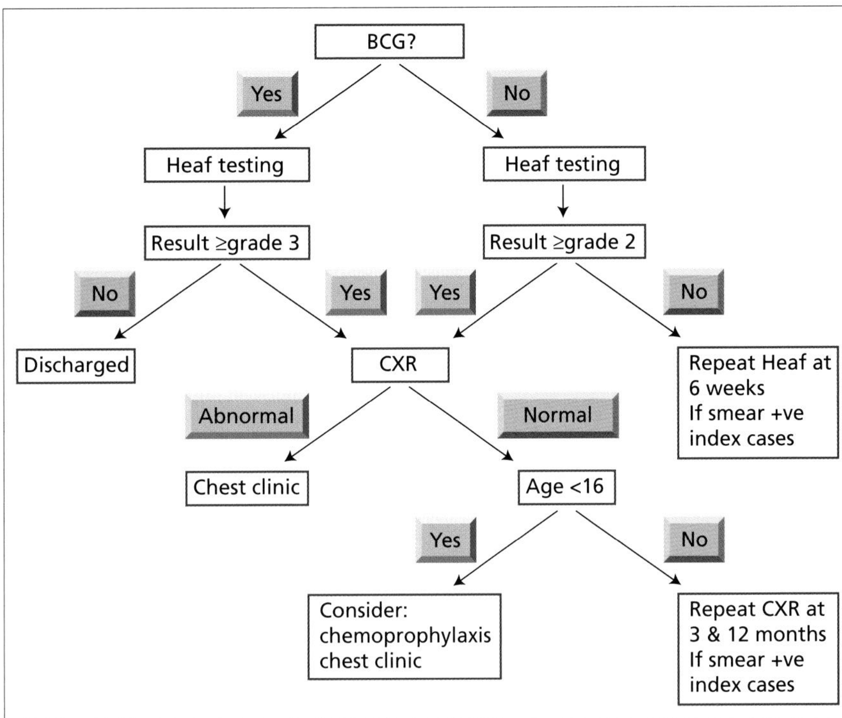

Fig. 58 Examination of contacts with pulmonary tuberculosis. BCG, Bacillus Calmette–Guérin; CXR, chest radiograph.

Approach to investigation and management

Management

You have a clear duty to public health and must take reasonable steps to track him down. At the same time, he may be quite vulnerable and find authority threatening. If possible, write to him or phone, explaining that it is important to attend. If this fails, talk to his GP. If he still fails to attend, notify the CCDC.

Non-compliant patients

Individuals likely to be non-compliant should be identified early and arrangements should be put in place to maximize compliance. In this case, the people to contact would usually be the TB specialist nurse for the region, who will initially be responsible for chasing the individual, and the CCDC. Possible strategies for improving compliance include the following:

- Education
- Initial or entire treatment course as an inpatient
- Supervised outpatient therapy: daily supervision, twice or three times weekly; this may involve trained staff in a hostel, outreach nurses, etc.
- Special drug packaging and other aids to memory
- Incentives such as transport to clinic, food, help with housing (e.g. hostel for the homeless).

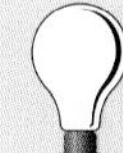

The law

An infectious patient who presents a risk to others can be compulsorily admitted to hospital on a magistrate's order, but cannot be compulsorily treated.

Contact tracing

Do not forget his contacts (Fig. 58). About 10% of TB cases are diagnosed by contact tracing and disease occurs in about 1% of contacts. Close contacts of patients with smear-positive pulmonary disease are at highest risk. Contacts of non-pulmonary TB are not usually examined. Examination of contacts may involve enquiry into BCG immunization, Heaf status (see Section 3.2, p. 151) and chest radiograph.

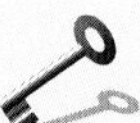

Tuberculosis and public health

- TB is a notifiable disease under the Public Health regulations of 1988 [2]
- TB is a disease of public health importance and has been highlighted by the Department of Health as an area of concern for prevention and control [3]
- Treatment, except in exceptional circumstances, is compulsory not optional
- Treatment of all cases of TB should be supervised by a consultant with appropriate experience (usually the respiratory or infectious disease consultant)
- Checks on patient compliance should be done as a routine
- Arrangements should be in place to follow up those who default from clinic attendance
- Contact tracing is an integral part of management of patients with TB.

See Section 1.5 and *Respiratory Medicine*, Sections 1.9 and 1.10

1 Septowitz KA. How contagious is tuberculosis? *Clinical Infectious Diseases* 1996; 23: 954–962.
2 Omerod LP, Watson JM, Poznia KA *et al.* Notification of tuberculosis: an update code of practice for England and Wales. *J R Coll Physicians Lond* 1997; 31: 299–303.
3 Interdepartmental Working Group on Tuberculosis. *The Prevention and Control of Tuberculosis in the United Kingdom.* London: Department of Health Jan 2000. Available on www.doh.gov.uk/tbguide.htm.

1.40 Penicillin allergy

Case history

A 30-year-old woman presents with community-acquired pneumonia and reports that she is allergic to penicillin (Fig. 59).

Clinical approach

You do not want to put this woman at risk of a serious drug reaction, but you need to ensure that she receives adequate therapy for her infection.

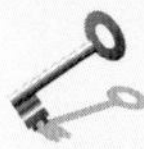

Suspected drug allergy

- What is the allergy?
- How severe?
- Was it documented?
- What disease is being treated?
- Is there an acceptable alternative?

History of the presenting problem

When, what and how bad?

Always clarify what is meant by 'allergy' (Table 37). A large proportion of patients are unable to give any further information—'my mother told me that I was allergic'—or report side effects of the drug that are not related to an allergic phenomenon, e.g. nausea, diarrhoea, headache.

Table 37 Manifestations of antibiotic allergy.

Clinical manifestation	Type of reaction (Gell and Coombs)	Onset
Anaphylaxis, urticaria	I (IgE)	0–24 h
Haemolytic anaemia, neutropenia, thrombocytopenia	II	>72 h
Drug fever, serum sickness	III	7–14 days
Contact dermatitis	IV	Variable
Rash (Fig. 59), fixed drug reactions, exfoliative dermatitis	V (idiopathic)	7–14 days

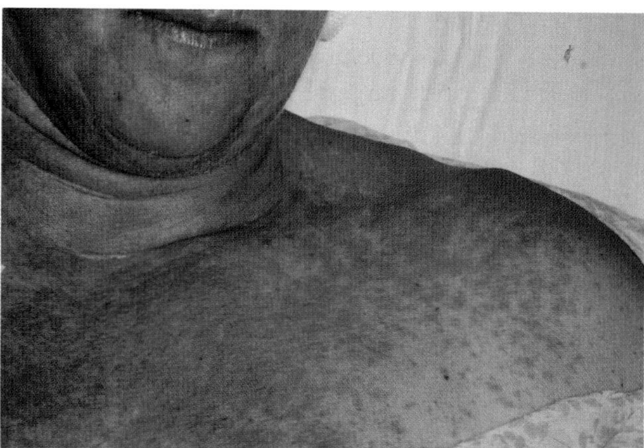

Fig. 59 Typical maculopapular rash of penicillin allergy.

The most important history to get is of anaphylaxis, severe skin disorders such as Stevens–Johnson syndrome (see *Dermatology*, Section 1.2), or other life-threatening reactions. You do not want to give an individual who has had one of these reactions another dose of the same antibiotic or a closely related one.

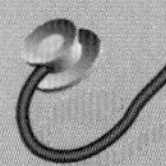

Penicillin allergy

The most common antibiotic allergy, reported to occur in 7–40/1000 penicillin treatment courses. Anaphylaxis occurs in 1/32 000–100 000 treatment courses.

Risk factors for β-lactam allergy

- Prior history of reaction to penicillins/β-lactam drugs: four to six times the increased risk of subsequent reaction, especially if the previous reaction was anaphylaxis or urticaria
- Risk is greater with parenteral than with oral therapy
- Children and elderly people appear to have fewer reactions
- Atopy is not an independent risk factor.

Approach to investigation and management

Investigations

IgE-mediated allergy to penicillin (severe immediate reactions) can be confirmed in some cases by skin-prick testing. This may be of help in individual cases but not as a general screening test.

Management

Need for penicillin

The choice of antibiotic should always be guided by suspected pathogens and the severity of disease. In this case the most likely agent is *Strep. pneumoniae*, but other pathogens also need to be considered (see Section 1.4, p. 10). The guidelines of the British Thoracic Society for the treatment of community-acquired pneumonia are that those with mild-to-moderate infection should be given oral treatment with an extended spectrum penicillin (amoxicillin), alone or plus a macrolide (erythromycin). In severe pneumonia, the recommendation would be for parenteral therapy with a second- or third-generation cephalosporin plus a macrolide (oral or intravenous).

Alternatives

MILD PNEUMONIA

The appropriate alternative to the standard regimen would be to use a macrolide alone and omit the amoxicillin.

MODERATE OR SEVERE PNEUMONIA

Could a cephalosporin be used? Patients with penicillin allergy often tolerate a cephalosporin, but these are also β-lactam drugs and there is 5–10% crossreactivity with penicillin allergies. If the previous reaction to penicillin was simply a rash, you should not be dissuaded from using a cephalosporin in this woman in this situation. It is more difficult to know what to do if the penicillin allergy were severe; the options most commonly taken would be to use high-dose (1 g four times daily) intravenous erythromycin alone, observing clinical progress very closely, or to give this together with a cephalosporin, monitoring carefully for side effects and treating these promptly should they arise.

Antibiotic allergy

There is usually an acceptable alternative antibiotic that you can prescribe. You must judge how likely a severe reaction is. If the history is not suggestive of allergy and you choose to give the drug in question or a related compound, advise the patient to report any adverse effects immediately. The first dose, particularly if intravenous, should be administered under supervision.

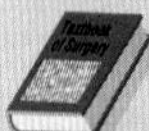

See *Clinical pharmacology*, Section 4.

1 Weiss ME, Franklin Adkinson N. Beta-lactam allergy. In: *Mandell, Douglas and Bennett's Principles and Practice of Infectious Diseases* (5th edn). New York: Churchill Livingstone, 1995: 272–278.
2 Penicillin allergy. *Drug Ther Bull* 1996; 34(11): 87–88.
3 Lin RY. A perspective on penicillin allergy. *Arch Intern Med* 1992; 152: 932–937.

Pathogens and management

2.1 Antimicrobial prophylaxis

Principle

In addition to treating established infection, antibiotics can, on occasion, be used to prevent infectious disease [1,2]:

• Primary prophylaxis is used when infection is not present but there is a high risk

• Secondary prophylaxis is used after an infection to prevent relapse or recurrence.

A difficult balance must be maintained between preventing infection and encouraging the emergence of antimicrobial resistance by injudicious antibiotic use. Prophylaxis should be reserved for infections with a risk of mortality or serious morbidity and where there is clear evidence of effectiveness.

Preventing infection

Preventing infection is not limited to antibiotic prophylaxis but includes the following:

• Infection control: see Section 2.3, p. 99

• Immunization or immunoprophylaxis: see Section 2.2, p. 97

• Lifestyle advice.

Practical details

When

Common situations where prophylaxis is of proven benefit are shown in Table 38. For each scenario the aim of therapy is to achieve therapeutic levels of the correct antibiotic for the period of risk. For surgical procedures, this means having high levels of antibiotic during the period from the initial incision until skin closure. An immunocompromised patient, however, may require prolonged prophylaxis until the period of immunosuppression is over.

Table 38 Uses of antimicrobial prophylaxis.

Situations	Examples
General population	Immunizations
Immunocompetent at high risk	Malaria prophylaxis
Procedures in a normal host	Perioperative antibiotic prophylaxis [3]
Procedures with an underlying cardiac defect	Infective endocarditis prophylaxis [4,5]
After exposure to specific pathogens	PEP following needlestick injury (see Section 1.25, p. 63) Anti-tuberculous prophylaxis (see Section 1.39, p. 92)
Block transmission from colonized hosts	*N. meningitidis* (see Section 1.38, p. 91) Selected cases of *Staph. aureus*
Recurrent infections	Urinary tract, rheumatic fever
Prevent infection in immunocompromised	PCP prophylaxis in HIV (see Section 1.26, p. 65)

PEP, postexposure prophylaxis; PCP, *Pneumocystis carinii* pneumonia; HIV, human immunodeficiency virus.

What

The choice of an individual prophylactic regimen is made using similar principles employed in selecting empirical therapy for established infection (see Section 1.1, p. 5). One needs to consider the likely infecting organisms, site of infection and host factors, e.g. in immunodeficiency the need for prophylaxis varies according to the host defect [6] (Table 39).

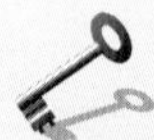

Factors in choosing antimicrobial prophylaxis

• Likely infecting organisms

• Site at risk of infection

• Exposure, e.g. tropical travel

• Patterns of local antimicrobial resistance

• Host factors, e.g. immunodeficiency, allergy, organ impairment

• Route of administration

• Cost-effectiveness.

Outcome

Antimicrobial prophylaxis can substantially reduce the morbidity and mortality associated with infection in high-risk situations. This has to be balanced against the risks of encouraging antimicrobial resistance, and resistance should always be considered where prophylaxis fails.

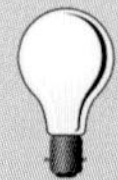

Lifestyle advice

• Boiling water reduces *Mycobacterium avium-intracellulare* (MAI) and cryptosporidiosis in AIDS

• Avoiding mosquito bites is as effective as antimalarial chemotherapy

• Marijuana may contain viable aspergillus spores

• Reptiles often carry salmonella

• Immunization will prevent many infections.

Table 39 Prophylactic regimens in immunodeficiency

Host defect	Infecting organisms	Consider prophylaxis with
Post-splenectomy or complement deficiency	Encapsulated bacteria, e.g. pneumococci, meningococci	Penicillin Immunize against pneumococci, *Haemophilus* spp. and meningococci
Antibody deficiency	Bacteria including pneumococci	Penicillin, e.g. Consider IVIG
Neutropenia	Bacteria including *Pseudomonas* spp. *Candida* spp. Herpes simplex	Quinolone Fluconazole Aciclovir
HIV/AIDS CD4 >200	Pneumococcal pneumonia Tuberculosis Herpes simplex, shingles	Pneumococcal immunizations Isoniazid in high-risk groups Aciclovir for recurrent disease
HIV/AIDS CD4 <200	PCP, toxoplasmosis *Candida* spp., cryptoccci	Co-trimoxazole Fluconazole
HIV/AIDS CD4 <75	Cytomegalovirus MAI	Ganciclovir (CMV) Azithromycin or rifabutin

IVIG, intravenous immunoglobulin; AIDS, acquired immune deficiency syndrome; PCP, *Pneumocystis carinii* pneumonia; CMV, cytomegalovirus; MAI, *Mycobacterium avium-intracellulare*.

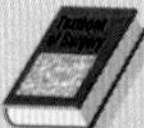

1 Osman DR. Antimicrobial prophylaxis in adults. *Mayo Clin Proc* 2000; 75: 98–109.
2 Lambert HP. Principles of chemoprophylaxis. In: O'Grady F, Lambert HP, Finch RG, Greenwood D (eds) *Antibiotic and Chemotherapy* (7th edn). London: Churchill Livingstone, 1997: 147–149.
3 Song F, Glenny AM. Antimicrobial prophylaxis in colorectal surgery: a systematic review of randomized controlled trials. *Br J Surg* 1998; 85: 1232–1241.
4 British Society for Antimicrobial Chemotherapy Working Party Report. The antibiotic prophylaxis of infective endocarditis. *Lancet* 1982; ii: 1323–1326.
5 Recommendations from the Endocarditis Working Party of the British Society for Antimicrobial Chemotherapy. Antibiotic prophylaxis of infective endocarditis. *Lancet* 1990; 335: 88–89.
6 Kovacs JA, Masur H. Prophylaxis against opportunistic infections in patients with human immunodeficiency virus infection. *N Engl J Med* 2000; 342: 1416.

2.2 Immunization

Principle

Immunization (synonym: vaccination) aims to induce long-term protective immunological memory (active immunization) [1,2]. This is done using a variety of strategies to present foreign antigens to the immune system. In this context, an antigen is any portion of the pathogen or its products that can be recognized by the immune system, e.g. a viral coat protein or bacterial toxin. Rarely, it is appropriate to give temporary immunization by passive transfer of preformed antibody.

Active immunization

Protective immunity involves humoral and cellular elements [3] (Fig. 60).

Humoral or B-cell memory

• Common type of immunity generated by antiviral vaccines (e.g. hepatitis B, influenza)
• Wanes over time if non-replicating pathogen, and may therefore require boosting
• Induces sterilizing immunity, i.e. circulating antibody prevents initial infection (neutralizing antibody)
• Protective only if directed against conserved surface antigens. Mutation of surface proteins within populations (influenza) or within individuals (HIV) may allow escape from these antibodies.

Cellular or T-cell memory

• $CD8^+$ or cytotoxic T lymphocytes (CTL) and $CD4^+$ or helper T lymphocytes
• Evoked by presentation of small viral peptides (epitopes) derived from any viral protein to HLA (human leucocyte antigen) molecules on specialized antigen-presenting cells
• $CD4^+$ cells help to sustain antibody responses, or provide direct protection against certain pathogens (e.g. BCG and TB)
• Epitopes recognized depend on the HLA type of the individual
• T cells recognize only cells that are already infected and cannot provide sterilizing immunity
• $CD8^+$ cells are active against persistent or non-cytopathic organisms, the intracellular position of which is protected against antibodies.

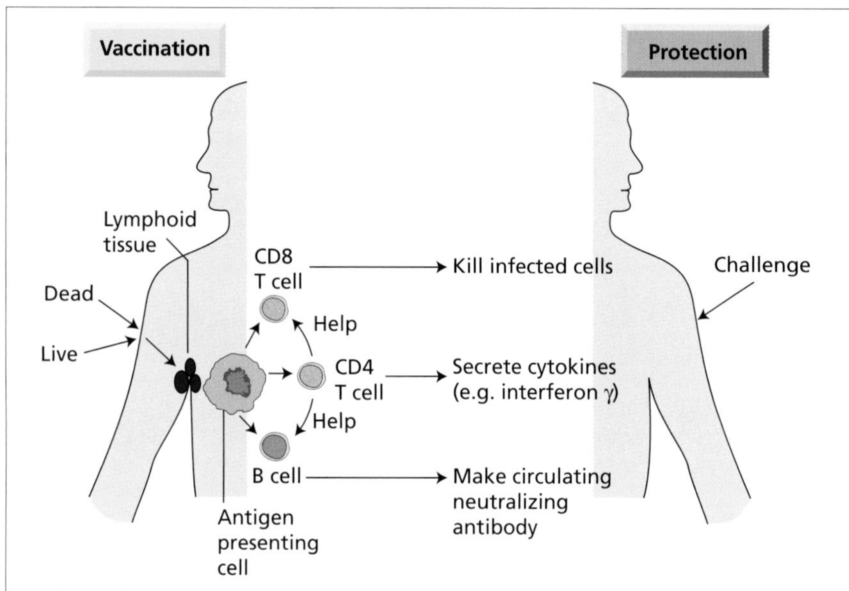

Fig. 60 Events following immunization.

Passive immunization

This involves the transfer of preformed antibody. The antibody confers immediate protection, but only for a limited time period, and is often combined with or followed by active immunization.

Chickenpox (herpes/varicella zoster)

This is given in cases where there has been significant exposure to a non-immune individual at high risk of life-threatening disease (newborn, pregnant or immunosuppressed) (see Section 1.19, p. 50). Non-immune status is confirmed by measuring specific antizoster antibody (lab report will indicate 'VZV IgG negative').

Hepatitis B

This is given where there has been exposure to infected blood from a known carrier (e.g. a needlestick injury) (see Section 1.25, p. 63) and there is no pre-existing antibody. This is combined with an accelerated hepatitis B vaccine schedule to stimulate long-term immunity.

Hepatitis A

Human immunoglobulin protects for 3 months and was routinely given to travellers to an endemic area. It has largely been replaced by active immunization, but it may still be needed where there is insufficient time for active immunization to work or for close contacts of a hepatitis A case.

Respiratory syncytial virus

There is evidence that specific anti-RSV antibodies improve morbidity and mortality when combined with ribavirin for the treatment of severe disease in young children.

Others

Specific immunoglobulin protects after rabies exposure and against tick-borne encephalitis (mainly eastern Europe and Austria; a killed vaccine is also available).

Inducing immunity

There are several methods of inducing protective immunity (Table 40).

Live attenuated vaccines

As these replicate they will induce cellular and humoral immunity, of appropriate specificity, at a high level which is maintained lifelong. In general, avoid in an immunocompromised host.

Antigen-only (dead) vaccines

These induce high antibody levels, although they may be short-lived and require boosting:
- Killed (e.g. polio-inactivated vaccine)
- Subunit vaccines (e.g. influenza vaccines)
- Recombinant vaccines (e.g. hepatitis B vaccine): use antigens made by artificial expression *in vitro*, rather than by growth of a whole virus.

Novel approaches

Vaccines that are simply strips of DNA encoding the relevant viral genes induce very effective antibodies and

Table 40 Methods of immunization.

Vaccine	Examples	Advantages	Disadvantages
Live attenuated organism	Oral polio Measles Rubella BCG	Sustained broad immunological response	Must be kept cold Risk of reversion to pathogenicity Avoid in immunosuppression
Killed	Inactivated polio HAV	Safe Good antibody response Long shelf-life	Booster often needed
Subunit	Tetanus		
Recombinant	HAV		
Passive	IVIG VZV Rabies HBV	Immediate action	Limited supply, potential risk of transmissible infection

HAV, hepatitis A virus; HBV, hepatitis B virus; IVIG, intravenous immunoglobulin; VZV, varicella-zoster virus

cellular immunity. They are effective in animal models and are entering human trials.

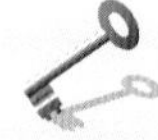

Future vaccine possibilities

- Recombinant vectors, e.g. vaccinia based
- DNA vectors [4]
- Monoclonal antibodies.

Contraindications

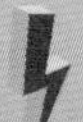

Check contraindications for each vaccine, but note the following:

- Most live vaccines are contraindicated in immunosuppressed patients
- Influenza immunization should be avoided if history of egg allergy
- MMR (mumps, measles, rubella) vaccine has been the subject of some controversy regarding a potential link with autism, but most other investigators have found no evidence for this association [5].

Do not forget patients going for splenectomy—who should receive vaccines against the capsulated organisms—pneumococci, *Haemophilus influenzae* and meningococci.

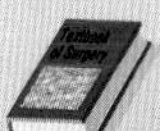

1 Salisbury D, Begg N, eds. *Immunization against Infectious Disease.* London: HMSO: 1996.
2 Nye FJ, Kennedy N. Update on vaccination guidelines. *Br J Hosp Med* 1997; 57: 313–318.
3 Zinkernagel RM. Immunology taught by viruses. *Science* 1996; 271: 173–178.
4 Gurunathan S, Klinman DM, Seder RA. DNA vaccines: immunology, application, and optimization. *Annu Rev Immunol* 2000; 18: 927–974.
5 Taylor B, Miller E, Farrington CP *et al.* Autism and measles, mumps, and rubella vaccine: no epidemiological evidence for a causal association. *Lancet* 1999; 353: 2026–2029.

2.3 Infection control

Principle

In the UK, about 10% of hospital admissions are the result of infection, with a further 10% of patients acquiring infection in hospital [1,2]. Furthermore, a recent Audit Commission report revealed that, in England and Wales, 5000 people die in hospital every year as a direct result of hospital-acquired infection (HAI) [3]. Reasons underlying HAI are complex, as illustrated in Fig. 61. Infection control tries to reduce infection rates in the following ways.

Universal precautions

This refers to the application of general measures to all patients irrespective of their infection status, and should protect patients and staff from contact and blood-borne infections.

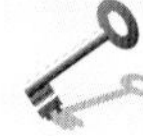

Universal precautions

- Handwashing: between all patient contact
- Protective clothing where indicated to prevent contamination with body fluids
- Gloves when possibility of contamination with body fluids.

Specific precautions

The second mechanism of control is through the isolation of patients with infections that pose particular problems. Recognizing who needs additional precautions depends on an understanding of the mechanisms involved in transmission of HAI. Routes of dissemination are predominantly by contact, droplets, air-borne or blood (Table 41).

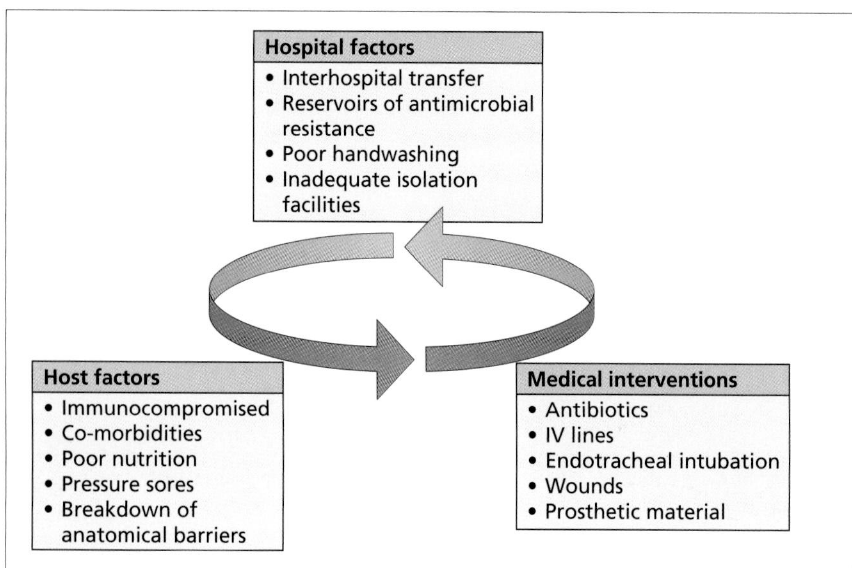

Fig. 61 Interrelationships in hospital-acquired infection.

Table 41 Routes of transmission of infection within hospital.

Route	Organisms	Response to prevent spread
Air-borne	TB Varicella-zoster virus Respiratory syncytial virus Smallpox	Isolation in an appropriately ventilated room Negative-pressure room recommended for TB Patient to wear mask outside room [4]
Droplet	*Neisseria meningitidis* *Haemophilus influenzae* Whooping cough Respiratory viruses Mumps Rubella	Cover mouth when sneezing Handwashing
Contact	*Staph. aureus* including MRSA Most other bacteria Enteric pathogens, including *Clostridium difficile* and *E. coli* 0157, RSV, herpes simplex, scabies	Handwashing, gloves, gowns and protective clothing where contamination likely [5]
Blood: via needlestick	Hepatitis B Hepatitis C HIV Ebola virus Malaria Trypanosomiasis	Universal precautions Postexposure prophylaxis
Unknown	New variant CJD	Risk unknown

RSV, respiratory syncytial virus; TB, tuberculosis; MRSA, methicillin-resistant *Staph. aureus*; CJD, Creutzfeldt–Jakob disease.

Infection control is everyone's responsibility—how often do you wash your hands?

Protective isolation

In some circumstances, an immunocompromised patient may be isolated to protect him or her from HAI. Handwashing still remains the most important means of reducing crossinfection. Nursing neutropenic patients in a filtered positive-pressure room reduces the risk of aspergillosis.

Practical details

Risk assessment

When assessing whether to take precautions, such as protective isolation, a risk assessment is made of the situation, taking the following factors into consideration:

• Nature of organism, e.g. potential route of spread, pathogenicity of the organism, potential for outbreaks, etc.
• Host factors, e.g. immune status, sputum production, diarrhoea, confusion
• At-risk population, e.g. immunocompromised or vulnerable patient
• Surroundings: are isolation rooms available, can the patient be safely nursed in isolation?

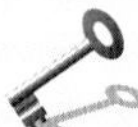

Elements of effective infection control

• Surveillance/audit of indicator infections such as wound or central line infections
• Infection control policy, including outbreak plan
• Training of staff, e.g. handwashing techniques
• Audit of infection control practices
• Support/resources.

Control of HAI

Infection control plays a central role in reducing the transmission of infection, but a sustained reduction in HAI needs a coordinated approach using the following:
• Infection control policies
• Staff education
• Antibiotic protocols and control [7]
• Surveillance at local, regional, national and international levels.

1 Barrett SP. Guidelines for nosocomial infection control in Britain. *J Hosp Infect* 1999; 43(suppl): S307–308.
2 Hospital Infection Society: www.his.org.uk.
3 National Audit Office: www.nao.gov.
4 Standing Medical Advisory Committee Subgroup on Antimicrobial Resistance. *The Path of Least Resistance*. London: Department of Health, 1998.
5 Centers for Disease Control. CDC guidance for isolation precautions in hospitals. *Am J Infect Control* 1996; 24: 24–52.
6 Interdepartmental Working Group on Tuberculosis. (UK Health Department). *UK Guidance on the Prevention and Control of Transmission of (1) HIV-related Tuberculosis and (2) Drug-resistant, including Multiple Drug-resistant, Tuberculosis*. London: Department of Health, 1998.
7 Cookson BD. Nosocomial antimicrobial resistance surveillance. *J Hosp Infect* 1999; 43(suppl): S97–103.

2.4 Travel advice

Principle

Most travellers experience no serious health problems. Simple steps can be taken to minimize the risk of travel-related illness [1]. Travellers can be educated how to treat simple conditions and to recognize the features of serious illness. You should tailor your advice taking account of the following:
• Geographical area to be visited—where, when and for how long?
• Special risks of the journey or visit
• General health of the traveller.

Practical details

Here is a brief list of subjects that you should consider when dispensing travel advice. Some advice requires specialized knowledge and up-to-date information. Seek help from an appropriate specialist if you are unsure.

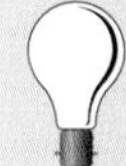

Travel-related mortality

• Cardiovascular disease is the most common cause of mortality
• Ensure that travellers at risk of cardiovascular disease are well controlled, have an ample supply of medication and take steps to avoid dehydration.

General advice

• Water and food: 'boil it, peel it or forget it'. Use treated water even for tooth brushing; avoid ice in drinks.
• Climate: dangers of dehydration and sunburn.
• Sex with new partners: increased risk when travelling; advise on safe sex and condom use.
• Avoiding insects and other nasty beasts. Use insect repellents and examine daily for ticks in an endemic area.
• Recommend taking out appropriate travel insurance.

First-aid kit

The contents will need to reflect the purpose of the trip, e.g. a remote trek as opposed to a hotel-based tour. As a minimum consider the following:
• Digital thermometer
• Antiseptic solution, bandages and plasters
• Scissors and tweezers
• Proprietary analgesic, antipyretic, antidiarrhoeal, antihistamine and a drug for motion sickness
• Consider taking needles and syringes (official letter of explanation for customs).

Aid workers and medical or nursing personnel may be at risk of needlestick injury far from help. Consider providing a supply of HIV postexposure prophylaxis, with specific advice on how to take it, and recommend review by an experienced physician as soon as possible after the event. (See Section 1.25, p. 63.)

Specific advice

Prevention of malaria

ANTIMOSQUITO MEASURES

The mosquito that transmits malaria bites at dusk and during the night. Wear long-sleeved shirts, long trousers and socks in the evening. Use a bed net, preferably impregnated with permethrin. Use a DEET-based insect repellent.

CHEMOPROPHYLAXIS

Although no regimen is completely effective, used correctly prophylaxis can reduce the risks of malaria. If you are not familiar with the area of travel, obtain up-to-date advice on recommended prophylaxis [2,3].

RECOGNITION OF SYMPTOMS AND SIGNS

Warn the patient that prophylaxis does not completely prevent malaria. Discuss the symptoms (see Section 1.20, p. 52) of disease so that the traveller can seek appropriate help when abroad. Stress that malaria can kill and not to delay until returning home.

Travellers' diarrhoea

Travellers' diarrhoea is the most common travel-related infection, affecting up to 50% of travellers to certain destinations. Although mortality is very low, there is significant associated morbidity and holiday upset. Symptoms are generally mild and resolve within 3–5 days. Oral hydration and symptomatic management are the mainstays of treatment, but occasionally severe disease requires antimicrobial therapy, particularly if a long way from medical help (Table 42). Advise to seek help if diarrhoea is associated with bloody stools, fever or abdominal pain.

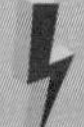

Patients with significant immunocompromise are at increased risk of severe salmonella and other bacterial infections. If travel is essential, warn of the risks and consider supplying a course of antibiotics to take if severe symptoms develop and cannot obtain medical help.

Fever is due to malaria in any patient from a high-risk area until proved otherwise (see Section 1.20, p. 52).

Table 42 Empirical therapy of diarrhoea in remote areas.

Syndrome	Therapy
Diarrhoea without fever or blood	Rehydration and antimotility agents
Diarrhoea with fever but no blood	Quinolone
Bloody diarrhoea with or without fever	Quinolone + metronidazole

Immunizations

Yellow fever is the only vaccine for which there is an international requirement before entering some countries. Yellow fever vaccine is contraindicated in pregnancy and those who are immunocompromised (you can issue an exemption certificate).

Other vaccines should be given as appropriate to the expected risk. Consider hepatitis A, hepatitis B, typhoid, meningococcal, Japanese B encephalitis and rabies where necessary [4–6].

Take the opportunity to update routine immunizations such as polio and tetanus.

Post-travel review

This is of limited benefit in asymptomatic travellers. Warn travellers to report any unusual symptoms, particularly fever, after their return.

1 The yellow book at www.cdc.gov/travel/index.htm—up-to-date and comprehensive guide to travel medicine.
2 Croft A. Extracts from 'Clinical Evidence'. Malaria: prevention in travellers. *BMJ* 2000; 321: 154–160.
3 Ryan ET, Kain KC. Health advice and immunizations for travelers. *N Engl J Med* 2000; 342: 1716–1725.
4 Thompson RF, Bass DM, Hoffman SL. Travel vaccines. *Infect Dis Clin North Am* 1999; 13: 149–167.
5 Dreesen DW, Hanlon CA. Current recommendations for the prophylaxis and treatment of rabies. *Drugs* 1998; 56: 801–809.
6 Engels EA, Lau J. Vaccines for preventing typhoid fever. *Cochrane Database Syst Rev* 2000; (2): CD001261.

2.5 Bacteria

Description of the organism

In the usual laboratory system of bacterial classification, the main groups of bacteria are distinguished by their morphology, staining reactions and growth requirements [1–4].

Morphology

Most bacteria can be classified as either:
- coccoid/spherical, or
- bacilli/rod like.

Staining characteristics

Differences on Gram stain reflect fundamental differences in cell wall structure and separate most bacteria into two main groups:
1 Gram-positive bacteria
2 Gram-negative bacteria.

Growth requirements

Strict aerobes require oxygen and strict anaerobes the absence of oxygen for optimal growth. However, there are many bacteria that can tolerate various environments.

Others

There are some groups of bacteria that do not fit neatly into the above scheme:
- Mycobacteria (see Section 2.6, p. 110) have a cell wall rich in mycolic acid and do not stain well by the Gram method, although if they do they are Gram positive.
- Spirochaetes (see Section 2.7, p. 114) stain as Gram negative but differ in morphology, being slender, spiral and motile.
- Rickettsiae and chlamydiae (see Section 2.8, p. 117) are obligate intracellular parasites that lack an outer cell wall.

2.5.1 GRAM-POSITIVE BACTERIA

Description of the organism

Using the scheme outlined above, medically important Gram-positive bacteria can be rapidly grouped as shown in Table 43.

Table 43 Medically important Gram-positive bacteria.

Morphology	Aerobic	Anaerobic
Cocci	Staphylococci Streptococci Enterococci	Anaerobic streptococci
Bacilli	*Corynebacterium* spp. *Bacillus* spp. *Listeria monocytogenes* *Nocardia asteroides*	*Clostridium* spp. *Lactobacillus* spp. *Actinomyces* spp.

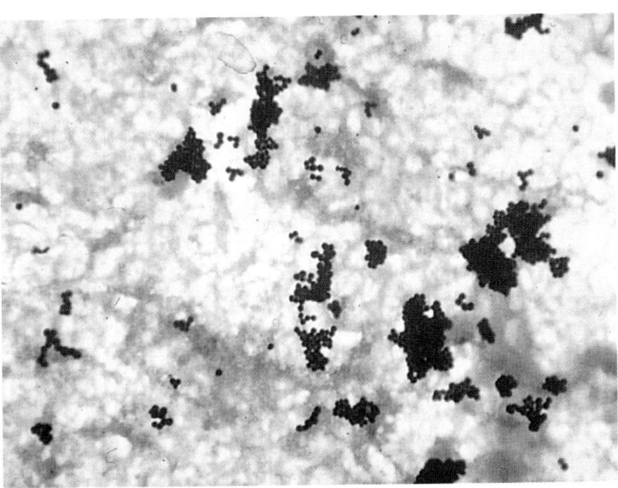

Fig. 62 *Staphylococcus aureus.*

Disease syndromes and therapy

Aerobic Gram-positive cocci

Staphylococci

Staphylococcus aureus [3] (Fig. 62) is a high-grade pathogen and may cause both community- and hospital-acquired infection (Table 44). Other staphylococcal species are less pathogenic and mainly encountered as opportunistic infections in the hospital setting.

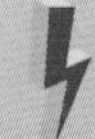

***Staphylococcus aureus* bacteraemia**

Staphylococcus aureus bacteraemia may seed to distant sites:
- Bone/joints
- Heart valves
- Prosthetic material.

Streptococci

Streptococci (Fig. 63) are traditionally classified by the type of haemolysis seen on blood agar (Table 45):
- Some produce a clear zone of haemolysis (β-haemolysis) and these can be further subdivided on the basis of cell wall antigens (Lancefield groups).
- Others produce a partial clearing of the agar and green coloration (α-haemolysis) or no obvious change in the agar around the colony.

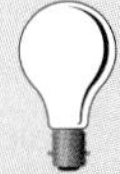

Pneumococcal immunization

- Elderly people
- Chronic respiratory/cardiovascular disease
- Diabetes or renal failure
- Immunocompromised individuals
- Hyposplenism.

Table 44 Staphylococci and their disease syndromes.

Organism	Epidemiology	Disease syndromes	Therapy
Staph. aureus (methicillin sensitive)	Asymptomatic carriage in the nasopharynx of up to 30% of the population May cause severe disease, particularly in diabetes and immunocompromised patients	Boils Wound infections Cellulitis Abscesses Bacteraemia Endocarditis (see Section 1.8, p. 20) Septic arthritis Osteomyelitis (see Section 1.6, p. 16) Pneumonia (uncommon, postinfluenza)	Mainstay of therapy is flucloxacillin High-dose intravenous therapy needed for bacteraemia, endocarditis (see Section 1.8, p. 20) and osteomyelitis Consider adding a second agent such as fusidic acid, rifampicin or gentamicin in serious infection Surgery for deep-seated abscess, osteomyelitis or prosthetic material
MRSA distinguished by resistance to methicillin	Increasing in the UK Outbreaks in high-risk areas such as ICU	Nosocomial infection at any site but commonly infection of wounds, intravenous lines and line prosthetic devices	Vancomycin, monitor levels
Toxin-producing *Staph. aureus*	Sporadic cases with occasional clusters Outbreaks of tampon-associated toxic shock syndrome	Food poisoning Toxic shock syndrome Scalded skin syndrome	Anti-staphylococcal antibiotics when appropriate plus supportive care Consider IVIG in toxic shock
Coagulase-negative staphylococci, e.g. *Staph. epidermidis*	The majority are normal skin commensals	Prosthetic valve endocarditis Long line infections Prosthetic joint infections Cerebrospinal shunt infections Peritoneal dialysis catheter infection	Removal of prosthetic material and/or prolonged intravenous therapy, commonly with glycopeptides
Staph. saprophyticus	Tend to occur in young women	Urinary tract infection	Guided by sensitivities Usually trimethoprim sensitive

MRSA, methicillin-resistant *Staphylococcus aureus*; IVIG, intravenous immunoglobulin

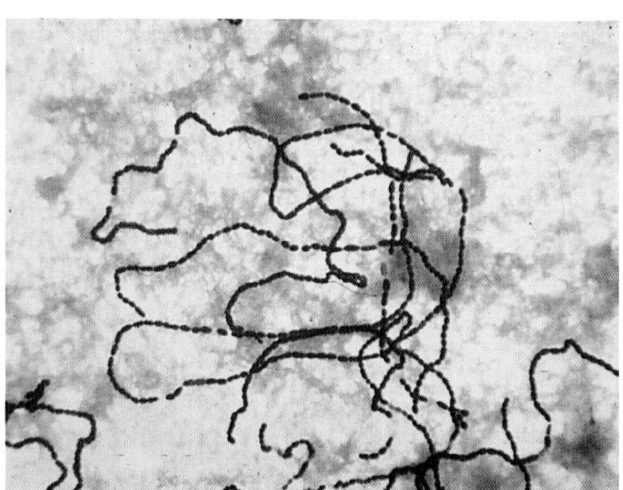

Fig. 63 Streptococci.

Aerobic Gram-positive bacilli

Gram-positive bacilli (Table 46) tend to be normal skin commensals or spore-forming, environmental organisms. They seldom cause disease, but there are some very important pathogens.

Anaerobic Gram-positive bacilli

These spore-forming organisms (Table 47) are generally found in soil. Improvements in immunization and public health have dramatically reduced the incidence of tetanus and botulism in the developed world, but they are still major cause of disease in other countries.

2.5.2 GRAM-NEGATIVE BACTERIA

Description of the organism

Gram-negative bacteria (Table 48) are characterized by the presence of endotoxin (lipopolysaccharide) in the outer leaflet of the bacterial cell wall. Endotoxin is a potent immune activator and has been strongly implicated in cases of severe sepsis and shock associated with Gram-negative bacterial infection.

Table 45 Streptococci and enterococci and their disease syndromes.

Haemolysis	Organism	Epidemiology/public health	Disease syndromes	Therapy
β-Haemolytic	Lancefield GAS (*Strep. pyogenes*)	May cause institutional outbreaks Long-term pharyngeal carriage can occur	Pharyngitis Cellulitis, impetigo Scarlet fever Necrotizing fasciitis Septic arthritis Rheumatic fever Glomerulonephritis	Penicillin Erythromycin or clindamycin in penicillin allergy Antibiotics as above Fasciitis requires aggressive débridement. Antibiotics to prevent recurrence
	Lancefield GBS (*Strep. agalacticae*)	Normal vaginal flora in 30% of women	Neonatal and peripartum infections Skin, soft tissue, bone and joint infections	Penicillin Neonatal meningitis requires 2–3 weeks' intravenous therapy
α-Haemolytic	*Strep. pneumoniae*	Colonizes the respiratory tract Invasive disease common in smokers, respiratory illness and immunodeficiency	Pneumonia Sinusitis and otitis media Empyema Bacteraemia Meningitis Septic arthritis Spontaneous peritonitis	Penicillin, if sensitive; second- or third-generation cephalosporin or a macrolide if sensitive Penicillin resistance increasing and now 5–15% in the UK; 50% in parts of southern Europe
	Viridans streptococci	Mouth commensals	Endocarditis Line infection in neutropenic host	Benzylpenicillin Add gentamicin in endocarditis (see Section 1.8, p. 23)
	Strep. milleri	Colonizes gastrointestinal tract	Abscess formation in brain, lung and abdomen	Penicillin sensitive, but infections are often polymicrobial requiring broad-spectrum antibiotics
	Enterococcus faecalis	Colonizes the gastrointestinal tract Occasional cause of community-acquired infection	UTI Endocarditis	Ampicillin or vancomycin Add gentamicin in endocarditis (see Section 1.8, p. 23)
	E. faecium	Hospital-acquired pathogen VRE are an increasing infection control concern	Intra-abdominal infection Septicaemia UTIs Wound infection Line infection Endocarditis	As above unless VRE VRE: seek expert advice

GAS, group A streptococcus; GBS, group B streptococcus; VRE, vancomycin-resistant enterococci; UTI, urinary tract infection.

Table 46 Aerobic Gram-positive bacilli and their disease syndromes.

Organism	Epidemiology/public health	Disease syndromes	Therapy
Corynebacterium spp.	Most corynebacteria (diphtheroids) are normal skin commensals	Occasional cause of central line infection in neutropenia	Penicillin or vancomycin
C. diphtheriae	Diphtheria is rare in most developed countries because of mass immunization It is still common in developing countries	Diphtheria Pharyngitis Toxin (cardio- and neurotoxic) Skin ulcers (less common)	Penicillin, erythromycin or tetracyclines Supportive care for the effects of the toxin Immunization of contacts
Bacillus spp.	Frequent skin commensals	Occasional cause of central line infection in neutropenia	Penicillin or vancomycin
B. anthracis	Zoonosis reported in Africa and Asia Human infection arises from inoculation injury Inhalation of spores can lead to rapidly fatal disease Potential use in bacterial warfare	Anthrax Malignant pustule Septicaemia Haemorrhagic pneumonia High case fatality in invasive disease	Penicillin Immunization requires annual boosters and hence only of use if serious risk of infection
B. cereus	Outbreaks related to poor reheating of cooked food	Food poisoning caused by preformed toxin	Supportive
Listeria monocytogenes	Found in various food stuffs, e.g. pâté, soft cheeses Invasive disease in immunocompromised people, including pregnant women	Septicaemia Neonatal disease Meningitis Endocarditis	Ampicillin + gentamicin
Nocardia spp.	Found in soil Inoculation infections in Africa and Asia Invasive disease in immunocompromised people	Skin and soft tissue, e.g. Madura foot Invasive, pulmonary, CNS and disseminated infection	Co-trimoxazole, amikacin or imipenem all have useful activity

CNS, central nervous system.

Table 47 Important anaerobic Gram-positive bacilli and their disease syndromes.

Organism	Epidemiology/public health	Disease syndromes	Therapy
Clostridium perfringens	Ubiquitous in soil; may colonize gastrointestinal tract	Gas gangrene Food poisoning	Penicillin or metronidazole + aggressive débridement
C. *tetani*	Ubiquitous in soil worldwide, infection following inoculation	Tetanus	Penicillin + antitoxin Débridement of wound Ventilatory support
C. botulinum	May contaminate food processing, particularly in tins where anaerobic conditions may exist	Botulism	Supportive care
C. difficile	Colonizes gastrointestinal tract Nosocomial pathogen particularly in elderly and debilitated patients	Antibiotic-associated and pseudomembranous colitis	Cessation of causative antibiotic Oral metronidazole or oral vancomycin
Actinomyces spp.	Found as part of oral flora Increased in poor dental hygiene May complicate intrauterine contraceptive device	Actinomycosis is a chronic suppurative infection with sinus formation Maxillofacial infections Pelvic Hand infection acquired from an adversary's teeth	Penicillin is the treatment of choice

Disease syndromes and therapy

Gram-negative cocci

Meningococci and gonococci are of clinical importance (Table 49). The majority of other *Neisseria* spp. are commensals of the upper respiratory tract and do not cause serious disease apart from rare cases of endocarditis.

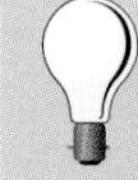

Meningococcal immunization

- Type A polysaccharide vaccine for travellers to at-risk areas
- No vaccine for type B
- Meningo-C conjugate vaccine introduced in 2000.

Table 48 Medically important Gram-negative bacteria.

Morphology	Aerobic	Anaerobic
Cocci	*Neisseria* spp.	–
Bacilli	Enterobacteriaceae Pseudomonads Coccobacilli Curved Gram-negative rods	*Bacteroides* spp. *Fusobacterium* spp.

Gram-negative bacilli

Enterobacteriaceae

The taxonomy of Gram-negative bacilli is very complicated. Enterobacteriaceae is the name given to a group of Gram-negative bacilli that fulfil certain laboratory-based criteria, based on biochemical testing (Table 50). It includes organisms often found in the gastrointestinal tract, many of which are associated with similar diseases.

Table 49 Medically important Gram-negative cocci.

Organism	Epidemiology/public health	Disease	Treatment
Neisseria meningitidis (meningococcus)	Subtyped by capsular polysaccharides, most common being A, B and C Types B and C are prevalent in Europe and the USA Type A is associated with epidemics in the meningitis belt of sub-Saharan Africa	Septicaemia Meningitis Septic arthritis Pneumonia or pericarditis is uncommon	Penicillin or third-generation cephalosporin (see Sections 1.2, p. 8 and 1.14, p. 38) Penicillin resistance emerging abroad Chemoprophylaxis for contacts (see Section 1.38, p. 91)
Neisseria gonorrhoeae (gonococcus)	Sexually transmitted disease Occasional mother–child transmission at delivery (ophthalmia neonatorum)	Urethritis, cervicitis Epididymo-orchitis, proctitis, PID Disseminated infection (arthritis–dermatitis syndrome) Perihepatitis (Fitz–Hugh-Curtis syndrome)	Options include: penicillin + probenicid, i.m. ceftriaxone, azithromycin, fluoroquinolones Antibiotic resistance patterns vary from region to region and resistance is a worldwide problem Resistance to penicillin is as high as 30–40% in south-east Asia

PID, pelvic inflammatory disease.

Table 50 Medically important Enterobacteriaceae.

Organism	Epidemiology/public health	Diseases	Treatment
Escherichia coli	Colonize the gastrointestinal tract Important nosocomial pathogen	UTI at all ages Septicaemia Intra-abdominal/biliary tract infection Pneumonia in debilitated or hospital-acquired. Meningitis in neonates or elderly patients	Guided by antimicrobial susceptibilities and local empirical guidelines
EPEC/ETEC	Contaminated food or water	Diarrhoea (see Section 1.23, p. 59) HUS complicating *E. coli* 0157	Rehydration, no evidence for role of antimicrobials, even in HUS
E. coli 0157	Occasional cause of community-acquired infection		Typically amoxicillin resistant
Klebsiella spp.	Nosocomial pathogen	Biliary and GI tract septicaemia Cavitating pneumonia Nosocomial infections	Multi-resistant strains in hospital Specific therapy is guided by susceptibilities
Proteus spp.	Colonize GI tract	UTI: association with renal stones	Specific therapy is guided by susceptibilities (see Section 1.12, p. 31)
Salmonella typhi	Tropical and subtropical distribution	Typhoid/enteric fever	Oral fluoroquinolones or intravenous ceftriaxone
S. paratyphi	Human-only pathogen Acquired via contaminated food or drink		Complicated by the emergence of resistant strains
Non-typhoidal *Salmonella* spp.	Sporadic cases and outbreaks related to poor hygiene	Food poisoning Rare cause of osteomyelitis or infected aneurysm	Normally self-limiting and does not require antibiotics Quinolones for invasive disease or immunocompromised patients
Shigella spp.	Faecal–oral spread More common in developing world	Common Diarrhoea/food poisoning	Normally self-limiting and does not require specific antimicrobial treatment
Yersinia pestis	Zoonotic infection Still found in many parts of the world, such as south-east Asia, central and southern Africa	Plague: bubonic involving regional lymph nodes and pneumonic forms may occur	First line: streptomycin or gentamicin Alternatives: chloramphenicol or tetracyclines
Yersinia enterocolitica and other *Yersinia* spp.	Worldwide distribution Iron overload states	Gastrointestinal infection Mesenteric adenitis Reactive arthritis Severe sepsis	Usually no specific antimicrobial treatment required Co-trimoxazole

EPEC, enteropathogenic *E. coli*; ETEC, enterotoxigenic *E. coli*; GI, gastrointestinal; HUS, haemolytic uraemic syndrome; UTI, urinary tract infection.

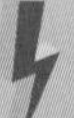

Antibacterial resistance in the Enterobacteriaceae

- Emergence of multiresistant strains as nosocomial pathogens
- Public health and infection control concern
- Resistance is usually the result of β-lactamase production
- Often transferable on plasmids
- Requires isolation and infection control precautions.

Pseudomonads

The pseudomonads include a mixture of aerobic Gram-negative rods (Table 51). The majority are environmental organisms often found in water and soil. Many are recognized as opportunistic pathogens, being responsible for severe nosocomial infections.

Gram-negative coccobacilli

These are short rods most commonly responsible for respiratory tract disease (Table 52).

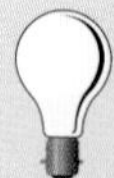

Invasive *Haemophilus influenzae* type b

- Uncommon now that immunization available
- Remains an important pathogen in the developing world
- Prophylaxis is given to non-immunized household contacts of cases with invasive Hib infection.

Curved Gram-negative bacilli

The importance of *Campylobacter* spp. and *Helicobacter* spp. in gastrointestinal disease has been recognized since the 1970s and 1980s (Table 53). *Vibrio* spp. are commonly found in aquatic environments, and historical importance has been almost exclusively related to pandemics and epidemics of cholera.

Anaerobes

Anaerobes are the predominant component of the gastrointestinal bacterial flora. As a result of their fastidious nature, they are difficult to isolate and are often overlooked (Table 54).

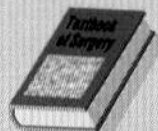

1. Koneman EW *et al. Color Atlas and Textbook of Diagnostic Microbiology*, 5th edn. New York: Lippincott Williams & Wilkins, 1997.
2. Murray PR, Barton EJ, Pfaller MA, Tenover F, Yolken RH. *Manual of Clinical Microbiology*, 6th edn. Washington DC: ASM Press, 1995.
3. Weiss ME, Franklin Adkinson N. *Mandell, Douglas and Bennett's Principles and Practice of Infectious Diseases*, 5th edn. New York: Churchill Livingstone, 1995: 272–278.
4. Armstrong D, Cohen J. *Infectious Diseases*. London: Harcourt Publishers, 1999.

Table 51 Medically important pseudomonads.

Organism	Epidemiology/public health	Diseases	Treatment
Pseudomonas aeruginosa	Hospital-acquired infection Risk factors include: burns prolonged hospital stay antibiotic usage neutropenia chronic suppurative lung disease diabetes	Septicaemia Nosocomial pneumonia Nosocomial UTI Line infections Wound infections Malignant otitis externa Keratitis Pneumonia complicating cystic fibrosis	Aminoglycosides Ceftazidime Carbapenems Fluoroquinolones Penicillins, e.g. piperacillin Dual therapy used in the neutropenic population Often resistant to disinfectants
Burkholderia cepacia	Nosocomial pathogen Colonizes respiratory tract in cystic fibrosis	Pneumonia particularly cystic fibrosis	Difficult to eradicate, often multidrug resistant
Burkholderia pseudomallei	Ubiquitous in soil and waterlogged areas in parts of Asia, Northern Australia, Africa and South America.	Melioidosis Septicaemia Pneumonia Suppurative disease	Ceftazidime i.v. for a prolonged course followed by long-term oral therapy

UTI, urinary tract infection.

Table 52 Medically important Gram-negative coccobacilli.

Organism	Epidemiology/public health	Diseases	Treatment
Haemophilus influenzae type b	Colonizes nasopharynx of 25–75% population.	Sinusitis Otitis media Meningitis Epiglottitis Cellulitis Septic arthritis Osteomyelitis	Third-generation cephalosporin for serious disease Erythromycin or co-amoxiclavulinic acid for localized respiratory disease β-Lactamase production in about 25% strains leads to ampicillin resistance
Non-type B *Haemophilus* spp.	Colonizes nasopharynx of 25–75% population Increased disease in smokers	Sinusitis Otitis media Acute exacerbation of COAD Pneumonia Endocarditis (rare)	Erythromycin or co-amoxiclavulinic acid for localized respiratory disease Seek advice in endocarditis
H. ducreyii	Sexually transmitted, endemic in tropical areas	Chancroid	Azithromycin
Bordetella pertussis	Of worldwide importance, but incidence in countries with active immunization programmes is low	Whooping cough	Erythromycin is the antibiotic of choice but often has little or no effect with established infection Erythromycin for 10–14 days.
Legionella pneumophila	Infection from inhalation of infected droplets Outbreaks linked to aerosols from: hot water, cooling towers, air-conditioning, spa baths and showers	Legionnaire's disease (atypical pneumonia) (see Section 1.4, pp. 10–12) Pontiac fever (self-limiting 'flu-like illness)	Consider adding rifampicin in severe disease
Brucella spp.	Zoonotic infection (*B. abortus* from cattle and *B. melitensis* from goats) Transmitted to humans by contact with infected animals or ingestion of unpasteurized dairy products Endemic to Mediterranean basin, North Africa, Central and South America and the Middle East Farmers and vets at increased risk	Acute disease: self-limiting 'flu-like illness Bacteraemia, septic arthritis, granulomatous hepatitis or endocarditis may occur Chronic disease: osteoarticular in 30–40% of cases Sacroilitis, vertebral osteomyelitis and monoarthritis Epididymo-orchitis or meningitis less common	Combination therapy with doxycycline and rifampicin or streptomycin is better than monotherapy Co-trimoxazole as second line Osteoarthritis requires 6–12 weeks' therapy

COAD, chronic obstructive airway disease.

Table 53 Medically important curved Gram-negative rods.

Organism	Epidemiology/public health	Diseases	Treatment
Campylobacter jejuni	Most common cause of acute infective diarrhoea in developed countries	Diarrhoea/food poisoning	Self-limiting and does not require antimicrobial treatment
Helicobacter pylori	Worldwide; higher prevalence in developing world	Acute and chronic gastritis Duodenal ulceration Possible link to gastric carcinoma and lymphoma	Eradication therapy requires multiple drug therapy for 7–10 days Typically two antibiotics plus an acid inhibitor
Vibrio cholerae	Epidemics and pandemics, spread through contaminated water Increased after natural disasters	Profuse watery diarrhoea: rice water stool (toxin-related disease)	Rehydration of paramount importance Tetracycline reduces excretion period
V. parahaemolyticus	Associated with shellfish	Diarrhoea	Supportive therapy
V. vulnificus	Warm salt water exposure	Cellulitis and sepsis	Tetracycline

Table 54 Medically important Gram-negative anaerobes.

Organism	Epidemiology/public health	Diseases	Treatment
Bacteroides spp.	Gut commensal Most common cause of non-clostridial anaerobic infections in humans	Intra-abdominal infections Decubitus ulcers Lung abscess	Metronidazole Co-amoxiclav and clindamycin are suitable alternatives
Fusobacterium spp.	Part of the normal oral flora	Head and neck infections	Drainage of pus Sensitive to penicillin and metronidazole

2.6 Mycobacteria

Description of the organism

The genus *Mycobacterium* includes a large number of bacteria with widely differing pathogenicity. They are described as acid- and alcohol-fast bacilli and all appear red when stained using the Ziehl–Neelsen stain (Fig. 64). This group of bacteria can be divided broadly into three groups:

1 *M. tuberculosis* complex which causes TB
2 *M. leprae*—the causative agent of leprosy
3 Opportunistic (environmental or atypical) mycobacteria.

2.6.1 *MYCOBACTERIUM TUBERCULOSIS*

Most cases of TB result from *M. tuberculosis*, although less commonly TB may be caused by other bacteria from the *M. tuberculosis* complex such as *M. bovis* and *M. africanum*.

Epidemiology

Approximately one-third of the world's population is infected with *M. tuberculosis* with humans as the only reservoir (cattle are the reservoir for *M. bovis*). Poverty and social deprivation are the most common factors associated with a high prevalence of TB. The incidence of TB in developed countries was decreasing steadily until the mid-1980s, when there was an upturn in notifications related in part to the HIV epidemic. Approximately 10% of those infected develop clinical disease. Transmission is by inhalation of tubercle bacilli and patients with smear-positive pulmonary TB are highly infectious. In the past, *M. bovis* infection, acquired through ingesting contaminated milk, was a common route of spread but this is now very rare.

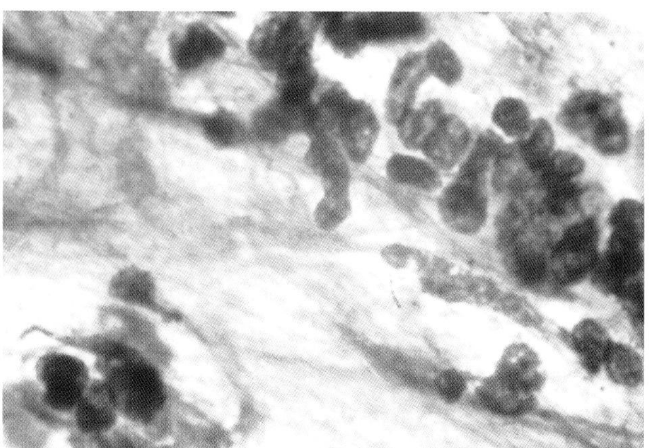

Fig. 64 Ziehl–Neelsen stain for mycobacteria. A red beaded bacterium, *Mycobacterium tuberculosis,* can be seen against a blue background.

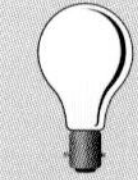

Tuberculosis is a notifiable disease in the UK.

Diagnostic tests

Imaging

• The most common finding on the chest radiograph in patients with pulmonary TB is upper lobe shadowing with or without cavitation (see Fig. 8, p. 14). In miliary TB, fine nodular shadows are seen throughout both lung fields (see Fig. 9, p. 14). Pleural TB in the absence of parenchymal lung disease may occur (see Fig. 10, p. 15).
• Ultrasonography, CT or MRI may be used to localize extrapulmonary disease and guide diagnostic procedures.

Cultures

• Sputum: three samples on consecutive days should be sent for acid-fast smear and TB culture. A minimum of 5000–10 000 mycobacteria/mL of sputum must be present to be detected on sputum smear. Culture and sensitivity testing may take 6–8 weeks on standard solid media, but this may be reduced to 2–3 weeks using liquid media such as the BACTEC system.
• Bronchoscopy: if sputum is not available, refer for bronchoscopy and send washings from affected individuals for microscopy and culture.
• Gastric washings: alternative to bronchoscopy in patients in whom sputum collection is not possible.

• Early morning urine: rarely positive on direct smear, but may culture TB if sterile pyuria is present.
• Blood: blood cultures on specific media may be positive in patients with AIDS.
• Bone marrow: smear and culture should be considered in patients with suspected miliary disease.
• PCR: the role of PCR in the diagnosis of pulmonary TB is limited. In sterile body sites such as the CSF, PCR has a sensitivity of 30–50%. The use of PCR to identify multidrug resistance is gaining acceptance.

Tuberculin testing

A Mantoux or Heaf test (see Section 3.2, p. 151) is often used in patients with suspected TB. The size of the tuberculin reaction relates to antituberculous cell-mediated immunity and is a marker of disease exposure. A strongly positive reaction gives additional weight to the diagnosis of TB. However, 20% of patients with TB may be negative on these tests and the test is often negative in severely immunocompromised individuals.

Histology

In the absence of any abnormal findings on chest radiograph, the diagnosis of extrapulmonary TB often depends on obtaining a sample of tissue. It is very important that, when this tissue is taken, it is split into two—one sample is sent in formalin for histology and the other in a sterile pot for TB culture. On histology, caseating or non-caseating epithelioid cell granulomas may be seen (Fig. 65).

Disease syndromes

Pulmonary TB

This accounts for about 75% of cases of TB. (See Section 1.5, p. 13.)

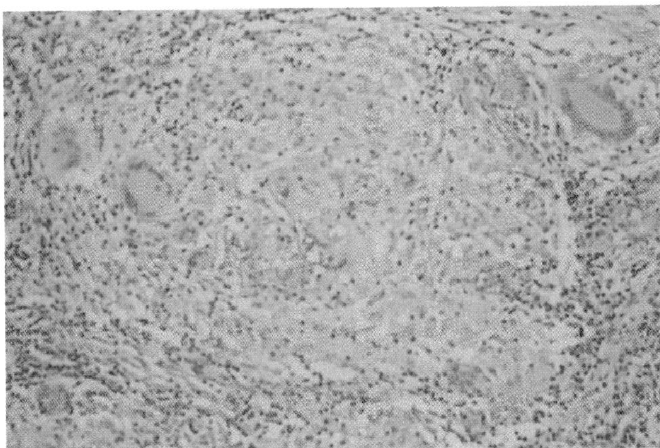

Fig. 65 Granuloma with multinucleate giant cells and central necrosis consistent with tuberculosis.

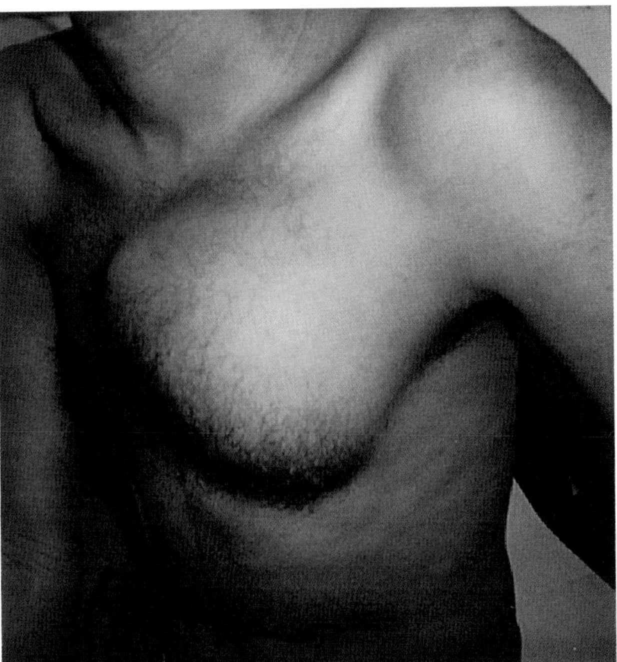

Fig. 66 Large tuberculous cold abscess on the chest wall.

Extrapulmonary disease

After primary infection, TB disseminates haematogenously. This may lead to miliary disease or to late reactivation at one or more body sites. Diagnosis is often delayed in extrapulmonary TB and there is a higher morbidity and mortality. Extrapulmonary disease is more common in the immunocompromised host, including AIDS. Typical sites include the following:
• Lymph nodes (see Fig. 12, p. 19)
• Abscesses (Fig. 66)
• Bone (particularly the spine—Pott's disease)
• Central nervous system (CNS) tuberculous meningitis (see Section 1.14, p. 36) and tuberculomas (Fig. 67)
• Pericardial
• Genitourinary
• Skin: lupus vulgaris.

Complications

Pulmonary disease

• Erythema nodosum is seen in some cases of primary TB
• Fibrosis and respiratory failure
• Pneumothorax
• Massive haemoptysis
• Aspergilloma in a healed TB cavity (see Section 2.9.2, p. 122).

Extrapulmonary disease

• Cranial nerve palsy and other neurological sequelae
• Spinal cord damage

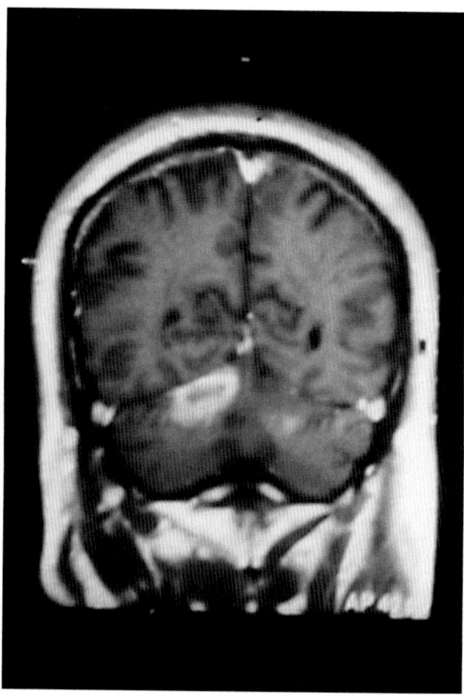

Fig. 67 MRI scan of a tuberculoma. A ring-enhancing lesion is present in the right cerebellum. This lesion enlarged during anti-TB treatment, necessitating corticosteroid use.

- Constrictive pericarditis
- Infertility as a result of fallopian tube blockage
- Interstitial nephritis.

Therapy

Drugs

All TB except CNS disease

Treatment is with rifampicin, isoniazid, pyrazinamide and ethambutol for 2 months, followed by rifampicin and isoniazid for a further 4 months [1].

CNS TB

Treatment is with rifampicin, isoniazid, pyrazinamide and ethambutol for 2 months, followed by rifampicin and isoniazid for a further 10 months, making a total of 12 months' therapy.

Corticosteroids

There is good evidence that these should be given in addition to antituberculous treatment for pericarditis and stage II (focal neurological signs) and III (reduced level of consciousness) TB meningitis. They may be beneficial in patients with TB lymphadenitis whose lymph nodes enlarge during treatment, in pleural effusions and in TB involving the ureter.

Advice

- Compliance is essential. Explain why and give practical help such as dosette boxes where needed.
- Rifampicin may render all bodily fluids, including urine, saliva and tears, orange.
- Rifampicin may render the oral contraceptive ineffective.
- Drug-induced hepatitis (rifampicin, isoniazid and pyrazinamide) may complicate therapy. Warn patients to contact the clinic immediately if they become jaundiced. This complication is more likely in elderly people or those with underlying chronic liver disease. Liver function tests (LFTs) should be checked regularly in these patients and before commencement of therapy in all patients [2].
- Ethambutol may occasionally cause visual impairment.

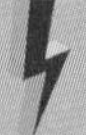

Ethambutol and the eye

- Check visual acuity using a Snellen chart
- Check colour vision using an Ishihara chart

Document the results in the case notes. Tell the patient to stop ethambutol and to contact you if he or she notices any change in vision.

Monitoring therapy

Monitor the following for clinical improvement:

- Symptoms, e.g. fever/cough
- Weight
- Inflammatory or other laboratory markers
- Chest radiograph.

Treatment failure

There are several possible reasons for treatment failure:

- Non-compliance: check urine for the orange colour associated with rifampicin.
- Multi-drug resistance: chase sensitivity results, consider PCR for rifampicin resistance. Seek specialist advice regarding the next regimen.
- Wrong diagnosis, e.g. sarcoidosis. Was an organism cultured?
- Malabsorption: the patient may have unsuspected small bowel TB. Rifampicin and isoniazid drug levels may help.
- Drug fever: the TB may be responding well and new symptoms are a result of a drug reaction—particularly common with rifampicin.

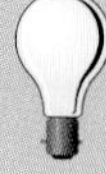

Directly observed therapy (DOT)

- Treatment of choice in suspected non-compliance
- Use a dosing regimen of two or three times a week
- Each dose to be given by a nurse at the clinic or at home.

Patient isolation

Patients in hospital with smear-positive pulmonary TB should be isolated in a negative-pressure room. Smear-positive cases of pulmonary TB residing within an institution (e.g. a nursing home) should be admitted for isolation until they have received 2 weeks of antituberculous therapy.

If the patient is moved around the hospital, he or she should wear a high-filter facemask.

Confirmed or suspected multidrug-resistant pulmonary TB cases should be admitted to hospital and isolated in a negative-pressure room.

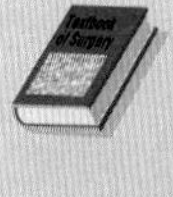

1 Joint Tuberculosis Committee of the British Thoracic Society. Chemotherapy and management of tuberculosis in the United Kingdom: recommendations 1998. *Thorax* 1998; 53: 536–548.
2 Ormerod LP, Skinner C, Wales J. Hepatotoxicity of antituberculous drugs. *Thorax* 1996; 51: 111–113.

2.6.2 *MYCOBACTERIUM LEPRAE*

This is the agent of leprosy or Hansen's disease.

Epidemiology

There are an estimated six million people with leprosy worldwide. It is endemic in Africa, Asia and South America. Spread is thought to be person to person through infected nasal droplets, but less than 10% of those exposed develop the disease.

Diagnostic tests

The organism cannot be grown *in vitro*. Diagnosis is clinical and confirmed by biopsy of a skin lesion or thickened nerve.

Disease syndromes

The majority of people exposed to *M. leprae* develop no clinical symptoms. In patients who develop disease, the clinical manifestations depend on the level of cell-mediated immunity (CMI) against the organism:

- Strong CMI response (Th1) (see *Immunology and immunosuppression*, Sections 3 and 4) is associated with tuberculoid leprosy
- Weak CMI response (Th2) is associated with lepromatous leprosy
- Intermediate response leads to borderline disease [1].

Tuberculoid leprosy

This presents with one to a few macules (pale on dark skin, red on white skin) with loss of sensation and sweating over them. A few nerves may be affected and thickened, with associated sensory or motor impairment. Few or no bacilli are seen on histology in these patients.

Lepromatous leprosy

Numerous skin lesions occur, mainly macules, infiltrating lesions and nodules. These are not anaesthetic or anhidrotic. As the disease progresses, the skin becomes thickened and the ears, lips and nose swell. Nerve thickening tends to be symmetrical and leads to peripheral neuropathy, neuropathic ulcers and deformity. Many bacilli are seen on biopsy.

Indeterminate leprosy

This is often the initial clinical manifestation and is characterized by a small macule without sensory loss. At this stage, the disease may progress to either of the types described above.

Complications

Tissue damage

Severe sensory neuropathy leads to deformity and loss of digits, tip of the nose and ears in lepromatous disease.

Erythema nodosum leprosum

This usually occurs in lepromatous or, less commonly, borderline leprosy after treatment has been commenced. Symptoms include fever and crops of painful red nodules that last for a few days. Other affected organs include the eyes (iridocyclitis), testes (orchitis), swollen joints and rarely an immune complex nephritis. Thalidomide is an effective treatment.

Reversal reaction

This occurs in borderline leprosy as the bacterial load is reduced with treatment. Skin lesions and affected nerves swell and may lead to severe nerve compression and damage within days. Treatment is with steroids, which may need to be continued for several months.

Therapy

- Tuberculoid leprosy (paucibacillary): rifampicin and dapsone for 6 months

• Lepromatous and borderline leprosy (multibacillary): rifampicin, dapsone and clofazimine for a minimum of 2 years or until skin-smear negativity occurs.

1 Gelber RH, Rea TH. *Mycobacterium leprae.* In: Mandell GL, Bennett JE, Dolin R (eds) *Principles and Practice of Infectious Diseases* (5th edn). Philadelphia: Churchill Livingstone, 2000: 2608–2616.

2.6.3 OPPORTUNISTIC MYCOBACTERIA

Epidemiology

These species of mycobacteria are widespread in the environment (soil, water, birds and animals) and person-to-person spread is very unusual. The prevalence of infection by individual species varies from country to country.

Diagnostic tests

Isolation of atypical mycobacteria may represent true infection or simply contamination, so always interpret culture results within the clinical context. Atypical mycobacteria often grow more quickly in culture than *Mycobacterium tuberculosis*. PCR- or DNA-based tests can rapidly distinguish between the *M. tuberculosis* group and other species.

Disease syndromes

There is a variety of disease syndromes caused by these mycobacteria, depending on age, level of immunocompromise and underlying lung disease (Table 55) [1]. *Mycobacterium avium intracellulare* (MAI) tends to be the predominant species causing disseminated disease in patients with AIDS.

Table 55 Principal disease site(s) of more common opportunistic mycobacteria.

Mycobacterial species	Site(s) of infection
M. kansasii	Pulmonary
M. malmoense	Pulmonary
M. xenopi	Pulmonary
M. avium intracellulare (MAI)	Pulmonary
	Lymph nodes: predominantly in children
	Disseminated infection in HIV-infected patients
M. fortuitum	Skin and soft tissue
M. chelonei	Skin and soft tissue
M. abscessus	Skin and soft tissue
	Pulmonary
M. marinum	Skin and soft tissue
M. ulcerans	Skin and soft tissue

Therapy

In general, atypical mycobacteria are inherently more drug resistant than *M. tuberculosis*. Recommended therapy varies according to site of infection, species of *Mycobacterium*, and presence or absence of immunocompromise. See the British Thoracic Society guidelines for detailed information on therapy [1]. In severely immunocompromised patients, the response to therapy is often poor unless the immune response can be improved.

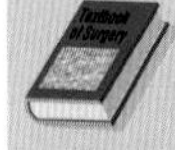

1 Subcommittee of the Joint Tuberculosis Committee of the British Thoracic Society. Management of opportunist mycobacterial infections: Joint Tuberculosis Committee Guidelines 1999. *Thorax* 2000; 55: 210–218.

2.7 Spirochaetes

Description of the organism

Spirochaetes are thin, helical, Gram-negative bacteria. They include *Treponema*, *Borrelia* and *Leptospira* spp. (Table 56).

2.7.1 SYPHILIS

Epidemiology

The majority of cases are sexually transmitted with increased incidence in gay men, commercial sex workers and the developing world. Syphilis can be transmitted transplacentally and via blood transfusion or needlestick injury.

Table 56 Important spirochaetes, their vectors and diseases.

Agent	Species	Vector	Human disease
Treponema	*T. pallidum* subsp. *Pallidum*	None	Syphilis
	T. pallidum subsp. *endemicum*	None	Bejel
	T. pallidum subsp. *pertenue*	None	Yaws
	T. pallidum subsp. *carateum*	None	Pinta
Borrelia	*B. burgdorferi*	Ixodes tick	Lyme disease
	B. recurrentis	Human louse	Louse-borne relapsing fever
	B. duttoni and other species	Soft tick	Tick-borne relapsing fever
Leptospira	*L. interrogans*	Rodent urine	Leptospirosis
	L. ictohaemorrhagicae		Aseptic meningitis

Table 57 Clinical features of syphilis.

Stage of disease	Timing	Site	Clinical features
Primary	3 days to 3 months (average 3 weeks)	Site of inoculation	Painless chancre Regional lymphadenopathy
Secondary ('the great imitator')	2–8 weeks after appearance of chancre	General	Diffuse lymphadenopathy Fever, malaise, arthralgia
		Skin	Maculopapular rash, involving palms and soles
		Genitalia	Condylomata lata
		Mouth	Snail-track ulcers Mucous patches
		CNS	Headache Meningism
Latent	Variable	–	Asymptomatic
Tertiary	Years	Skin, mucosa and skeletal system	Gumma: 15% untreated cases
		Cardiac	Aortitis/aneurysm formation in 10% of untreated cases
		CNS	Argyll Robertson pupil Tabes dorsalis Charcot's joints Psychiatric manifestations.
Congenital	Early	General	Osteochondritis Rash Anaemia Hepatosplenomegaly
	Late	General	Saddle nose Frontal bossing Hutchinson's teeth

Clinical presentation

See Table 57.

Diagnostic tests

- Clinical picture and serology (see Sections 1.33, p. 81 and 1.35, p. 86)
- Identification can be made from primary lesions by dark field microscopy.

Disease syndromes

Local infection at the site of inoculation is followed by dissemination (secondary syphilis). There follows a long period of clinical latency before late-stage end-organ disease.

Therapy

Parenteral long-acting benzylpenicillin is preferred at all stages of syphilis. The dosage and duration of therapy depend on the clinical stage. (See Section 1.35, p. 86.)

1 Singh AE, Romanowski B. Syphilis: review with emphasis on clinical, epidemiologic, and some biologic features. *Clin Microbiol Rev* 1999; 12: 187–209.

2.7.2 LYME DISEASE

Epidemiology

Lyme disease occurs throughout the USA, Europe and the former Soviet Union. There are small foci of disease in the New Forest, Exmoor and other areas of the UK. Deer and rodents serve as the most common hosts for the ticks. Campers and hikers are at particular risk [1]. Infection can be prevented by removing ticks within 24 h.

Diagnostic tests

The diagnosis is usually made on serology in association with a suitable clinical picture. Serology may be difficult to interpret in people from an endemic area. In CNS disease, PCR for *Borrelia burgdorferi* can be performed on the CSF.

Disease syndromes

The illness is characterized by three stages.

Localized early

Onset is from 3 days to 1 month after tick bite. There is a

spreading rash with central clearing, erythema chronicum migrans, at the site of the bite. This clears after 2–6 weeks.

Early disseminated

Secondary skin lesions, malaise, arthralgia and lymphadenopathy are common and may start within a few days of the initial lesion. Aseptic meningitis may occur.

Late, persistent infection

Late manifestations (months–years after initial infection) occur in 20–50% of untreated patients.

- Arthritis: large-joint mono- or oligoarthopathy, often as recurrent attacks over months–years. Polyarthritis is unusual.
- Carditis: occurs in 10%; more commonly seen in the USA and manifests as dysrhythmias or heart block.
- CNS manifestations: in 10–15% of cases, including lymphocytic meningitis, cranial nerve palsies, encephalopathy, neuropathy and radiculopathy.
- Skin: acrodermatitis chronicum atrophicans (skin discoloration and swelling at original erythema chronicum migrans site).

Therapy

Stage 1 and mild cases at stage 2 can be treated with 2–3 weeks of doxycycline or amoxicillin. Serious complications usually require intravenous ceftriaxone.

1 Nadelman RB, Wormser GP. Lyme borreliosis. *Lancet* 1998; 352: 557–565.

2.7.3 RELAPSING FEVER

Epidemiology

Louse-borne relapsing fever

This is endemic in the highlands of Ethiopia, Yemen, Peru and Bolivia. The disease thrives where people live in crowded conditions [1].

Tick-borne relapsing fever

This has a worldwide distribution. *Borrelia duttoni* is prevalent in parts of east, central and South Africa.

Diagnostic tests

The spirochaetes can be seen on blood films taken as for malaria (see Section 3.2, p. 151). They are less easily detected in tick-borne disease. Serology is helpful: there is crossreactivity with *B. burgdorferi*.

Disease syndromes

Louse-borne relapsing fever

- Severe febrile illness, single relapse
- Haemorrhagic complications in 50%, hepatitis, myocarditis
- Mortality rate of 10–70% in epidemics.

Tick-borne relapsing fever

- Milder febrile illness is followed by multiple relapses
- Mortality is lower, but neurological complications in 5–10%.

Therapy

Treatment with tetracycline or erythromycin to eliminate spirochaetes may be complicated by a Jarisch–Herxheimer reaction in 30–100% of people. This is characterized by rigors, delirium and shock a few hours after antimicrobial administration, and is thought to be principally related to release of tumour necrosis factor (TNF). Monitoring and support through a Jarisch– Herxheimer reaction are essential.

1 Cook GC. Other spirochaetal diseases. In: Cook GC (ed) *Manson's Tropical Diseases* (20th edn). London: WB Saunders: 1996: 951–962.

2.7.4 LEPTOSPIROSIS

Epidemiology

Leptospirosis has a worldwide distribution. *Leptospira* spp. are excreted in rodent urine, the rat being the most common vector, and humans are infected from environmental contact through skin abrasions or the mucosa. Risk factors include farming, sewage work, veterinary medicine and recreational freshwater exposure.

Diagnostic tests

Diagnosis relies on suspicion from the clinical picture and relevant exposure history (see Section 1.20, p. 52). The organism can be cultured from blood or urine in acute disease, but this is beyond the capability of routine microbiology laboratories. The diagnosis is confirmed retrospectively by serology.

Disease syndromes and complications

There is a range from asymptomatic infection, a 'flu-like illness 7–14 days after infection, to severe illness in about 10% of those with clinical disease. Severe disease (Weil's disease) is characterized by liver failure, conjunctival suffusion, renal failure, haemorrhages, impaired consciousness, myocarditis and shock, and has a mortality rate approaching 10%. *Leptospira* spp. can also cause aseptic meningitis without hepatic or renal involvement.

Therapy

Penicillin is active against *Leptospira* spp. and should be administered, if possible, early in disease, although there are conflicting data on whether antibiotics improve outcome [1]. Tetracycline is suitable in penicillin allergy. Supportive care in serious illness is the most important factor in determining outcome.

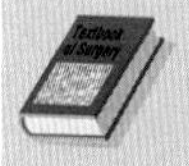

1 Guidugli F, Castro AA, Atallah AN. Antibiotics for treating leptospirosis. *Cochrane Database Syst Rev* 2000; (2): CD001306.

2.8 Miscellaneous bacteria

2.8.1 *MYCOPLASMA* AND *UREAPLASMA*

Description of the organism

Mycoplasmas and ureaplasmas lack a cell wall and are the smallest free-living organisms known. They require special media for culture and do not stain using Gram stain. Many species have been described with a few of clinical importance, the most significant of these being *Mycoplasma pneumoniae.*

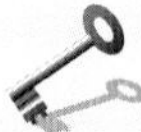

Mycoplasmas and ureaplasmas of clinical importance

- *Mycoplasma pneumoniae*
- Genital mycoplasmas, e.g. *Mycoplasma hominis, Mycoplasma genitalum*
- *Ureaplasma urealyticum.*

Epidemiology

Mycoplasma pneumoniae

Worldwide distribution transmitted by respiratory droplets from an infected case. There are sporadic cases with epidemic outbreaks every 3–5 years. Children and young adults are particularly likely to acquire infection.

Genital mycoplasmas and ureaplasma

These are found worldwide as common colonizing organisms in the female genital tract. There is an epidemiological association with genital and pelvic disease [1].

Diagnostic tests

Mycoplasma pneumoniae

Blood tests

- WCC: usually normal or slightly raised ($<15 \times 10^9$/L).
- Cold agglutinins: present in about 50% of patients with *M. pneumoniae* infection. Although not specific (may occur in EBV, CMV and some lymphomas), their detection is highly suggestive of the diagnosis in the correct clinical setting.
- Serology: confirmation of the diagnosis is based on the demonstration of a fourfold rise in antibody titre between acute and convalescent (10–14 days) samples.

Imaging

Chest radiograph may reveal consolidation at lung bases, but is not diagnostic; pleural effusion is uncommon.

Genital mycoplasmas and ureaplasma

Culture from relevant genital specimens requires specific techniques and is not routinely practised. *Mycoplasma hominis* can occasionally be isolated from blood in severe infection.

Disease syndromes

Mycoplasma pneumoniae

The most common site of infection with *M. pneumoniae* is the respiratory tract [2] (see Section 1.4, p. 10). The majority of cases are limited to the upper respiratory tract but pneumonia develops in 5–10% of patients. *Mycoplasma pneumoniae* is the second most common cause of community-acquired pneumonia in young adults. There is an insidious onset with fever, headache and malaise. Cough is initially dry, but may become productive. Pleuritic chest pain or pleural effusion is rare in *M. pneumonia*. As with the other atypical organisms, auscultation of the chest may reveal no or only minimal abnormality.

Genital mycoplasmas and ureaplasma

Females

Mycoplasma hominis and *U. urealyticum* are implicated in some cases of salpingitis, endometritis and pelvic inflammatory disease. Both may cause chorioamnionitis and can be isolated in septic abortion, postpartum sepsis and some cases of neonatal meningitis. Systemic spread with septic arthritis has rarely been reported for both organisms.

Males

The role of genital mycoplasmas in non-gonococcal urethritis is controversial. *Ureaplasma urealyticum* can cause urethritis, epididymo-orchitis and prostatitis.

Complications

Mycoplasma pneumoniae

- Rashes: often macular but erythema multiforme and erythema nodosum described
- Bullous myringitis
- Arthralgia and, rarely, arthritis
- Myocarditis and pericarditis
- Meningitis and encephalitis
- Raynaud's phenomenon related to cold agglutinins
- Haemolytic anaemia.

Therapy

Mycoplasma pneumoniae

Upper respiratory tract infections with *M. pneumoniae* do not require antibiotics. Pneumonia is usually self-limiting but 10–14 days with a macrolide antibiotic can shorten the duration of illness. Tetracyclines are also effective.

Genital mycoplasmas and ureaplasma

Doxycycline 100 mg twice daily is the drug of choice. Clindamycin is the choice in children. Macrolides are useful against resistant organisms.

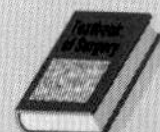

1 File TM Jr, Tan JS, Plouffe JF. The role of atypical pathogens: *Mycoplasma pneumoniae, Chlamydia pneumoniae*, and *Legionella pneumophila* in respiratory infection. *Infect Dis Clin North Am* 1998; 12: 569–592.
2 Cassel G, Wiates K, Taylor-Robinson D. Genital mycoplasmas. In: Morse SA, Moreland AA Holmes KK (eds) *Atlas of sexually transmitted diseases and AIDS* (2nd ed). London: Mosby-Wolfe, 1996: 119–132.

2.8.2 RICKETTSIAE

Description of the organism

Rickettsiae are small, Gram-negative, obligate intracellular parasites.

Epidemiology

Rickettsiae are zoonoses and are transmitted to humans by a number of arthropods (Table 58). Rickettsial infections are distributed throughout the world [1].

Diagnostic tests

The diagnosis is initially made on clinical grounds and confirmed by serological tests. Significant crossreactivity is encountered. PCR of blood, if available, may be helpful.

Disease syndromes

General features include fever, headache and rash. Many are associated with an eschar at the site of the bite with associated regional lymphadenopathy. The severity varies from epidemic louse-borne typhus, which has a mortality rate reported as high as 40%, to rickettsialpox which is usually a self-limiting illness.

The tetracyclines are the drugs of choice.

1 Cowan GO. Rickettsial infections. In: GC Cook (ed) *Manson's Tropical Diseases* (20th edn). London: WB Saunders, 1996: 797–816.

Table 58 Disease syndromes and epidemiology of the more common rickettsioses.

Group	Disease syndrome	Organism	Vector	Geographical distribution
Typhus	Epidemic typhus	*R. prowazeki*	Body louse	South America, Africa, Asia
	Endemic murine typhus	*R. typhi*	Flea	Worldwide
	Scrub typhus	*R. tsutsugamushi*	Larval trombiculid mite	South-east Asia, South Pacific
Spotted fever	Rocky Mountain spotted fever	*R. rickettsii*	Tick	USA
	Boutonneuse fever	*R. conori*	Tick	Africa, Mediterranean
	Rickettsialpox	*R. akari*	Mite	USA, Africa, Asia

2.8.3 *COXIELLA BURNETII* (Q FEVER)

Epidemiology

Coxiella burnetii is a zoonotic rickettsiosis reported throughout the world [1]. Cattle, sheep and goats are the main animal reservoirs. Spread is by inhalation of aerosolized particles from infected animals or their contaminated environment. Farmers, veterinarians and abattoir workers are particularly at risk.

Diagnostic tests

• Serology is the usual method of confirming diagnosis. Acute infection can be distinguished from chronic infection based on antibody responses to phase I and phase II antigens.
• White cell count is usually normal or slightly raised.
• Liver function tests: a slight elevation of the transaminases occurs in most patients.

Disease syndromes

Acute Q fever

The majority of infections are either asymptomatic or present as a flu-like illness. Common presentations of acute Q fever include atypical pneumonia or hepatitis.

Chronic Q fever

- Endocarditis, usually with a prosthetic heart valve
- Meningoencephalitis
- Hepatitis
- Osteomyelitis.

Therapy

• Acute Q fever: doxycycline 200 mg daily for 14 days. A quinolone may be used as an alternative.
• Q fever endocarditis: the optimal drugs are uncertain but some authors recommend doxycycline combined with chloroquine for at least 18 months. Doxycycline combined with rifampicin or ciprofloxacin has also been successful.

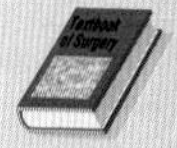

1 Maurin M, Raoult D. Q fever. *Clin Microbiol Rev* 1999; 12: 518–553.

2.8.4 CHLAMYDIAE

Description of the organism

Chlamydiae are small obligate intracellular parasites. There are three species causing human disease:

- *Chlamydia trachomatis*
- *Chlamydia pneumoniae*
- *Chlamydia psittaci*.

Epidemiology

Chlamydia trachomatis

C. trachomatis can spread from eye to eye by direct contact, fingers or shared cloths/sheets. The prevalence of genital chlamydial infection is high in young sexually active women (up to 10–25%) making *C. trachomatis*, spread by sexual intercourse, the most common STD and probably the single most common cause of tubal infertility.

Chlamydia pneumoniae

This is a common respiratory pathogen worldwide. Spread is by the respiratory route and infections occur particularly in children and young adults. Epidemiological links to heart disease have not been proven.

Chlamydia psittaci

Avian infection is transmitted to humans from infected birds by the respiratory route.

Diagnostic tests

The main diagnostic methods are serology, antigen detection, PCR and culture. Screening urine samples for subclinical genital *C. trachomatis* by sensitive DNA-amplification techniques is becoming available [1].

Clinical syndromes

A wide range of clinical manifestations may occur (Table 59).

Complications

Chlamydiae may cause tissue damage and subsequent scarring
• Blindness in trachoma
• Fallopian tube scarring and infertility
• Lymphoedema and rectal strictures in lymphogranuloma venereum (LGV).

Therapy

• Trachoma or conjunctivitis caused by *C. trachomatis* may be treated with topical tetracycline eye ointment and/or oral tetracycline or azithromycin
• Genital infections caused by *C. trachomatis* may be treated with doxycycline or azithromycin [2]

Table 59 Clinical syndromes caused by *Chlamydia species.*

Species	Affected group	Disease syndrome
C. trachomatis	Young children	Trachoma in developing world
	Men and women	Inclusion body conjunctivitis Reactive arthritis
	Genital infection in men	Urethritis Epididymo-orchitis Prostatitis
	Genital infection in women	Cervicitis and urethritis Endometritis Pelvic inflammatory disease Perihepatitis
	Perinatal infection	Ophthalmia neonatorum Pneumonia
C. trachomatis	Sexually active men and women	Lymphogranuloma venerum (LGV)
C. pneumoniae	Children and young adults	Upper respiratory tract infection Atypical pneumonia
C. psittaci	Contact with birds	Psittacosis

• *C. psittaci* and *C. pneumoniae* pneumonia require a tetracycline or macrolide for 2–3 weeks.

1 Stamm WE. *Chlamydia trachomatis* infections: progress and problems. *J Infect Dis* 1999; 179(suppl 2): S380–383.
2 Clinical Effectiveness Group (Association of Genitourinary Medicine and the Medical Society for the Study of Venereal Diseases). National guideline for the management of *Chlamydia trachomatis* genital tract infection. *Sex Transm Infect* 1999; 75(suppl 1): S4–8.

2.9 Fungi

Fungi are an important cause of disease in both immunocompetent and immunocompromised hosts. The more serious consequences of fungal infection, however, are most often encountered in patients with significant immune defects [1].

2.9.1 *CANDIDA* SPP.

Description of the organism

Candida spp. are budding yeasts that may form pseudohyphae during tissue invasion. They are ubiquitous and common commensals of mucosal surfaces and the gastrointestinal tract.

Epidemiology

Candida spp. are opportunistic pathogens taking advantage of breakdown in local or systemic defences to cause disease. Mucosal protection may be impaired by trauma or by antibiotics altering normal bacterial flora. Impaired cell-mediated immunity predisposes to mucocutaneous infection and neutropenia to disseminated candidiasis. Most infections are endogenous but nosocomial spread has been described [2].

Diagnostic tests

Candida spp. grow readily on simple laboratory media and can be isolated from blood cultures. The germ tube test rapidly distinguish *C. albicans* (produces germ tubes) from other *Candida* spp. Culture cannot always distinguish colonization from invasive disease and tissue biopsies may be required where budding yeasts and pseudohyphae are seen. There is no reliable serological test for invasive candidiasis, although a number are under evaluation.

Disease syndromes and complications

Mucocutaneous disease

Mucosal disease, either oral or vaginal, is the most common manifestation of candidiasis; it is seen in immunocompetent individuals and with a greater frequency in immunodeficiency. Cutaneous candidal infection occurs in moist skin creases and is a common cause of nappy rash. More serious mucocutaneous disease including chronic nail infection (onychomycosis) and oesophageal disease (Fig. 68) may complicate cell-mediated immunodeficiency. Urinary infection with *Candida* is seen in people with diabetes and patients with indwelling urinary catheters.

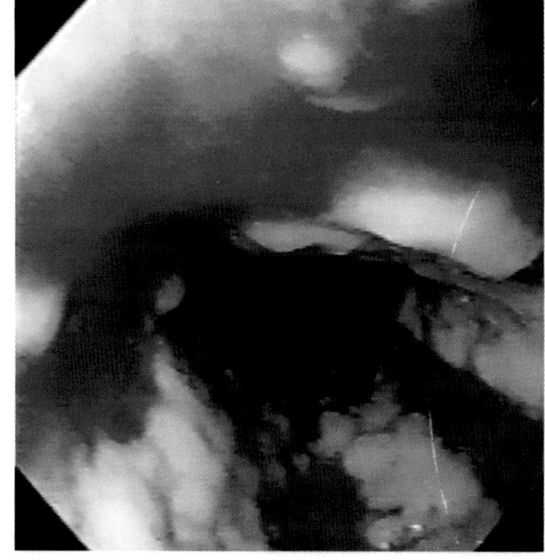

Fig. 68 Severe oesophageal candidiasis in a patient with AIDS and a CD4 count of 50 cell/μL.

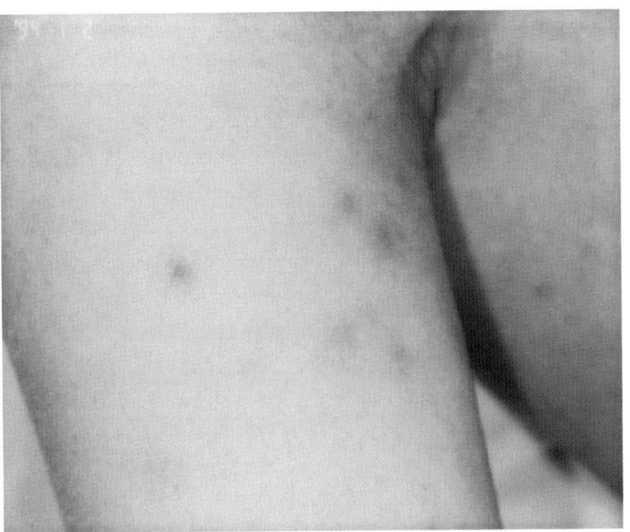

Fig. 69 Disseminated cutaneous candidiasis in a neutropenic patient.

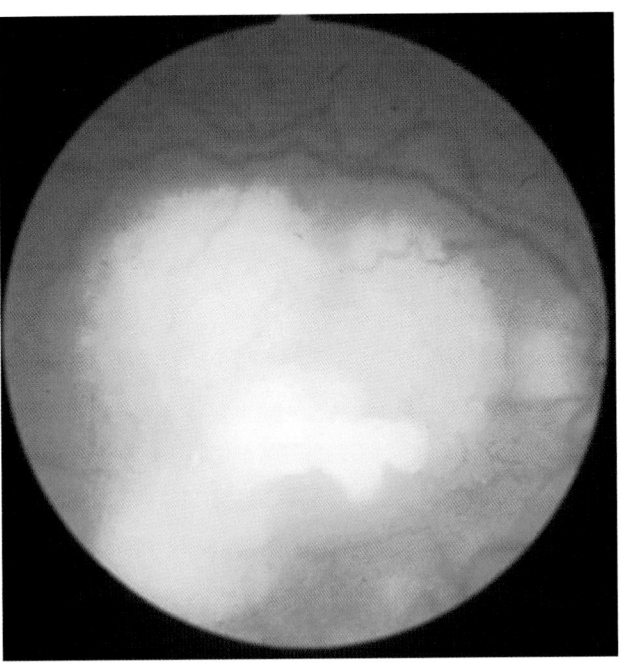

Fig. 70 Candida retinitis with white exudate extending into the vitreous. Intravitreal satellite lesions can be seen on slit-lamp examination. (Courtesy of Professor S Lightman.)

Disseminated disease

Invasive candidiasis is seen in patients with neutropenia, intravenous drug users and long-term central venous cannulation, particularly in intensive care. Manifestations include candidaemia, endocarditis, and invasion of liver/spleen, skin (Fig. 69), eyes or lungs.

Candidaemia

- May be complicated by endophthalmitis or endocarditis.
- Patients with candidaemia should have a full ophthalmic evaluation. Candidal infection appears as white patches on the retina (Fig. 70).
- Consider endocarditis in intravenous drug users and persistent fungaemia.

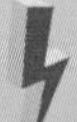

Amphotericin B

- May cause fever, rigors and hypotension, which can be prevented with hydrocortisone
- Dose-related renal toxicity with increased creatinine, hypokalaemia and hypomagnesaemia
- Encapsulating amphotericin in lipid vesicles reduces toxicity, but there are no data that lipid preparations are more effective than the conventional agent.

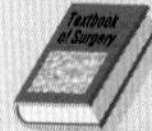

1 Warnock DW. Fungal infections in neutropenia: current problems and chemotherapeutic control. *J Antimicrob Chemother* 1998; 41 (suppl D): 95–105.
2 Viscoli C *et al.* Candidemia in cancer patients: a prospective, multicentre surveillance study by the Invasive Fungal Infection Group (IFig) of the European Organization for Research and Treatment of Cancer (EORTC). *Clin Infect Dis* 1999; 28: 1071–1079.

Therapy

Antifungal therapy (Table 60) should be complemented by management of the underlying predisposing factors, e.g. diabetes, neutropenia or poor dental hygiene.

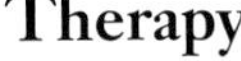

Table 60 Therapy of candidiasis.

Organism	Disease syndrome	Therapy
Candida albicans (most common cause of candidiasis)	Uncomplicated mucosal disease e.g. oral/vaginal	Topical therapy with nystatin, amphotericin B, azole Systemic therapy if fails
	Mucosal disease in immunocompromised host	Systemic therapy: azole first line, e.g. fluconazole Amphotericin B for resistant disease
	Urinary tract infection	Fluconazole
	Disseminated infection	Intravenous fluconazole or amphotericin B
	Endocarditis/meningitis	Amphotericin B + 5-flucytosine
	Endophthalmitis	Fluconazole penetrates eye well Intraocular amphotericin
Non-*albicans Candida* spp.	May cause all of the above but less frequently than *C. albicans*	Increased azole resistance Use azoles for mucosal disease but amphotericin B for initial therapy of systemic infections, e.g. *C. glabrata, C. kruseii, C. parapsilosis*

2.9.2 *ASPERGILLUS*

Description of the organism

Most human infections are caused by *Aspergillus fumigatus* which is a spore-forming mould (Fig. 71). *Aspergillus* spp. are ubiquitous and predominantly transmitted by inhalation of spores [1,2].

Epidemiology

Aspergillus sp. causes invasive disease in severely immunocompromised patients, particularly those with prolonged neutropenia. Outbreaks resulting from aerosolization of aspergillus spores have been described in association with building works in hospitals. Air filters can reduce the incidence of invasive disease in neutropenic patients.

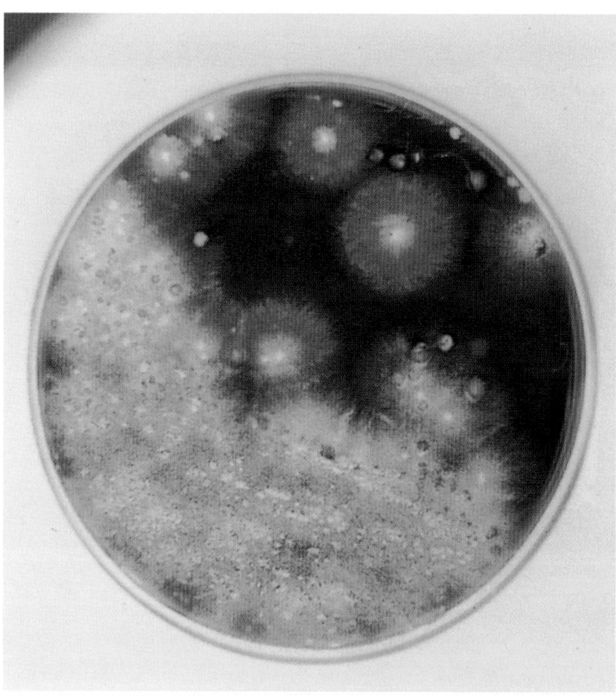

Fig. 71 *Aspergillus fumigatus* growing on chocolate agar. The mould produces numerous spores that easily aerosolize.

Diagnostic tests

- Invasive aspergillosis is confirmed by identifying typical fungal hyphae in tissue specimens
- Positive culture of respiratory material may only indicate colonization, but is strongly associated with invasive disease in severely immunocompromised hosts
- Cutaneous hypersensitivity reactions to aspergillus preparations and the detection of serum aspergillus precipitins help to establish the diagnoses of allergic disease and aspergilloma.

Disease syndromes and therapy

Disease may occur as a result of tissue invasion or a hypersensitivity reaction to aspergillus colonization of the respiratory tract (Table 61).

1 www.aspergillus.com—contains up-to-date information on disease manifestation diagnosis and therapy.
2 Denning DW. Invasive aspergillosis. *Clin Infect Dis* 1998; 26: 781–803.

2.9.3 *CRYPTOCOCCUS NEOFORMANS*

Description of the organism

This is an encapsulated yeast carried by avian species and acquired by inhalation.

Epidemiology

Distribution is worldwide with the most serious disease being seen in cell-mediated immune deficiency. *Cryptococcus neoformans* var. *gatti* has a subtropical distribution and may be more pathogenic to immunocompetent hosts.

Table 61 Types of aspergillosis and therapy.

Disease syndrome	Clinical presentation	Therapy
Aspergilloma (colonization of a pre-existing lung cavity)	Haemoptysis, fever and malaise, fungal ball inside cavity on chest radiograph	Surgery is the only definitive treatment
Allergic bronchopulmonary aspergillosis (ABPA)	Airflow obstruction, eosinophilia, pulmonary infiltrates, proximal bronchiectasis, positive aspergillus precipitins	Corticosteroids
Invasive aspergillosis	Pulmonary: pleurisy, haemoptysis, focal infiltrate Disseminated: fungaemia, brain abscess, liver/spleen	Amphotericin B is the only proven therapy but high mortality Itraconazole may have a role in prophylaxis

Diagnostic tests

Diagnosis is by microscopy, using India ink to outline the capsule, and culture of the organism. The capsular polysaccharide can be detected by ELISA in CSF/blood (cryptococcal antigen).

Disease syndromes

Manifestations are rare in the immunocompetent host; in immunocompromised individuals, the following disease patterns are seen.

Pneumonia

After inhalation pulmonary invasion is often asymptomatic, but a diffuse pneumonitis may be seen.

Meningitis

Haematogenous dissemination leads to meningitis, which is the most common presentation. Meningitis is accompanied by CSF lymphocytosis and low CSF glucose, but in severely immunocompromised patients the CSF may have no inflammatory cells. Meningitis may be complicated by cryptococcal abscess (cryptococcoma) and raised intracranial pressure resulting from impaired CSF reabsorption.

Cutaneous

Nodules or shallow ulcers may be a sign of disseminated disease. Rarely, there is isolated cutaneous disease after inoculation.

Therapy

Therapy has been best defined for patients with AIDS [1]. Induction treatment is with amphotericin B and 5-flucytosine for 2–4 weeks until the CSF has been sterilized. Blood levels of flucytosine should be checked. Secondary prophylaxis is continued with fluconazole while the CD4 count remains <200 cells/mL. Note that itraconazole has poor CNS penetration and is not used.

1 Van der Horst CM, Saag MS, Cloud GA *et al.* Treatment of cryptococcal meningitis associated with the acquired immunodeficiency syndrome. *N Engl J Med* 1997; 337: 15–21.

2.9.4 DIMORPHIC FUNGI

Description of the organism

Dimorphic fungi are not endemic to the UK. They exist in the soil as mycetes (filamentous) and are acquired through inhalation. During human infection they take on a yeast form. They all have primary infection via the respiratory tract which is asymptomatic in many cases. Dissemination can occur in immunocompetent hosts but is more common in cell-mediated immunodeficiency states [1].

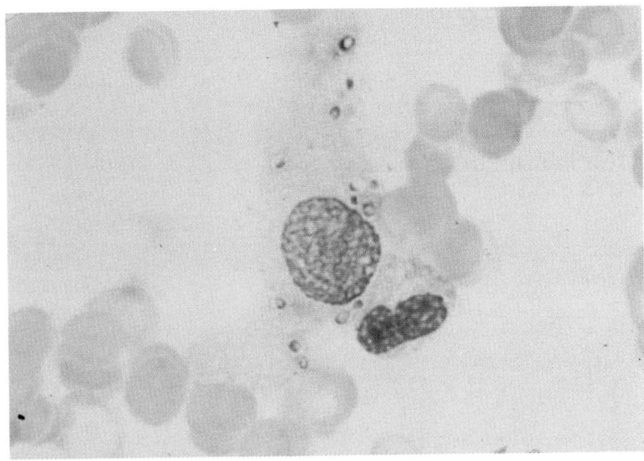

Fig. 72 Giemsa-stained peripheral blood smear from an AIDS patient with disseminated histoplasmosis. The intracellular organisms appear as small spherical inclusions with white cells. (Courtesy of B Viner.)

Diagnostic tests

Identification of typical yeast forms in tissue specimens. In disseminated disease, *Histoplasma capsulatum* may be seen in peripheral mononuclear cells (Fig. 72). Specific serological tests are available but are difficult to interpret in endemic areas.

Epidemiology, disease syndromes and therapy

Dimorphic fungi are most prevalent in river valleys in parts of the USA, central and South America (Table 62). Most infections in the immunocompetent individuals are subclinical but a significant minority experience clinical disease. Wide dissemination may occur in the immunocompromised host even many years after initial exposure [2,3].

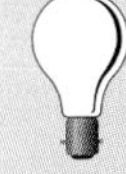

Consider disseminated infection with dimorphic fungi in immunocompromised patients who have lived/travelled in an endemic area and present with pneumonia, PUO or meningitis.

2.9.5 MISCELLANEOUS FUNGI

Description of the organism

A number of other fungal species are relatively common causes of minor cutaneous disease and rarely life-threatening or disfiguring illness (Table 63).

Table 62 Infections caused by dimorphic fungi.

Disease	Organism	Epidemiology	Syndromes	Therapy
Blastomycosis	*B. dermatidis*	Central/Southern USA	Chronic cutaneous disease Disseminate to: lung, skin, bones	Azole or amphotericin B
Coccidioidomycosis	*C. immitis*	South-western USA, Mexico	'Flu-like illness, pulmonary nodules, meningitis, osteomyelitis	Azole or amphotericin B
Histoplasmosis	*H. capsulatum*	Central/South USA, central and South America, Caribbean	Fever, erythema nodosum, hilar lymphadenopathy, pulmonary nodules (may calcify) Disseminated: skin, liver, spleen, bone marrow, lung and brain	Azole or amphotericin B
	H. capsulatum var. *duboisii*	Central Africa	Disseminated disease	
Paracoccidioidomycosis	*P. braziliensis*	Central and South America	Cutaneous, pulmonary, and disseminated forms	Sulphonamides, azoles or amphotericin B

Table 63 Features and therapy of specific fungal infections.

Disease	Organism	Disease syndromes	Therapy
Mucormycosis	*Mucor mycetales* (+ other zygomycetes)	Rhinosinusitis and intracranial spread in immunocompromised patients particularly diabetes mellitus	Surgical débridement, high-dose amphotericin B; high mortality
Fusariosis	*Fusarium* spp.	Local infection at sites of inoculation Disseminated disease in neutropenia	Responds poorly to amphotericin B
Penicilliosis	*Penicillium marneffi*	Endemic to south-east Asia Cutaneous and disseminated disease in AIDS	Acute therapy with amphotericin B Maintenance with itraconazole
Chromomycosis	Various pigmented fungi	Chronic subcutaneous disease with scarring	5-Flucytosine or azole therapy
Sporotrichosis	*Sporothrix schenckii*	Cutaneous, bone or joint infection at sites of inoculation Disseminated disease in immunocompromised patients	Potassium iodide or azoles Heat is effective for local lesions
Superficial skin and nail infections	*Malassezia* spp. *Trichophyton* spp. *Microsporum* spp.	Tinea (ringworm), chronic nail infection (onychomycosis)	Topical therapy with an azole Systemic therapy with terbinafine, itraconazole or griseofulvin Treatment directed by skin scraping results

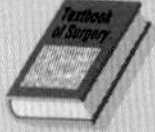

1 Bradsher RW. Histoplasmosis and blastomycosis. *Clin Infect Dis* 1996; 22(suppl 2): S102–111.
2 Lortholary O, Denning DW, Dupont B *et al.* Endemic mycoses: a treatment update. *J Antimicrob Chemother* 1999; 43: 321–331.
3 Warnock DW. Antifungal agents. In: O'Grady F, Lambert HP, Finch RG, Greenwood D (eds) *Antibiotic and Chemotherapy* (7th edn). London: Churchill Livingstone, 1997.

2.10 Viruses

Description of the organism

Viruses are the smallest living organisms that replicate through nucleic acids. They are classified according to their genome and structure [1]. A detailed knowledge of their classification is not required to understand them in a clinical context, but some idea of their relatedness is useful (Fig. 73). In general, DNA viruses have more stable genomes than RNA viruses and mutate less rapidly.

Diagnostic tests

Direct viral tests

Various methods are used to visualize, detect or culture viruses (Table 64).

The future is likely to see expansion of the use of rapid diagnostic tests for the detection and identification of viral infections. This will be essential to allow rational use of the next generation of antiviral agents.

Serological methods

The antibody response to viruses is often used to establish the diagnosis (Fig. 74). In general, detection of

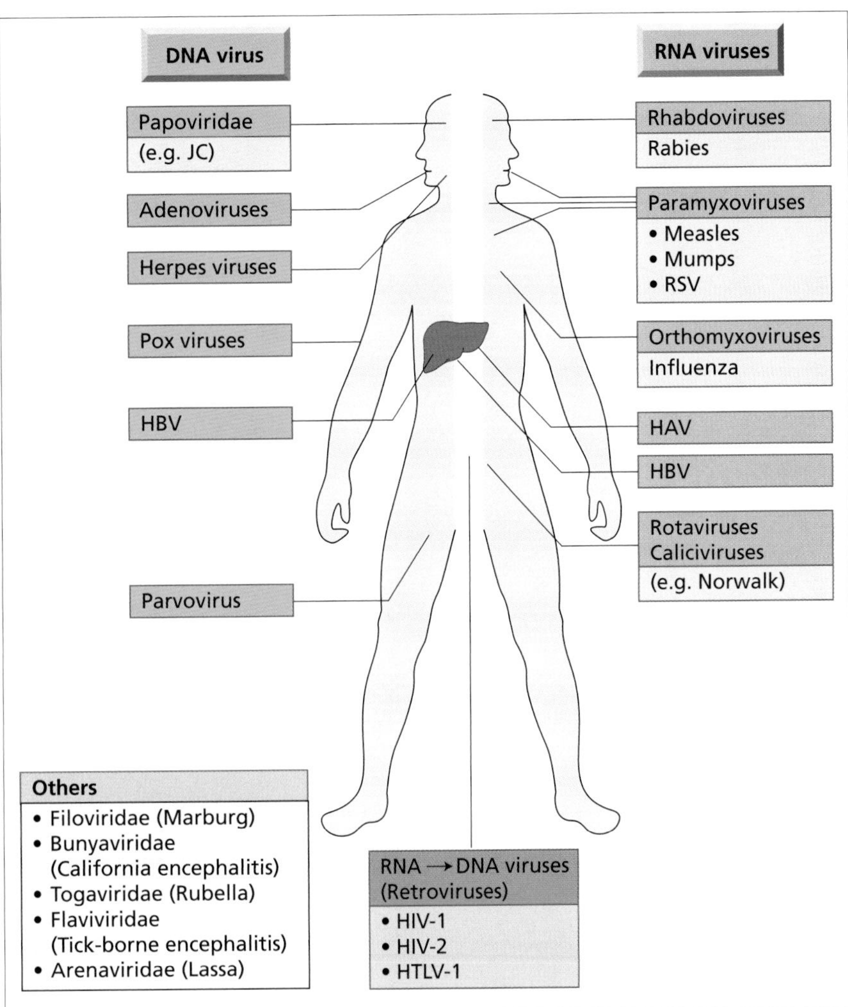

Fig. 73 Medically important viruses. HAV, hepatitis A virus; HBV, hepatitis B virus; HCV, hepatitis C virus; RSV, respiratory syncytial virus; HIV, human immunodeficiency virus; HTLV, human T-cell lymphotrophic virus.

Table 64 Viral detection methods.

Method	Example	Advantages	Disadvantages
Electron microscopy	Herpes viruses	Rapid	Operator dependent Cannot type or speciate
Viral culture	Adenovirus Herpes viruses	Generic Can allow sensitivity testing	Slow, labour intensive Requires viable virus
Antigen detection by ELISA	HBV	Rapid	May be insensitive
Antigen detection by immunofluorescence	RSV Influenza	Rapid	Operator dependent
PCR	Herpes viruses HIV, HCV	Sensitive May allow quantitative estimates	Expensive Contamination may lead to false positives Availability
Nucleic acid sequencing	HIV, HBV	Detect mutations associated with drug resistance	Slow Expensive

ELISA, enzyme-linked immunosorbent assay; RSV, respiratory syncytial virus; PCR, polymerase chain reaction; HBV, hepatitis B virus; HCV hepatitis C virus; HIV, human immunodeficiency virus.

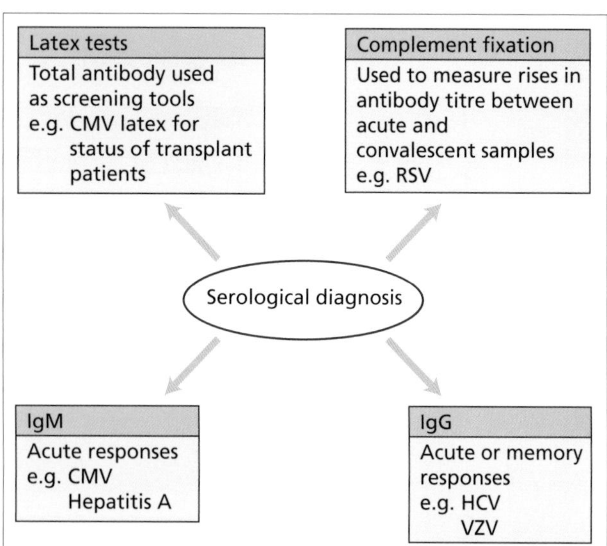

Fig. 74 Different serological methods used in viral diagnosis. Fourfold or greater rise in titre determines significance. CMV, cytomegalovirus; HCV, hepatitis C virus; VZV, varicella-zoster virus; RSV, respiratory syncytial virus.

organism-specific IgM antibody or a rising IgG titre signifies recent infection.

Pitfalls in diagnostic serology

- Antibodies arise slowly, so early tests may be negative. Always note date of onset/exposure when requesting serology to avoid false reassurance.
- IgM antibodies persist for variable lengths of time. Parvovirus B19 antibodies of IgM class are present for only a week or so, while those against CMV persist for months.
- IgM antibodies in particular may crossreact (especially between CMV and EBV).
- Severely immunocompromised patients may fail to mount an antibody response.
- Serology is of little value in identifying reactivation of disease (such as CMV).
- Crossreactive antibodies limit usefulness in some situations, e.g. diagnosing enterovirus infection.

1 Fields B, Knipe D, eds. *Virology*. New York: Lippincott-Raven, 1996.

2.10.1 HERPES SIMPLEX VIRUSES

Herpes viruses

- Large enveloped DNA viruses
- Complex genome allowing them to evade immune responses
- Latency leading to persistent infection
- Over 150 described but only 8 of clinical importance (Fig. 75)
- Gamma herpes viruses are oncogenic in immunosuppressed patients.

Herpes simplex virus types 1 and 2

HSV pathogenesis

The virus enters through mucosal surfaces and breaks in the skin. HSV-1 commonly enters through the buccal muosa and HSV-2 through genital mucosa, but they can invade either region causing local inflammation and vesicles. Virus attaches to and enters cutaneous sensory nerves followed by retrograde transport to the nucleus. Latency is established without expression of viral proteins, which means that immune responses are unable to detect these cells. Virus may then re-emerge causing recurrent disease.

Epidemiology

HSV-1 and -2 are found worldwide, affecting over 70% of the population. Person-to-person transmission is by direct contact with no animal reservoir. HSV-2 has traditionally been considered a sexually transmitted disease but HSV-1 may also cause genital disease [1].

Diagnostic tests

This is largely clinical. Herpes-like virus particles can be readily detected by electron microscopy of vesicle fluid. Specific immunofluorescence will detect virally infected cells, e.g. from a vesicle base. PCR can distinguish between HSV-1 and -2. CSF PCR is both sensitive and specific in the

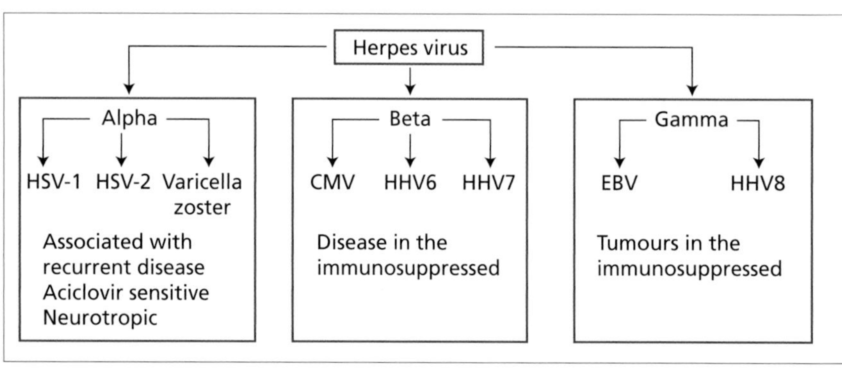

Fig. 75 Medically important herpes viruses. HSV, herpes simplex virus; CMV, cytomegalovirus; HHV, human herpes virus; EBV, Epstein–Barr virus.

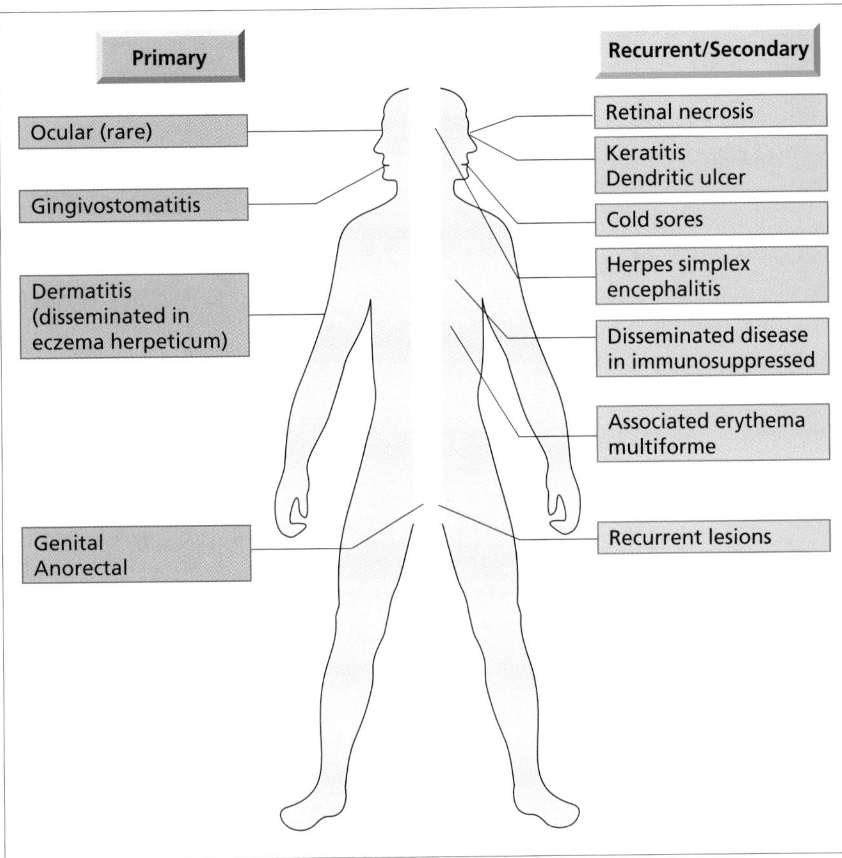

Fig. 76 Clinical manifestations of herpes simplex infection.

diagnosis of HSV encephalitis (see Section 1.15, p. 40). Serology may confirm exposure but plays little role in disease diagnosis.

Disease syndromes

Most primary infections in childhood are mild or asymptomatic. In addition, there are a variety of clinical syndromes associated with primary or recurrent disease (Fig. 76).

Complications

The most severe of these are the following:

- Acute retinal necrosis
- Herpes simplex encephalitis (see Section 1.15, p. 39)
- Neonatal encephalitis if the mother has active genital herpes at delivery
- Postherpetic erythema multiforme
- Radiculopathy in immunocompromised patients.

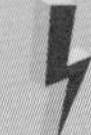

Eczema herpeticum is a severe disseminated form of HSV in patients with underlying eczema. It is frequently misdiagnosed at presentation as vesicles are often not visible.

Therapy

Aciclovir and related drugs (valaciclovir, famciclovir) may be used in either acute treatment or prevention of recurrent disease. High-dose intravenous aciclovir is required for treatment for encephalitis or severe disease in the immunocompromised [2].

1 Stanberry L, Cunningham A, Mertz G *et al.* New developments in the epidemiology, natural history and management of genital herpes. *Antiviral Res* 1999; 42: 1–14.

2 Keating MR. Antiviral agents for non-human immunodeficiency virus infections. *Mayo Clin Proc* 1999; 74: 1266–1283.

2.10.2 VARICELLA-ZOSTER VIRUS

Epidemiology

There is ubiquitous distribution with most people acquiring primary disease as a child. After primary infection the virus enters latency in the sensory dorsal root ganglion, leading to a life-long risk of reactivation disease.

Diagnostic tests

The clinical picture allows accurate diagnosis and supportive tests are not needed in uncomplicated disease. Serology can establish past exposure and risk of primary infection (see Section 1.19, p. 50). Viral culture, immunofluorescence and PCR are useful in some circumstances.

Disease syndromes and complications

Primary

Infection enters through the respiratory tract and is clinically silent for 2–3 weeks. A brief 'prodrome' (fever, headache) is followed by eruption of a blistering rash starting on the face and trunk. Lesions are sparse on the limbs but may occur on the mouth and palate. Vesicles come in crops, turn into pustules and then crust. When all lesions are crusted the patient is considered non-infectious. Pneumonia, hepatitis or encephalitis may complicate primary infection, particularly in the immunocompromised.

Secondary

Herpes zoster (shingles) occurs in a dermatomal distribution (Fig. 77), heralded by pain. A few vesicles may be seen elsewhere but extensive spread suggests immunodeficiency. Postherpetic neuralgia and ocular involvement are the main complications in people with normal immunity [1]. Disseminated disease, retinal necrosis and transverse myelitis may occur in immunocompromised individuals.

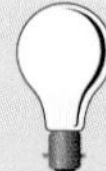

Postherpetic neuralgia

- More common as age increases, rare under 50
- More frequent with facial zoster
- May be reduced by early antiviral therapy
- Acute pain helped by amitriptyline.

Therapy

Aciclovir, valaciclovir and famciclovir are all active.

Primary

Uncomplicated primary infection does not need treatment, but high-dose aciclovir is indicated in varicella pneumonia, in immunocompromised individuals and pregnant women (see Section 1.19, p. 50). Zoster-immune globulin (ZIG) can be used to prevent infection in vulnerable hosts but is ineffective in treating active disease.

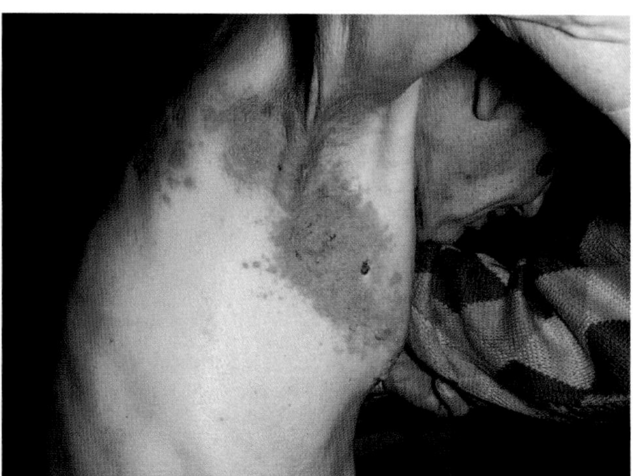

Fig. 77 Typical dermatomal distribution of herpes zoster.

Secondary

In herpes zoster antiviral therapy should be considered within the first 72 h if there is a high risk of postherpetic neuralgia. All patients with ocular disease and those who are immunocompromised should be treated.

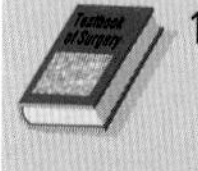

1 Snoeck R, Andrei G, De Clercq E. Current pharmacological approaches to the therapy of varicella zoster virus infections: a guide to treatment. *Drugs* 1999; 57: 187–206.

2.10.3 CYTOMEGALOVIRUS

Epidemiology

There is ubiquitous distribution with most people acquiring primary disease as a child. Seroprevalence in the UK population is around 65%, higher in at-risk groups including gay men. The main burden of disease is in immunocompromised individuals [1].

Diagnostic tests

Primary disease is diagnosed serologically (IgM). Recurrence is diagnosed by a mixture of clinical suspicion and detection of virus by PCR or direct antigen detection in blood, or more formally by histology of infected tissue. Fetal infection is associated with excretion of virus in the urine.

Disease syndromes and complications

Primary CMV infection is often silent, but may cause a 'glandular fever'-type illness, including hepatitis. The most significant consequences of infection are in severely immunosuppressed individuals, e.g. organ and bone-marrow transplant recipients and those with HIV infection.

Severe primary infection may result if a seropositive organ is given to a seronegative donor (see Section 1.17, p. 44). CMV reactivation in transplant recipients may present with diffuse disease affecting the gut, lungs, liver or CNS.

In AIDS the virus replicates widely with the principal syndromes of retinitis, gastrointestinal disease and encephalitis (see Section 1.27, p. 68).

Congenital infection may complicate primary CMV during pregnancy, resulting in fetal malformations.

Therapy

Disease in immunosuppressed people is usually treated with intravenous ganciclovir or foscarnet (see Section 1.27, p. 68). Therapy will not eradicate disease while the patient remains immunocompromised and increasing antiviral resistance may be encountered.

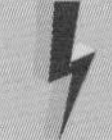

Adverse reactions to foscarnet

- Hypocalcaemia, hypomagnesaemia
- Renal failure
- Penile ulceration.

1 Sia IG, Patel R. New strategies for prevention and therapy of cytomegalovirus infection and disease in solid-organ transplant recipients. *Clin Microbiol Rev* 2000; 13: 83–121.

2.10.4 EPSTEIN–BARR VIRUS

Epidemiology

Epstein–Barr virus is distributed worldwide, but there are variations in the prevalence of EBV-related disease, particularly malignancy.

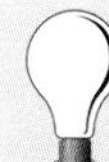

EBV-associated malignancy

- Burkitt's lymphoma in Africa
- Nasopharyngeal carcinoma in the Far East
- Non-Hodgkin's B-cell lymphoma in immunocompromised individuals.

Diagnostic tests

Serology is the mainstay of diagnosis (see Section 1.13, p. 33). The Paul–Bunnell (or Monospot) test provides a rapid diagnosis that can be confirmed with measurement of a specific EBV IgM. CSF PCR for EBV is often positive in AIDS-related cerebral lymphoma.

Disease syndromes and complications

Infection in childhood is usually asymptomatic, but 'glandular fever' commonly complicates infection in adolescence or adult life. Other manifestations of EBV are shown in Fig. 78 [1].

Therapy

Epstein–Barr virus is poorly sensitive to current antiviral agents. Specific therapy is rarely required, although corticosteroids are sometimes used in severe pharyngitis or hepatitis.

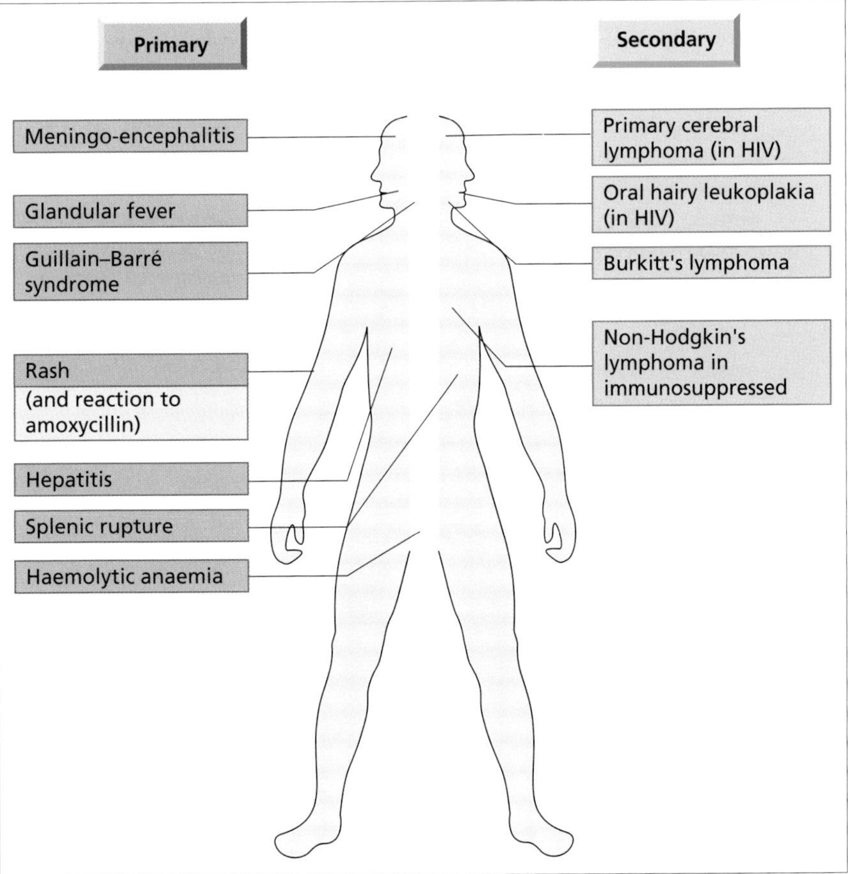

Fig. 78 Epstein–Barr virus-related disease.

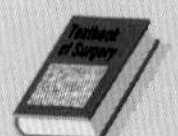

1 Faulkner GC, Krajewski AS, Crawford DH. The ins and outs of EBV infection. *Trends Microbiol* 2000; 8: 185–189.

2.10.5 HUMAN HERPES VIRUSES 6 AND 7

Epidemiology

These are very widespread viruses, affecting almost the entire population. They infect T cells and establish life-long latency [1].

Diagnostic tests

Specific diagnostic tests are not usually required. PCR can detect the virus and serology past exposure.

Disease syndromes

• Herpes virus 6 (HHV6) causes roseola infantum (exanthem subitum) in infants. HHV6 has been linked with multiple sclerosis, although a causal relationship is not proven. HHV7 causes a similar disease, but less commonly.
• Reactivation of both viruses has been described in immunosuppressed people, but their role in disease is not understood.

Therapy

None is currently available.

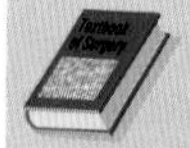

1 Clark DA. Human herpesvirus 6. *Rev Med Virol* 2000; 10: 155–173.

2.10.6 HUMAN HERPES VIRUS 8

Epidemiology

Human herpes virus 8 (HHV8) is also known as Kaposi's sarcoma-associated herpes virus (KSHV). It is found worldwide and is mainly of interest by association with certain malignancies [1].

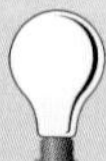

Kaposi's sarcoma

• Elderly Mediterranean men, usually on the lower leg
• Severe cell-mediated immunosuppression, e.g. AIDS or transplantation
• Endemic form in Africa.

Diagnostic tests

HHV8-associated malignancies are suspected clinically and confirmed on histology. Serological tests and PCR have been used in research.

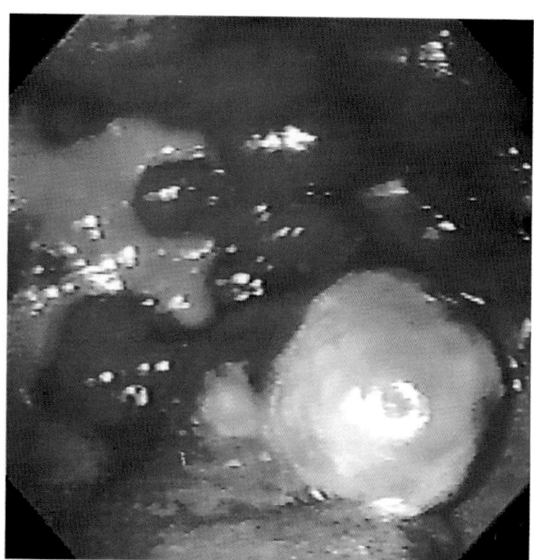

Fig. 79 Kaposi's sarcoma in the stomach of a patient with AIDS and a CD4 count of 10 cell/μL. Partial remission was induced with chemotherapy and antiretroviral therapy was started. Four years later, the Kaposi's sarcoma is in complete remission without chemotherapy and CD4 count is over 300 cells/μL.

Disease syndromes

HHV8 is associated with three tumours:
1 Kaposi's sarcoma, most commonly on the skin (see Section 1.28, p. 70), but may involve the lung or gut
2 Primary effusion lymphoma (a rare B-cell lymphoma in AIDS)
3 Multicentric Castleman's disease.

Therapy

• No specific antiviral therapy, although aciclovir and ganciclovir have anti-HHV8 activity
• Chemotherapy is used to control the malignancy but long-term remission can be achieved only by improving immunological function (Fig. 79).

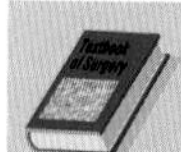

1 Levy JA. Three new human herpesviruses (HHV6, 7, and 8). *Lancet* 1997; 349: 558–563.

2.10.7 PARVOVIRUS

Epidemiology

Parvovirus B19 is a DNA virus and the only parvovirus known to infect humans. A related DNA virus, transfusion transmitted virus (TTV), is not clearly associated with any clinical syndrome and is almost universally carried.

Diagnostic tests

Parvovirus is diagnosed clinically but may be confirmed (and distinguished from rubella) by detection of IgM.

Table 65 Important features of hepatitis viruses.

Virus	Genome	Diagnosis	Hepatitis	Complications	Therapy
HAV	RNA	HAV IgM	Acute	Fulminant hepatic failure (rare)	Supportive
HBV	DNA	HBsAg and HBeAg detect active viral replication	Acute	Fulminant hepatic failure	Supportive
		HB core IgM first detectable antibody	Chronic	Hepatoma Cirrhosis	Interferon-α + lamivudine
HCV	RNA	Serology, PCR to detect viraemia	Chronic	Hepatoma Cirrhosis Cryoglobulinaemia Glomerulonephritis Porphyria cutanea tarda	Interferon-α + ribavirin
HDV	RNA (viroid)	HDV IgM	Acute in patients with active HBV	Cirrhosis	As for HBV
HEV	RNA	HEV IgM	Acute	Fulminant hepatic failure in pregnancy	Supportive

HAV, hepatitis A virus; HBV, hepatitis B virus; HCV, hepatitis C virus; HDV, hepatitis D virus; HBsAg, hepatitis B surface antigen; HBeAg, hepatitis B 'e' antigen.

Parvovirus DNA can be directly identified by hybridization in blood from chronically infected, immunocompromised patients.

Disease syndromes

- Infection with parvovirus B19 in childhood is usually subclinical, but may cause an acute illness characterized by a high fever and bright red face—'slapped cheek disease'. Other, less common disease syndromes are related to decreased red blood cell production as a result of the effects of parvovirus on the bone marrow [1]:
- Arthritis: in adults pain, swelling and stiffness of the small joints often complicate parvovirus B19. There is no clear evidence that this is associated with chronic rheumatological disease.
- Red cell crises (severe anaemia) in those with compromised red cell production (e.g. sickle cell).
- Chronic anaemia in severely immunosuppressed patients.
- Transplacental infection can cause hydrops foetalis and fetal loss.

Therapy

Treatment is supportive in most cases; intravenous immunoglobulin (IVIG) may benefit immunocompromised patients with chronic infection.

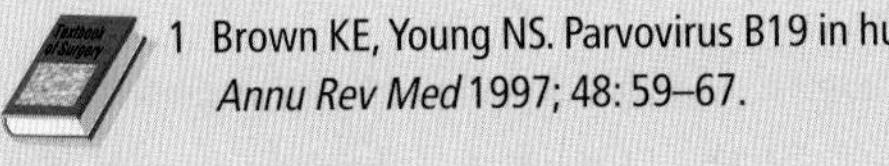

1 Brown KE, Young NS. Parvovirus B19 in human disease. *Annu Rev Med* 1997; 48: 59–67.

2.10.8 HEPATITIS VIRUSES

Description of the organism

Although linked to similar clinical syndromes, virologically these are quite distinct (Table 65).

Epidemiology

These viruses cause very common human infections:

- Faecal–oral transmission: hepatitis A (HAV) is endemic throughout the world, with prevalence closely related to standards of sanitation. Hepatitis E (HEV) is mainly found in the developing world where it is responsible for both endemic and epidemic jaundice.
- Body fluid transmission: over a third of the world's population has been infected with hepatitis B (HBV), predominantly acquired through heterosexual contact or vertical transmission. The global prevalence of hepatitis C (HCV) is unknown, but estimated at 200 million. Approximately 1.7% of the population of the USA are infected and around 0.1–0.2% of people presenting to donate blood in the UK.

See Section 1.23 and *Gastroenterology and hepatology*, Sections 2.9 and 2.10.

Diagnostic tests

Serology is the mainstay of making a specific diagnosis in viral hepatitis (see Table 65). PCR detection and quantification of viraemia is being increasingly used to guide management in chronic HBV and HCV. (See *Gastroenterology and hepatology*, Section 2.10.)

Hepatitis B serology

In acute disease hepatitis B surface antigen (HBsAg) is present and accompanied by IgM antibodies (to core). Patients presenting with such serology should be followed to watch for the disappearance of HBsAg.

In chronic carriage, HBsAg persists and may be either:

• high level, in which case it is accompanied by hepatitis B 'e' antigen (HBeAg), or

• low level, in which case HBeAg is absent (and HBe antibody is detected).

Hepatitis B precore mutants

• Fail to make HBe antigen

• Infectivity and disease progression are similar to HBeAg-positive patients

• Rare in the UK, but increasingly common worldwide

• Diagnosis requires quantification of HBV DNA.

Treatment

In general treatment of acute disease is supportive. Specific antiviral therapy for chronic hepatitis (see Table 65) may clear some but by no means all patients [1,2]. (See *Gastroenterology and hepatology*, Section 2.10.)

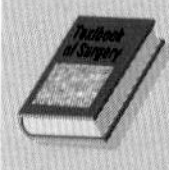

1 Torresi J, Locarnini S. Antiviral chemotherapy for the treatment of hepatitis B virus infections. *Gastroenterology* 2000; 118: S83–103.

2 Davis GL. Current therapy for chronic hepatitis C. *Gastroenterology* 2000; 118: S104–114.

2.10.9 INFLUENZA VIRUS

Description of the organism

Influenza is an RNA virus organized as shown schematically in Fig. 80. Three serogroups—A, B and C—are responsible for human disease [1].

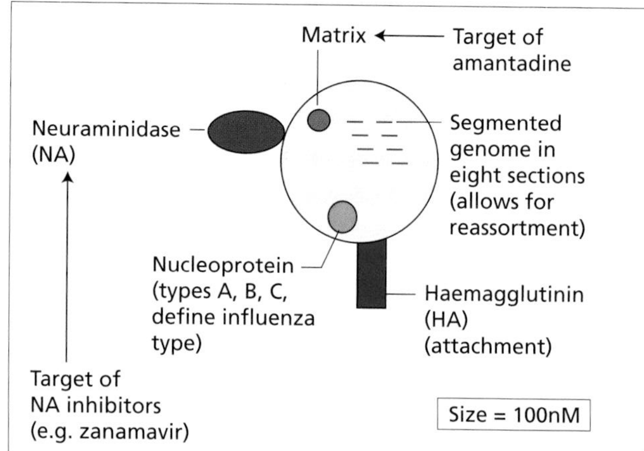

Fig. 80 Schematic representation of influenza. HA, haemagglutinin; NA, neuraminidase.

Epidemiology

Influenza A and B cause disease sporadically, in epidemics or pandemics. Influenza A appears to be the more virulent strain and is linked most closely to mortality from influenza. Influenza C causes mild endemic disease. The virus can evolve through small mutations ('drift') associated with partial loss of herd immunity and, in a more dramatic way, by reassorting its segmented genome ('shift'), leading to complete loss of herd immunity and the potential for a pandemic.

Diagnostic tests

Diagnosis is predominantly clinical, aided by the demonstration of a rise in antibody titres or direct immunofluorescence or culture of virus.

Disease syndromes and complications

In most cases these infections are self-limiting, but significant morbidity and mortality occurs in elderly people, those with underlying lung disease and immunocompromised individuals. There is no systemic spread of the virus and, in most cases, severe complications are the result of secondary bacterial pneumonia, particularly pneumococci and *Staph. aureus*.

Therapy

Treatment is symptomatic. Prophylaxis and treatment with amantidine are effective but rarely used. The neuraminidase inhibitor zanamavir is the first of a new class of specific anti-influenza agents. Zanamavir is highly effective, but only when started within the first 36 h of symptoms. It reduces the duration of fever on average only by about 1 day, and so its widespread use has not been recommended [2]. The National Institute for Clinical Excellence (NICE) has issued guidance on the use of Zanamavir in vulnerable groups in the UK [3].

1 Zambon MC. Epidemiology and pathogenesis of influenza. *J Antimicrob Chemother* 1999; 44(suppl B): 3–9.

2 Colman PM. A novel approach to antiviral therapy for influenza. *J Antimicrob Chemother* 1999; 44(suppl B): 17–22.

3 http://www.nice.org.uk/pdf/NiceZANAMIVAR15guidance.pdf

2.10.10 PARAMYXOVIRUSES

Description of the organism

Paramyxoviruses are RNA viruses, including measles, mumps and respiratory syncytial virus (RSV).

Epidemiology

Measles and mumps are now much less common in the UK as a result of effective immunization, but worldwide measles remains an important disease with high morbidity and mortality in young children. RSV is a common respiratory pathogen in children and elderly people, for which there is no effective vaccine. RSV also has the potential to cause severe outbreaks within paediatric units.

Diagnostic tests

Clinical diagnosis is very unreliable as a result of the non-specific rashes and the overlap with other viral infections. Mumps virus can be isolated from saliva, but measles and mumps are usually confirmed serologically. RSV may be rapidly identified directly from a nasopharyngeal aspirate or bronchial lavage by immunofluorescence.

Disease syndromes

Measles

Measles classically has two phases:
1 Pre-eruptive: associated with fever, coryza, conjunctivitis and Koplik's spots (grey on a red base opposite the second molar).
2 Eruptive: associated with a maculopapular rash especially over the face, becoming confluent.

Systemic spread involving many organs, but especially the lungs, may occur. Measles may be complicated acutely by bacterial infection and late complications include subacute sclerosing panencephalitis (SSPE).

Mumps

Mumps causes parotid swelling and, rarely, meningitis or encephalitis, orchitis and pancreatitis.

Respiratory syncytial virus

RSV is associated with upper and lower respiratory tract infection. Most infections are mild. Severe and sometimes fatal disease may be seen in neonates, very young children and the immunocompromised adult [1].

Therapy

Therapy is supportive in most cases.
• Vitamin A supplementation is considered of benefit for malnourished children with measles.
• RSV is sensitive to ribavirin, which can be administered via a small particle nebulizer for severe disease in neonates or the immunocompromised individual. Specific anti-RSV antibody may also have a role in paediatric practice.

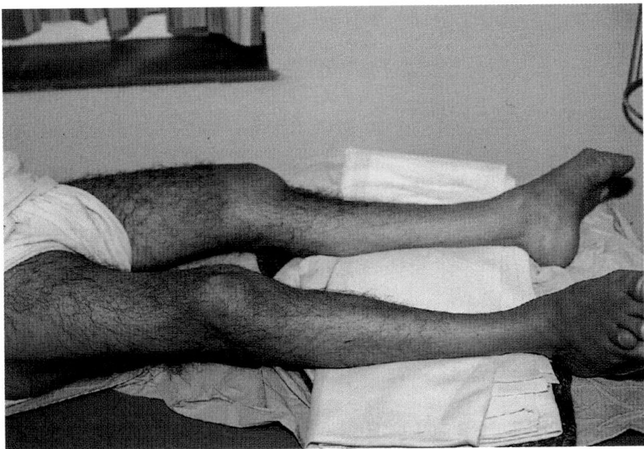

Fig. 81 Severe wasting and shortening of the legs as a result of childhood polio.

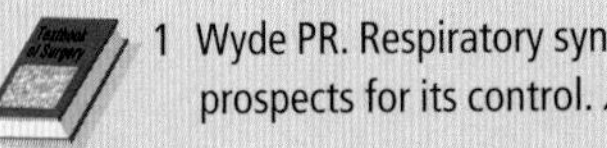

1 Wyde PR. Respiratory syncytial virus (RSV) disease and prospects for its control. *Antiviral Res* 1998; 39: 63–79.

2.10.11 ENTEROVIRUSES

Description of the organism

This is a very large group of related RNA viruses (family of picornaviruses). Poliovirus (Fig. 81), previously the most important organism in this group, is heading towards global eradication following a WHO immunization programme.

Enteroviruses enter the body via the gastrointestinal tract and are spread by the faecal–oral route. Despite the name, they are generally associated with mucosal, neurological, muscular or cardiac disease rather than diarrhoea.

Diagnostic tests

Enteroviruses may be cultured from stool early in an acute infection. Diagnosis is often serological but there is much crossreactivity in this group. PCR is being increasingly used, e.g. of the CSF in meningitis.

Disease syndromes

A wide variety of illnesses has been associated with enteroviruses (Fig. 82).

Therapy

No specific antiviral therapy is available. Immunization against polio has dramatically decreased global disease.

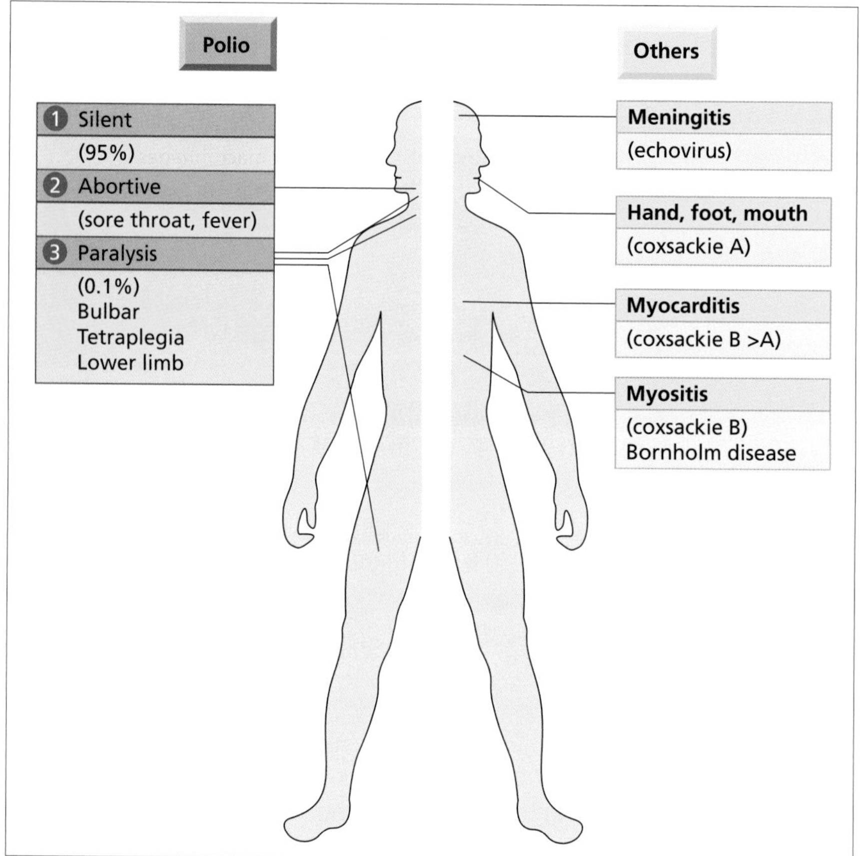

Fig. 82 Diseases associated with enteroviruses.

Prevention of exposure within families relies on good hygiene and is particularly important when there is a newborn in the house because infection may be very severe.

2.11 Human immunodeficiency virus

Description of the organism

Human immunodeficiency virus (HIV) is a retrovirus (family of lentiviruses) [1]. Retroviruses are RNA viruses that replicate by converting RNA into DNA using the enzyme reverse transcriptase. The HIV virion contains two strands of RNA stabilized by packaging proteins and surrounded by a lipid membrane (Fig. 83).

Surface proteins

Glycoproteins Gp120 and Gp41 are important polymorphic proteins involved in attachment and entry into target cells. Gp120 binds to CD4 and Gp41 interacts with chemokine receptors (such as CCR5) to mediate cell entry (Fig. 84).

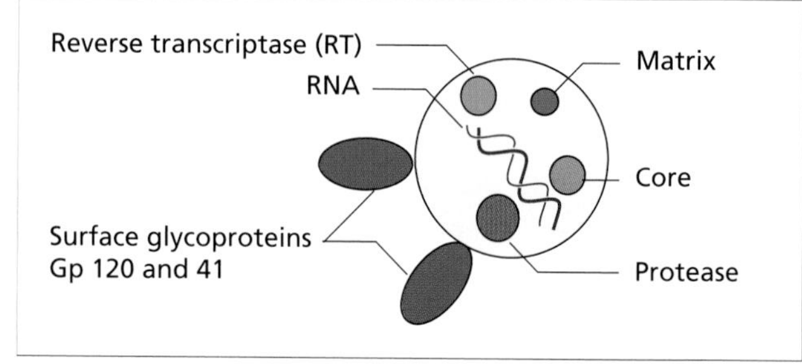

Fig. 83 Schematic representation of components of an HIV virion.

Core proteins

P24 antigen and matrix (p17) are involved in packaging HIV RNA and transporting to the nucleus.

HIV RNA

RNA is present within the virion in two linear strands. HIV RNA is highly polymorphic as a result of its high turnover rate, accompanied by lack of 'proofreading capacity' of the viral reverse transcriptase enzyme. This degree of variation means that HIV exists as a swarm of closely related strains or 'quasi-species'.

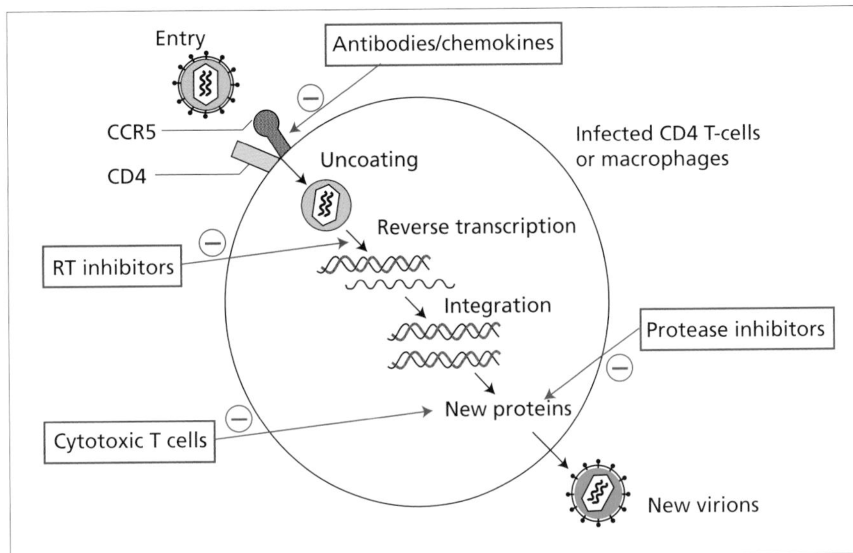

Fig. 84 HIV replication cycle showing sites where replication can be blocked by the immune system or drugs.

Reverse transcriptase

This enzyme is required for the transformation of viral RNA into double-stranded DNA. The active site of this enzyme is conserved between retroviruses and is a major therapeutic target.

Protease and integrase

Protease is required for maturation of the viral particle after release. Particles in which protease is inactivated are not infectious. Integrase is essential for integration of HIV DNA into the host genome.

Regulatory genes

HIV encodes genes (importantly *tat* and *nef*) for regulatory proteins that control upregulation of transcription and virulence. *Nef*-deficient viruses are less pathogenic in animal models and human infection.

Epidemiology

Over 36 million people are living with HIV/AIDS infection with the highest burden in sub-Saharan Africa [2]. In the UK, there have been over 35 000 reported cases and approximately 15 000 deaths related to HIV infection. HIV is spread through sex, needle sharing, blood products and from mother to child.

Diagnostic tests

HIV antibody tests

Serology forms the basis of detecting HIV infection. Following a seroconversion illness, antibody is usually detectable by ELISA within 2–4 weeks (see Section 1.24, p. 61). However, serology may remain negative for up to 3 months, particularly after asymptomatic primary infection.

P24 antigen

This antigen is detectable in high levels by ELISA during HIV seroconversion. In stable disease P24 assays were used to monitor disease but have been supplanted by PCR.

Polymerase chain reaction

Several methods are available to amplify and quantify plasma and cell-associated HIV nucleic acid. Current generation tests can detect as few as 20–50 copies of HIV RNA/mL. The level of the HIV circulating viral load (VL) can predict the rate of disease progression and is used to monitor therapy. (See Sections 1.28, p. 70 and 1.29, p. 73.)

HIV resistance testing

By amplifying and sequencing the reverse transcriptase and protease genes, it is possible to detect mutations associated with resistance to antiretroviral drugs [3].

Immunological function

The CD4 T-lymphocyte count is assayed by flow cytometry.

Disease syndromes

Pathogenesis of AIDS

HIV causes acquired immune deficiency syndrome (AIDS) through infection of CD4-positive T lymphocytes and macrophages, leading to immunological deterioration and increased susceptibility to infections.

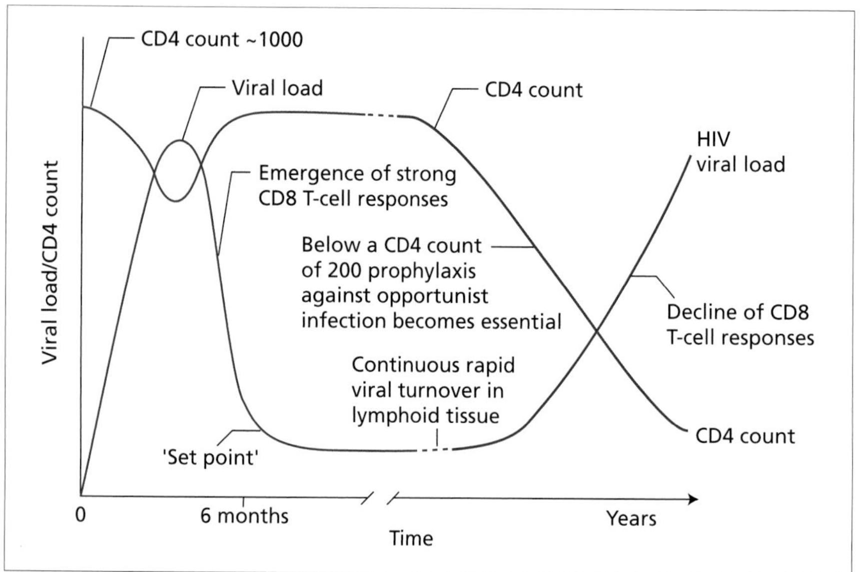

Fig. 85 Host immune response and progression of HIV disease.

Life cycle of the virus

An overview of the HIV replication cycle is shown in Fig. 84.

CELL ENTRY

HIV enters cells through specific surface receptors, including the chemokine receptors CCR5 (macrophages) and CXCR4 (lymphocytes). Patients with polymorphisms in CCR5 show protection against infection and also slower progression to AIDS [4]. CD4 acts as a co-receptor increasing the susceptibility of CD4-positive cells. Dendritic cells play a key role in transferring infectious virions from the mucosae to lymphoid organs.

TURNOVER

Once in the cell, the virus is reverse transcribed by its own reverse transcriptase, integrated and may either remain latent if the cell is quiescent, or start to replicate. Once replicating, the turnover of the virus is very fast (half-life of 8 h in the blood), and most infected cells die rapidly. A small proportion of cells may remain dormant, containing latent proviral DNA.

HOST IMMUNE RESPONSE

After infection, cytotoxic T lymphocytes are the most important component of the host response [5]. These kill infected cells and secrete chemokines which block infection through CCR5. Cytotoxic T lymphocytes recognize infected cells through peptides presented by HLA class I molecules, and the HLA type of the patient affects the progression of infection. Antibody responses are present but less effective as a result of the variability in HIV GP120.

COURSE OF DISEASE

Primary HIV infection is accompanied by a clinical 'seroconversion illness' or 'acute retroviral syndrome' (fever, lymphadenopathy, rash ± meningism) in 30–70% (see Section 1.24, p. 61). After acute infection, the HIV viral load is controlled to a set point, which determines the subsequent rate of disease progression (Fig. 85). A minority of patients control HIV to below detectable levels and remain stable for many years without a decline in CD4 count. At some point, most patients suffer a decline in CD4 count and a rise in viral load. Why the immune response ultimately fails to control the virus is not understood.

Complications of HIV/AIDS

Complications may be the result of opportunistic infection, malignancy or the direct effect of HIV on organ function (Fig. 86). Opportunistic infections relate to the degree of immunosuppression and environmental exposure (e.g. *Penicillium marneffei* in south-east Asia). Effective combination ART may lead to 'immune reconstitution' and reduce the risks of infection.

Therapy

Antiretroviral therapy

The principles of how to select and use antiretroviral drugs are described in Sections 1.28, p. 70 and 1.29, p. 73. There are three current drug classes (Fig. 87) targeting two key HIV enzymes [6,7]:

- Reverse transcriptase inhibitors
- Protease inhibitors.

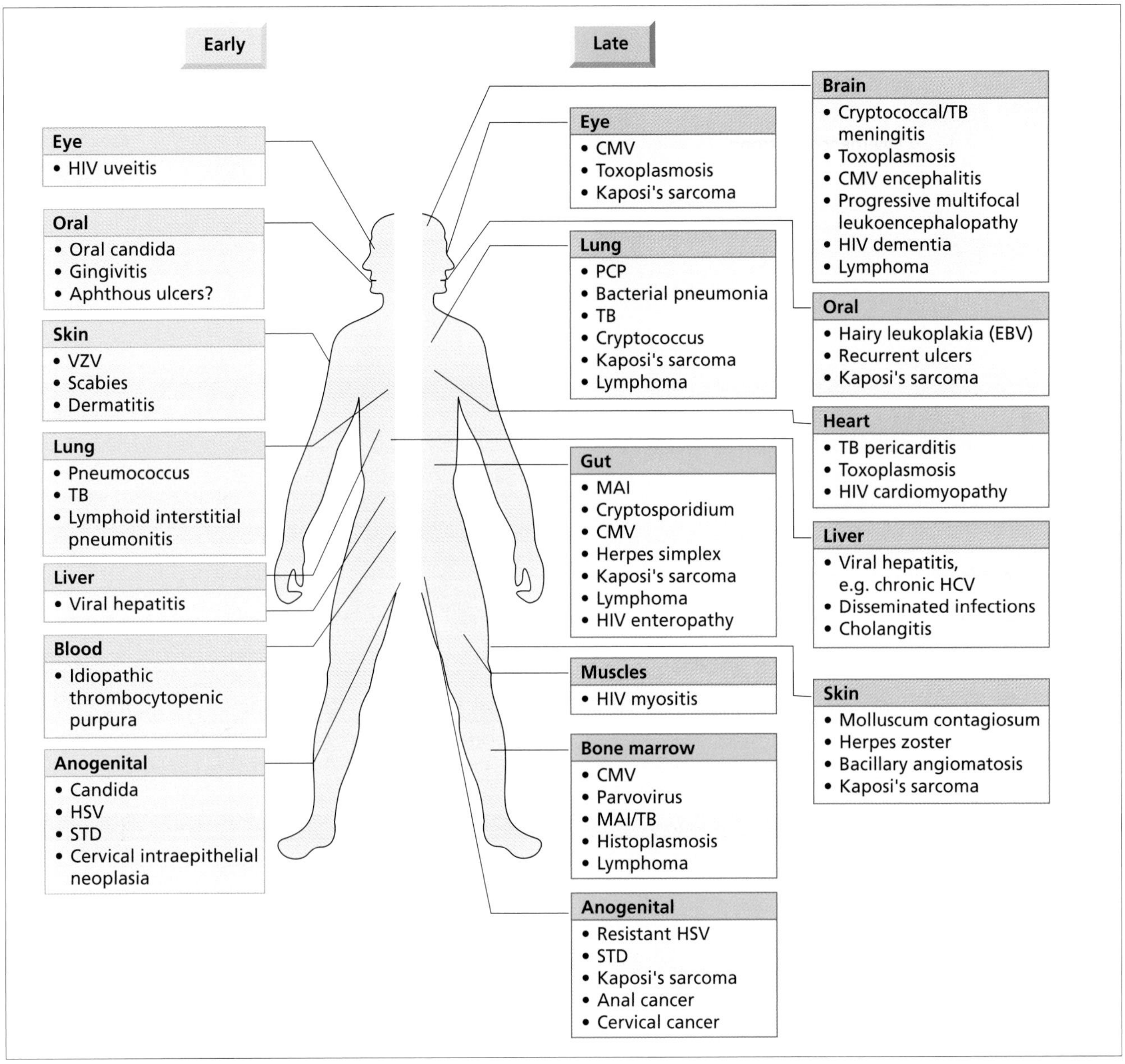

Early

Eye
- HIV uveitis

Oral
- Oral candida
- Gingivitis
- Aphthous ulcers?

Skin
- VZV
- Scabies
- Dermatitis

Lung
- Pneumococcus
- TB
- Lymphoid interstitial pneumonitis

Liver
- Viral hepatitis

Blood
- Idiopathic thrombocytopenic purpura

Anogenital
- Candida
- HSV
- STD
- Cervical intraepithelial neoplasia

Late

Eye
- CMV
- Toxoplasmosis
- Kaposi's sarcoma

Lung
- PCP
- Bacterial pneumonia
- TB
- Cryptococcus
- Kaposi's sarcoma
- Lymphoma

Gut
- MAI
- Cryptosporidium
- CMV
- Herpes simplex
- Kaposi's sarcoma
- Lymphoma
- HIV enteropathy

Muscles
- HIV myositis

Bone marrow
- CMV
- Parvovirus
- MAI/TB
- Histoplasmosis
- Lymphoma

Anogenital
- Resistant HSV
- STD
- Kaposi's sarcoma
- Anal cancer
- Cervical cancer

Brain
- Cryptococcal/TB meningitis
- Toxoplasmosis
- CMV encephalitis
- Progressive multifocal leukoencephalopathy
- HIV dementia
- Lymphoma

Oral
- Hairy leukoplakia (EBV)
- Recurrent ulcers
- Kaposi's sarcoma

Heart
- TB pericarditis
- Toxoplasmosis
- HIV cardiomyopathy

Liver
- Viral hepatitis, e.g. chronic HCV
- Disseminated infections
- Cholangitis

Skin
- Molluscum contagiosum
- Herpes zoster
- Bacillary angiomatosis
- Kaposi's sarcoma

Fig. 86 Complications of HIV infection. VZV, varicella-zoster virus; TB, tuberculosis; HSV, herpes simplex virus; STD, sexually transmitted disease; PCP, *Pneumocystis carinii* pneumonia; CMV, cytomegalovirus; HCV, hepatitis C virus.

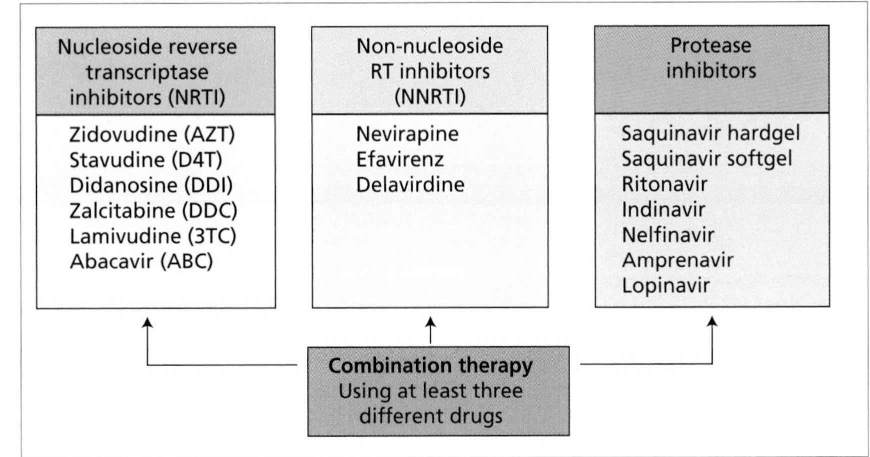

Fig. 87 Drugs currently available in the UK for the treatment of HIV. Zidovudine (AZT) and stavudine (D4T) should not be combined because of antagonism. RT, reverse transcriptase.

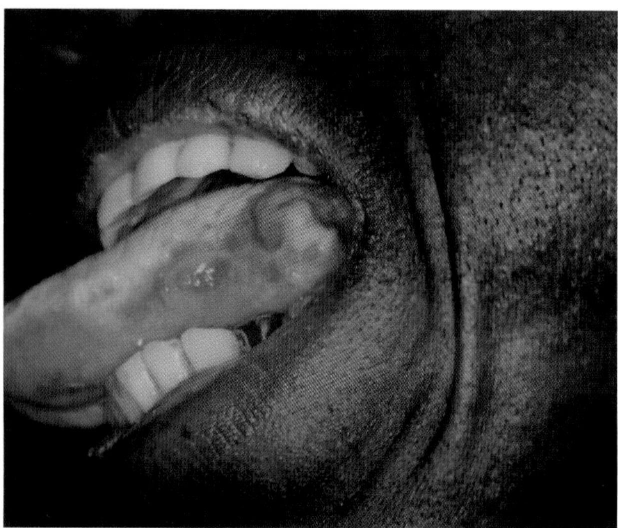

Fig. 88 Severe mouth ulcers caused by zalcitabine.

Table 66 Adverse effects of antiretroviral drugs.

Class	Side effects	Drugs
NRTI	Bone marrow suppression	AZT, 3TC
	Nail discoloration	AZT
	Peripheral neuropathy	D4T, DDC DDI (less commonly)
	Mouth ulcers (Fig. 88)	DDC
	Pancreatitis	DDI
	Lactic acidosis and hepatic steatosis [8]	Probably all
	Lipodystrophy	Probably all
	Hypersensitivity	ABC
NNRTI	Hypersensitivity	All agents
	Hepatic failure	
	Vivid dreams and psychological disturbances	Efavirenz
PI	Renal stones, nephropathy	Indinavir
	Gastrointestinal Lipodystrophy [9] Diabetes mellitus Lipid abnormalities Ingrowing toenails Impotence	All agents

AZT, zidovudine; 3TC, lamivudine; D4T, stavudine; DDC, zalcitabine; DDI, didanosine; ABC, abacavir; NRTI, nucleoside reverse transcriptase inhibitors; NNRTI, non-nucleoside reverse transcriptase inhibitors; PI, protease inhibitors.

In the near future, additional drugs may become available that inhibit HIV integrase or are targeted at viral entry into cells (chemokine receptor blockers). Anti-HIV drugs are toxic and patients require close monitoring for side effects (Fig. 88; Table 66).

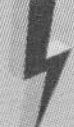

Hypersensitivity to abacavir (approx. 3%)

- Rash uncommon
- Fever, myalgia and abdominal pain
- May be fatal on rechallenge
- Warn patients.

Immunotherapy

Following successful anti-HIV therapy the CD4 count may rise, but in some patients it remains <200 cells/mL placing them at risk of opportunistic infections. Interleukin 2 (IL2), given subcutaneously, is recommended for this group. The role of IL2 in patients with higher CD4 cell counts is being investigated.

Prophylaxis

To prevent the predictable emergence of opportunistic infections as disease progresses, there are various strategies for prophylaxis (Fig. 89). After a robust response to antiviral therapy it may be possible to discontinue some prophylaxis, although the experience with this is limited.

Vigilance is required to detect and treat infectious and non-infectious complications of HIV (Fig. 90).

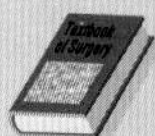

1 Daar ES. Virology and immunology of acute HIV type 1 infection. *AIDS Res Hum Retroviruses* 1998; 14(suppl 3): S229–234.
2 Padian N, Buve A. AIDS 1999. Epidemiology: overview. *AIDS* 1999; 13(suppl A): S59–60.
3 Harrigan PR, Cote HC. Clinical utility of testing human immunodeficiency virus for drug resistance. *Clin Infect Dis* 2000; 30(suppl 2): S117–122.
4 Michael N, Lovie LG, Rohrbaugh AL *et al.* The role of CCR5 and CCR2 polymorphism in HIV-1 transmission and disease progression. *Nature Med* 1997; 3: 1160–1162.
5 Price DA, O'Callaghan CA, Whelan JA *et al.* Cytotoxic T lymphocytes and viral evolution in primary HIV-1 infection. *Clin Sci* 1999; 97: 707–718.
6 Harrington M, Carpenter CC. Hit HIV-1 hard, but only when necessary. *Lancet* 2000; 355: 2147–2152.
7 Flexner C. HIV-protease inhibitors. *N Engl J Med* 1998; 338: 1281–1292.
8 Miller KD, Cameron M, Wood LV *et al.* Lactic acidosis and hepatic steatosis associated with use of stavudine: report of four cases. *Ann Intern Med* 2000; 133: 192–196.
9 Carr A. HIV protease inhibitor-related lipodystrophy syndrome. *Clin Infect Dis* 2000; 30(suppl 2): S135–142.

2.12 Travel-related viruses

2.12.1 RABIES

Description of the organism

Rabies is an RNA virus belonging to the family Rhabdoviridae [1]. Most human infections are from dog bites. The virus travels retrogradely along peripheral nerves to the CNS, where viral replication occurs causing fatal meningoencephalitis.

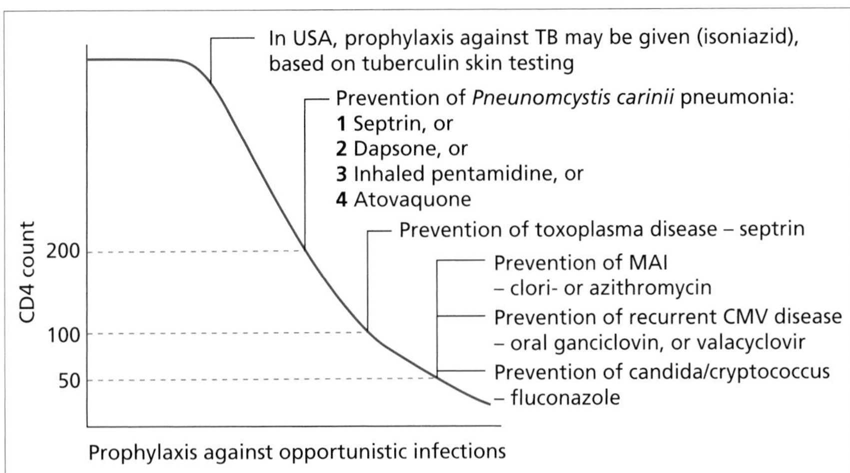

Fig. 89 Prophylaxis and immune function in HIV.

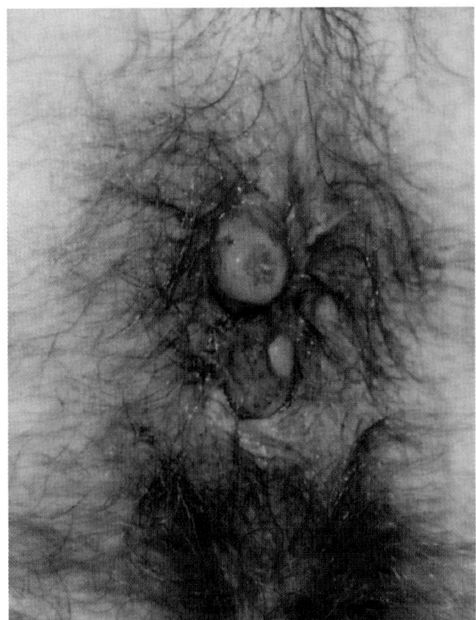

Fig. 90 Early anal carcinoma complicating HIV infection.

Epidemiology

Rabies is a zoonosis and remains endemic in most parts of the world. Exceptions include the British Isles, most of Scandinavia and Oceania. There are many thousands of human cases per year worldwide.

Diagnostic tests

- If possible, the brain of the suspect animal is examined for rabies antigen
- Detection of viral antigen in nerve endings in skin biopsy.

Disease syndromes and complications

Incubation period is usually between 20 and 90 days, but rarely can be very prolonged (up to several years). The incubation period tends to be shorter after bites on the face compared with bites on the limbs. Prodromal symptoms are common and include general malaise, fever, irritability and local symptoms (paraesthesiae, itching, pain) at the site of the healed bite wound.

- Furious rabies is the most common presentation and is caused by brainstem encephalitis. It is characterized by paroxysms of generalized arousal and terror and, in most cases, the diagnostic symptom of hydrophobia with inspiratory muscle and laryngeal spasm provoked by attempts to drink water. Within days, the patient lapses into a coma with generalized flaccid paralysis.
- Paralytic rabies is less common. It is characterized by ascending flaccid paralysis, usually starting in the bitten limb.

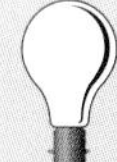

Rabies

- Any unexplained encephalitis in a person who has travelled in the past year
- Rabies risk in any returning traveller with an animal bite.

Therapy

Rabies encephalitis

Once the encephalitic stage is reached, rabies is almost universally fatal and intensive care is not generally recommended for confirmed cases. Only four cases of recovery have ever been documented. The prognosis is virtually hopeless.

Give sedation and analgesia and notify public health urgently.

Bite of a suspected rapid animal

Pre-exposure immunization does not obviate the need for postexposure prophylaxis, but shortens the course and increases efficacy. Start PEP as soon as possible after the bite:

- Clean wound
- Passive immunization with rabies immune globulin
- Active immunization with a course of rabies vaccine.

Postexposure prophylaxis can be stopped if either the suspect animal remains healthy for 10 days or the animal's brain is negative for rabies antigen.

1 Warrell MJ, Warrell DA. Rhabdovirus infections in man. In: Porterfield JS, Tyrell DAJ, (eds) *Handbook of Infectious Diseases*, Vol. 3, *Exotic Viral Infections*. London: Chapman & Hall Medical, 1995.

2.12.2 DENGUE

Description of the organism

Dengue viruses are RNA viruses belonging to the family Flaviviridae [1]. Dengue is transmitted from infected to susceptible humans by day-biting *Aedes aegypti* mosquitoes.

Epidemiology

Dengue is transmitted throughout the tropical and subtropical regions of the world. The most intense transmission occurs in south-east Asia, the Caribbean and central and southern America with areas of infection in West Africa. *Aedes aegypti* is found throughout the world and the dengue range is gradually extending with cases recently described in North America. There are approximately 100 million infections per year worldwide.

Diagnostic tests

- During the febrile phase: detection of viral genome by reverse transcriptase PCR (RT-PCR), or viral culture
- Retrospective diagnosis: paired serology.

Disease syndromes and complications

Dengue causes more illness and death than any other arboviral infection. After an incubation period of 5–10 days, there is sudden onset of fever, headache (often with retro-orbital pain) and severe myalgia. A faint, blanching maculopapular rash is often a clue to the diagnosis (see Section 1.20, p. 52). Typical laboratory findings are normal WCC, low platelets and mildly abnormal liver function.

In most cases, the illness resolves spontaneously after 5–7 days. A small proportion of cases develop bleeding and vascular leak (dengue haemorrhagic fever/dengue shock syndrome [DHF/DSS]).

Therapy

Treatment is symptomatic and supportive. DHF/DSS soon resolves if patients are supported appropriately. No special barrier precautions are needed. Viral haemorrhagic fevers are notifiable diseases.

1 Rigau-Perez JG, Clark GG, Gubler DJ *et al.* Dengue and dengue haemorrhagic fever. *Lancet* 1998; 352: 971.

2.12.3 ARBOVIRUS INFECTIONS

Description of the organism

More than 100 different arboviruses (arthropod-borne viruses) produce clinical and subclinical infection in humans [1]. They are transmitted by mosquitoes, ticks, sandflies and midges. They belong to many different virus families, but this classification is not of great importance to a clinician.

Epidemiology

Most arboviruses are zoonoses and infection in humans is accidental. For a few (e.g. dengue—Section 2.12.2, see above), humans are the principal source of virus amplification and infection. Arboviruses are transmitted in most parts of the world, but the distribution is often very localized. Sudden outbreaks may occur if the range of the animal host changes, bringing the infection to a new population.

Diagnostic tests

The diagnosis is usually made by serological testing, but there is much crossreactivity. PCR-based tests are more accurate for speciation but not readily available.

Disease syndromes

The incubation period is usually short (up to 10 days). There are four main clinical syndromes:

1 Acute, benign fever
2 Acute CNS disease: ranges from mild aseptic meningitis to encephalitis with coma and death
3 Haemorrhagic fevers
4 Polyarthritis and rash.

Therapy

- Symptomatic and supportive
- Standard barrier precautions
- Notify encephalitis or haemorrhagic fever to public health.

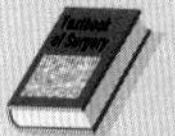

1 Benenson A, ed. *Control of Communicable Diseases in Man*, 14th edn. Washington: American Public Health Association, 1985.

2.13 Protozoan parasites

2.13.1 MALARIA

Description of the organism

Four parasite species that infect red blood cells cause human malaria. *Plasmodium falciparum* is the most important because it may cause rapidly progressive, life-threatening disease (see Section 1.20, p. 52). The other species (*P. vivax*, *P. ovale*, *P. malariae*) do not result in serious complications in most cases. Malaria is transmitted by anopheline mosquitoes, which bite at dusk and during the night.

Epidemiology

Malaria is the most important tropical disease and cause of fever in travellers. It is distributed throughout the tropical and subtropical regions of the world.

Diagnostic tests

• Thick film (see Section 3.2, p. 152) (Fig. 91): most sensitive, but speciation is difficult and parasitaemia cannot be assessed. Often not available outside reference laboratories.

• Thin film (see Section 3.2, p. 152) (Fig. 92): most widely used. Parasitaemia can be counted and species identification is easier.

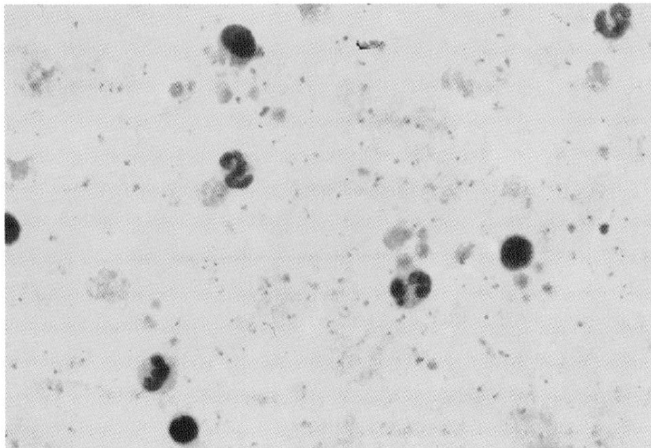

Fig. 91 Thick film in a case of *Plasmodium falciparum* malaria. The red blood cells have been lysed and abundant trophozoites can be seen.

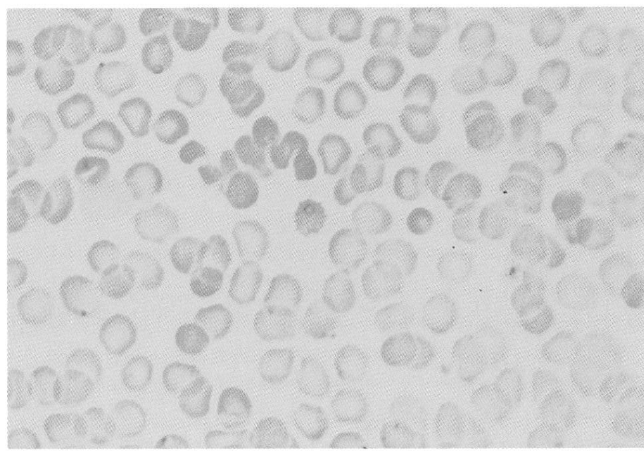

Fig. 92 Thin film from the same case as Fig. 91. *Plasmodium falciparum* trophozoites can be seen within red blood cells (5% parasitaemia).

• Rapid diagnostic tests: blood dipstick tests that detect malaria antigens are valuable adjuncts in the diagnosis of malaria.

• Serology is of no value in establishing an acute diagnosis.

Disease syndromes and complications

Incubation period

In 75% of cases, *P. falciparum* malaria presents within 1 month of exposure, in 90% by 2 months. Presentation beyond 6 months is uncommon. By contrast, disease resulting from the other species can develop even years after exposure.

Clinical features

No clinical features accurately predict malaria. Malaria commonly presents as fever of abrupt onset, with no localizing symptoms or signs (see Section 1.20, p. 52). However, in many cases, there are potentially confusing features such as abdominal discomfort, diarrhoea or jaundice. Typical laboratory findings in uncomplicated malaria are normal WCC and low platelets; there may be mild anaemia and elevation of bilirubin. The importance of *P. falciparum* lies in its capacity to cause severe disease (Table 67).

Therapy

Always seek specialist advice if you are unsure or if the patient is seriously ill [1].

Plasmodium falciparum

Disease can progress after the start of treatment, so admission to hospital is recommended.

Table 67 Complications of severe *P. falciparum* malaria.

Organ system	Complication
Neurological (cerebral malaria)	Impaired higher cerebral function Impaired consciousness Seizures
Haematological	Severe anaemia Macroscopic haemaglobinuria Disseminated intravascular coagulation
Renal	Acute renal failure
Pulmonary	Pulmonary oedema Adult respiratory distress syndrome
Cardiovascular	Shock
Metabolic	Metabolic acidosis Hypoglycaemia

For practical purposes, *P. falciparum* should be considered to be chloroquine resistant, so the usual choice for treatment is quinine. Quinine is given orally (600 mg 8-hourly for 7 days, followed by Fansidar 3 tablets as a single dose or doxycycline 200 mg daily for 7 days) unless there are serious complications (see Table 67), the patient is vomiting or the parasitaemia is >2%, which is a risk for development of complications. In these circumstances, intravenous quinine is used (loading dose 20 mg/kg (1.4 g maximum) over 4 h, followed by 10 mg/kg (700 mg maximum) over 4 h three times daily).

Hypoglycaemia and cardiac dysrhythmias are side effects of intravenous quinine. Monitor blood glucose (BMstix) hourly and consider cardiac monitoring in older patients, patients with known cardiac disease or patients with a prolonged QT interval. Daily blood films (until negative) are recommended to help monitor progress. The patient can be discharged when afebrile and well with a negative blood film.

Plasmodium vivax, P. ovale, P. malariae

Serious complications are rare and most patients can be managed without admission.

Chloroquine is the drug of choice for treatment (600 mg orally immediately; 300 mg 6 h later; followed by two 300 mg doses at 24-h intervals) but does not eradicate the dormant liver form of *P. vivax* and *P. ovale* that is responsible for late recurrences. To treat this exoerythrocytic form, chloroquine treatment of these species is followed by a course of primaquine. It is essential to check glucose-6-phosphate dehydrogenase (G6PD) status before prescribing primaquine and to seek advice in G6PD-deficient individuals.

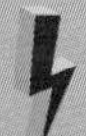

If in doubt as to the species treat for *P. falciparum*

See *Emergency medicine*, Section 1.27.

1 Winstanley P. Malaria: treatment. *J R Coll Physicians Lond* 1998; 32: 203.

2.13.2 LEISHMANIASIS

Description of the organism

Leishmaniasis is a zoonosis that is transmitted to humans by the bite of sandflies. The parasite is found within cells of the reticuloendothelial system.

Epidemiology

Visceral leishmaniasis is endemic in three main geographical areas: a belt that surrounds the Mediterranean basin and extends across the Middle East and Central Asia into parts of northern and eastern China; rural Sudan and Kenya; and parts of South America, particularly Brazil. Epidemic visceral leishmaniasis (kala-azar) occurs in addition in north-east India, Bangladesh and surrounding areas.

Diagnostic tests

- Parasitological diagnosis: parasites may be found in bone marrow, splenic aspirates or buffy coat
- Serological diagnosis: detection of antileishmanial antibody
- Skin sensitivity testing: by definition the leishmanin skin test is negative in established visceral leishmaniasis, reflecting a failure of cell-mediated immunity that allows the infection to progress.

Disease syndromes

The incubation period is generally 2–8 months. The following are classic features:
- Fever.
- Abdominal swelling.
- Weight loss.
- Splenomegaly, which may be massive, with or without hepatomegaly. Anaemia is characteristic, often with low white cells and platelets. Liver function tests are usually near normal. There is a polyclonal increase in immunoglobulins.
- Visceral leishmaniasis is associated with advanced HIV infection and may develop many years after initial exposure. Fever and splenomegaly are typical. In this setting, serology is often negative but parasites are abundant.

Complications

Secondary infections, caused by suppressed immunity, are common and potentially serious, accounting for many deaths in visceral leishmaniasis.

Therapy

Liposomal amphotericin B is the drug of choice because it is the least toxic effective treatment. It is very expensive [1].

In resource-poor countries, sodium stibogluconate and aminosidine are alternatives.

1 Olliaro P, Bryceson ADM. Practical progress and new drugs for changing patterns of leishmaniasis. *Parasitol Today* 1993; 9: 323.

2.13.3 AMOEBIASIS

Description of the organism

Entamoeba histolytica is an obligate parasite that resides in the large bowel. It is transmitted by ingestion of cysts in contaminated water or food. These develop into trophozoites (adult amoebae) which can invade tissues and cause disease. Only a small proportion of infections result in clinical disease [1].

Epidemiology

Amoebic infection occurs in all parts of the world where sanitation is poor and is much commoner in tropical countries.

Diagnostic tests

Asymptomatic intestinal amoebiasis

- Microscopy of stool for cysts.

Invasive intestinal amoebiasis

- Microscopy of fresh stool for amoebic trophozoites
- Amoebic serology is positive in approximately 75% of cases.

Amoebic liver abscess

- Amoebic serology is positive in >95% of cases
- Microscopy of liver aspirate: typically it is thick, pinkish-brown ('anchovy sauce') and odourless; microscopy shows no or few neutrophils and trophozoites may be seen in the final part of the aspirate; bacterial culture is negative
- Imaging: hepatic ultrasonography and CT (see Fig. 33b, p. 54).

Disease syndromes

Disease can arise weeks, months or even years after infection.

Invasive intestinal amoebiasis

The clinical features vary from mild diarrhoea to severe dysentery. Onset is usually gradual and constitutional upset is mild. Abdominal pain is not usually severe. A relapsing course is common.

Amoebic liver abscess

Most patients do not give an antecedent history of dysentery. The dominant features are fever and sweating, weight loss and right upper quadrant pain. Hepatomegaly and localized tenderness are often found; jaundice is rare. Neutrophilia is typical; liver function is often normal. A raised right hemidiaphragm or right basal lung changes are commonly seen on the chest radiograph. Ultrasonography or CT demonstrates a filling defect in the liver, which is usually solitary.

Complications

Invasive intestinal amoebiasis

- Fulminant colitis, especially in pregnancy or complicating steroid therapy
- Perforation of the colon
- Amoeboma, which is a localized inflammatory mass that may be confused with carcinoma.

Amoebic liver abscess

- Rupture into right chest, pericardium (Fig. 93) or peritoneum
- Haematogenous spread to lung, brain, etc.

Therapy

The mainstay of treatment of invasive amoebic disease

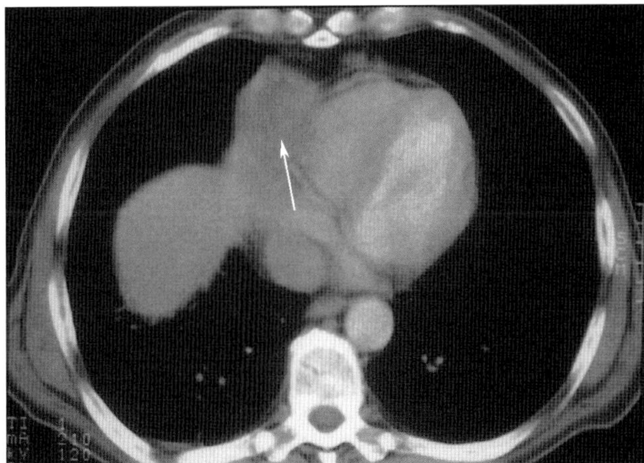

Fig. 93 CT scan showing an amoebic abscess extending up to the pericardium (arrow), placing the patient at high risk of rupture into the pericardium.

is metronidazole, which is a potent tissue amoebicide. Diloxanide furoate is used to kill amoebae in the bowel lumen.

1 Li E, Stanley SL. Protozoa. Amebiasis. *Gastroenterol Clin North Am* 1996; 25: 471.

2.13.4 TOXOPLASMOSIS

Description of the organism

Toxoplasma gondii exists in three forms:
1 Oocyst: excreted in cat faeces
2 Tachyzoite: invasive form which multiplies intracellularly
3 Cyst: the result of intracellular multiplication, containing thousands of parasites (bradyzoites) [1].

Epidemiology

Toxoplasma gondii is ubiquitous with the domestic cat as the definitive host. The prevalence of antitoxoplasma antibodies is high in most populations (approximately 30% of UK adults). Cysts containing viable parasites persist in the brain and striated muscle for life. Humans are usually infected by ingesting cysts in undercooked meat or from soil contaminated by cat faeces.

Diagnostic tests

• Serology: there are many different methods and so laboratory reports usually include interpretation. It is often difficult to distinguish past from acute infection.
• Culture: *T. gondii* can be isolated from bone marrow in acute disease, but this is available only in a few centres.
• PCR: this can be used on amniotic fluid to assess fetal risk if the mother develops toxoplasmosis in pregnancy.
• Histology: this may be needed to diagnose focal disease, e.g. brain abscess.

Disease syndromes and complications

Infection is usually asymptomatic. The characteristic feature of clinical disease is lymphadenopathy, either localized or generalized. Headache, myalgias, low-grade fever and prolonged fatigue may occur. Acute toxoplasmosis is a cause of atypical lymphocytosis. Severe complications (neurological, ocular and myocardial involvement) are very rare in immunocompetent patients, however:
• Toxoplasmosis relapses in immunosuppressed patients especially affecting the brain (Fig. 94), lung and eye.

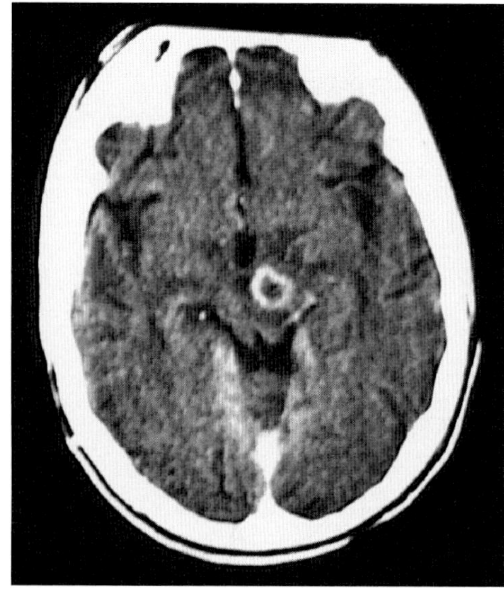

Fig. 94 Toxoplasma brain abscess complicating AIDS.

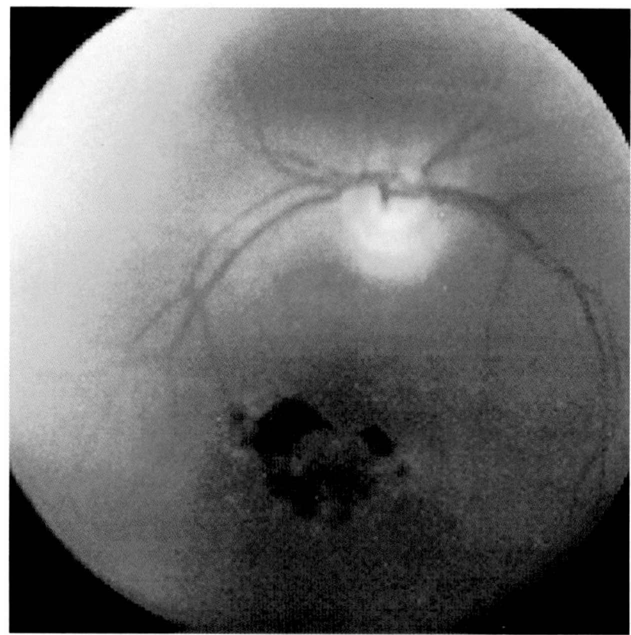

Fig. 95 Old toxoplasma chorioretinitis: retinal scarring often persists for life.

• Toxoplasmosis can cause serious congenital infection in infants born to mothers who acquired acute infection during pregnancy.
• Toxoplasmosis is the most common cause of choroidoretinitis (Fig. 95), usually as a result of relapse of congenitally acquired infection.

Therapy

Acute infection in an immunocompetent patient is not usually treated unless there are organ-specific complications or the symptoms are unusually severe or prolonged. Pyrimethamine and sulphadiazine are the main drugs used for treatment when indicated, e.g. in immunocompromised patients. Clindamycin can be substituted in sulphonamide hypersensitivity.

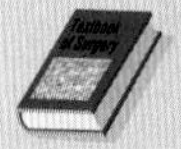

1 Couvreur J, Thulliez P. Toxoplasmosis. In: Weatherall DJ, Ledingham GG, Warrell DA (eds) *Oxford Textbook of Medicine*. Oxford: Oxford University Press, 1996: 865.

2.14 Metazoan parasites

2.14.1 SCHISTOSOMIASIS

Description of the pathogen

Schistosoma spp. are parasitic blood flukes. Three major species infect humans:

1 *Schistosoma haematobium*
2 *S. mansoni*
3 *S. japonicum*.

Humans are infected by contact with fresh water—the parasite penetrates intact skin. Water snails act as intermediate hosts. Human schistosomiasis is also known as bilharzia.

Epidemiology

It is estimated that 200 million people are infected with *Schistosoma* spp., most of these being in Africa (Table 68).

Diagnostic tests

• Identification of viable eggs: microscopy of terminal urine (*S. haematobium*) or stool (*S. mansoni* or *japonicum*). Eggs from all three species may be detected on rectal biopsy (see Fig. 35, p. 56).
• Serology: a positive result does not distinguish current active infection from past infection.

Disease syndromes and complications

Many infected individuals have a low worm burden and are asymptomatic. Eosinophilia is typical.

Table 68 Distribution of schistosomiasis.

Species	Geographical distribution
S. haematobium	North Africa, Middle East, sub-Saharan Africa
S. mansoni	Sub-Saharan Africa, Middle East, Brazil, Venezuela, parts of the Caribbean
S. japonicum	China, The Philippines, Indonesia

Invasion

Penetration of the skin can be associated with dermatitis ('swimmer's itch'). Migration through the lungs a few days after exposure can be associated with transient fever, cough and pulmonary infiltrates [1].

Acute schistosomiasis ('Katayama fever')

The development of adult worms and early stages of egg deposition, days to weeks after infection, may cause a severe systemic reaction causing fevers, rigors, myalgia, urticaria, lymphadenopathy and hepatosplenomegaly. High eosinophilia is typical.

Established infection

The main pathological process is granuloma formation around eggs.

• *S. haematobium*: eggs are deposited in the bladder and ureters, which may cause haematuria and other urinary symptoms.
• *S. mansoni* and *S. japonicum*: eggs are deposited in the bowel and liver, which is usually asymptomatic.

Late infection

This phase of infection causes the most clinical disease. Late complications occur as a result of fibrosis.

• *S. haematobium*: causes obstructive uropathy; infection is associated with squamous cell carcinoma of the bladder.
• *S. mansoni* and *S. japonicum*: the most severe manifestation is hepatic fibrosis with portal hypertension.

Chronic intestinal disease is a cause of bloody diarrhoea. Less commonly, egg deposition occurs at other sites. CNS involvement (myelopathy or focal epilepsy) and pulmonary hypertension are well recognized.

Therapy

Specialist advice is needed regarding treatment. Praziquantel is the drug of choice for all species. In the treatment of Katayama fever, steroids are also used.

1 Mahmoud AAF. Trematodes (schistosomiasis) and other flukes. In: *Mandell, Douglas and Bennett's Principles and Practice of Infectious Diseases* (5th edn). New York: Churchill Livingstone, 1995: 2538.

2.14.2 STRONGYLOIDIASIS

Description of the organism

Strongyloides stercoralis is a worm that lives in the small bowel of humans [1]. Humans are infected via penetration of intact skin. Infection may persist for many years as a result of a cycle of autoinfection, in which infectious larvae reinfect the same host by penetrating perianal skin or the gut wall.

Epidemiology

Strongyloides stercoralis is widely distributed in the tropical and subtropical regions of the world. It remains endemic in southern USA, Japan and parts of southern Europe.

Diagnostic tests

- Microscopy of stool for larvae
- Serology.

Disease syndromes and complications

Nearly all *S. stercoralis* infections are asymptomatic. Vague intestinal symptoms may occur, mimicking irritable bowel syndrome. A pathognomonic sign is larva currens—an intensely itchy, serpiginous, evanescent weal on the trunk or thighs.

Hyperinfection syndrome

Strongyloidiasis is important because overwhelming autoinfection can occur if host defences are impaired, e.g. by steroid or cytotoxic chemotherapy, malignancy, diabetic ketoacidosis or malnutrition. The features include diarrhoea (which may be bloody), cough, wheeze and haemoptysis, and Gram-negative septicaemia. Eosinophilia is absent. Mortality is high.

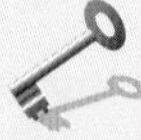

Strongyloides hyperinfection syndrome

- Triggered by immunosuppression
- May occur many years after parasite exposure
- Eosinophilia absent
- High mortality.

Therapy

Albendazole or ivermectin is used; seek specialist advice if hyperinfection is suspected.

1 Mahmoud AA. Strongyloidiasis. *Clin Infect Dis* 1996; 23: 949.

2.14.3 CYSTICERCOSIS

Description of the organism

The beef tapeworm, *Taenia saginata*, and the pork tapeworm, *Taenia solium*, are transmitted to humans by ingestion of undercooked meat containing the encysted larval stage (cysticercus). Adult tapeworms in the human gut, which are usually asymptomatic, release eggs. These are excreted via the faeces and develop into cysticerci if ingested by the appropriate animal host. Eggs of *T. solium* (but not *T. saginata*) can develop into cysticerci if ingested by humans and cause the disease cysticercosis [1,2].

Epidemiology

T. solium is found where undercooked pork is eaten. Eggs may contaminate other foodstuffs (faecal–oral transmission) and so avoiding pork does not protect against the disease.

Diagnostic tests

Serology

This can help to establish the diagnosis but is difficult to interpret in an endemic area.

Imaging

- Plain radiographs: cysticerci calcify and can be detected in plain radiographs of muscle
- CT of brain: active lesions show up as hypodense areas, inside which the scolex may be seen. Old lesions calcify and are often multiple (Fig. 96).

Disease syndromes and complications

Cysticerci can invade any organ, with the major sites involved being the CNS, eye and soft tissues. It may be asymptomatic.

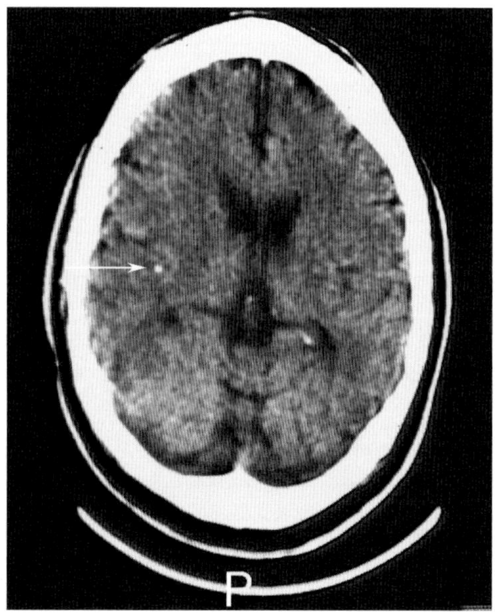

Fig. 96 CT brain of a patient with epilepsy, revealing a small calcified nodule (arrow) caused by past cysticercosis.

- Neurocysticercosis: epilepsy is the most common manifestation, but there is a wide range of neurological presentations, depending on the site and number of cysts. Obstructive hydrocephalus has occurred as a result of cysticerci within the ventricular system.
- Subcutaneous and muscular cysticercosis: the patient may notice subcutaneous nodules.
- Ocular disease: may lead to blindness.

Therapy

Specialist advice should be sought:

- Symptomatic, e.g. anticonvulsant therapy.
- Specific: praziquantel and albendazole are active against *T. solium* but efficacy is uncertain. Induction of therapy may lead to an intense inflammatory reaction and aggravate symptoms, requiring adjunctive corticosteroid use.

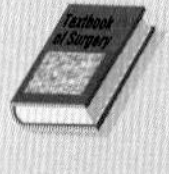

1 Cook GC. Taeniasis and cysticercosis. *J R Soc Med* 1998; 91: 534.
2 White AC. Neurocysticercosis: a major cause of neurological disease worldwide. *Clin Infect Dis* 1997; 24: 101.

2.14.4 FILARIASIS

Description of the organism

Four filarial species commonly cause disease in humans (Table 69; Fig. 97) [1]. Many more individuals are infected without disease. Filariasis is a cause of eosinophilia.

Fig. 97 Microfilaria of *Loa loa*. Microfilaria migrate through many tissues. This is from a cervical smear. (Courtesy of B Viner.)

Therapy

Specialist advice is needed regarding treatment. Ivermectin is increasingly used.

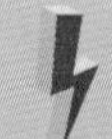

Diethylcarbamazine, and less commonly ivermectin, may induce an intense inflammatory reaction around microfilaria. In onchocerciasis this may damage vision.

1 Grove DI. Tissue nematodes (trichinosis, dracunculiasis, filariasis). In: *Mandell, Douglas and Bennett's Principles and Practice of Infectious Diseases* (5th edn). New York: Churchill Livingstone, 1995: 2531.

Table 69 Features of filariasis.

Pathogen	Vector	Distribution	Diagnostic tests	Disease and complications
Wuchereria bancrofti	Mosquitoes	Indian subcontinent, Central and S. America, Caribbean, E. Africa	Night blood for MF Filarial serology	Asymptomatic microfilaraemia Acute lymphatic filariasis Fever, lymphadenitis, lymphangitis Chronic lymphatic filariasis Lymphoedema (see Fig. 34). Tropical pulmonary eosinophilia.
Brugia malayi	Mosquitoes	South-east Asia		
Loa loa	Chrysops flies	West and Central Africa	Microscopy of day blood for MF (Fig. 97)	Calabar swellings Transient subcutaneous nodules, often on the arm Irritation of eye as an adult worm traverses the sclera
Onchocerca volvulus	Blackflies	Equatorial Africa (Central and S. America, Yemen)	Skin snips for MF	Chronic pruritis and excoriation Eye involvement, with gradual impairment of vision

MF, microfilariae.

2.14.5 TRICHINOSIS

Description of the organism

Humans are infected by eating undercooked pork and occasionally other meats. Adult worms in the intestine produce larvae, which disseminate in the blood stream, and penetrate and encyst in striated muscle [1].

Epidemiology

Infection is endemic in many parts of the world where pork is consumed. There is little infection in western Europe.

Diagnostic tests

- Serology
- Calcified nodules may be seen on plain radiographs
- Muscle biopsy.

Disease syndromes and complications

Light infections are usually asymptomatic. Heavy infections may manifest distinct stages:

- Invasion: abdominal pain, nausea, vomiting, diarrhoea, fever.
- Migration: myalgia, muscular tenderness, swelling of face and periorbital tissues, fever. A high eosinophil count is typical. Complications caused by migration in the heart, lungs and CNS can arise.
- Encystment: gradual recovery from symptoms of migration is typical. Serological tests become positive.

Therapy

Spontaneous recovery is usual. Steroids have been used to treat severe myalgia and complications during migration. Albendazole may be used for specific treatment.

1 Grove DI. Tissue nematodes (trichinosis, dracunculiasis, filariasis). In: *Mandell, Douglas and Bennett's Principles and Practice of Infectious Diseases* (5th edn). New York: Churchill Livingstone, 1995: 2531.

2.14.6 TOXOCARIASIS

Description of the organism

Humans are infected by ingestion of eggs of *Toxocara canis* or *T. catis* in contaminated soil. Most infections occur in children. Eggs hatch into larvae, the migration of which causes the clinical disease visceral (or ocular) larva migrans [1].

Epidemiology

Infections occur wherever there are significant dog and cat populations.

Diagnostic tests

- Serology.

Disease syndromes and complications

Most infections are asymptomatic. There are two important clinical syndromes:

1 Visceral larva migrans (VLM): myalgia, lassitude, cough, urticaria, hepatosplenomegaly and lymphadenopathy. Eosinophilia is typical.

2 Ocular toxocariasis: generalized manifestations of VLM may not be present, but ocular involvement may cause visual impairment. Eosinophilia may be absent.

Therapy

Specialist advice is needed regarding treatment. Many cases recover without specific therapy. Visible larvae in the eye can be photocoagulated.

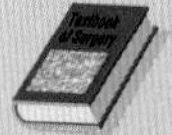

1 Overgaauw PA. Aspects of Toxocara epidemiology: Human toxocarosis. *Crit Rev Microbiol* 1997; 23: 215.

2.14.7 HYDATID DISEASE

Description of the organism

Echinococcus spp. are small tapeworms of canines. Infected canines excrete eggs in the faeces. Eggs ingested by sheep or cattle develop into cysts. Cysts can also develop in humans (an accidental host) if eggs are ingested, most commonly by consuming contaminated vegetables or after handling dogs with contaminated hair [1].

Epidemiology

Echinococcus infections occur in Europe, Asia, northern and eastern Africa, western South America, Australia and Canada. Human infections occur mostly associated with sheep or cattle rearing and close proximity to dogs.

Diagnostic tests

- Imaging of the affected area: plain films (Fig. 98) and CT may strongly suggest the diagnosis

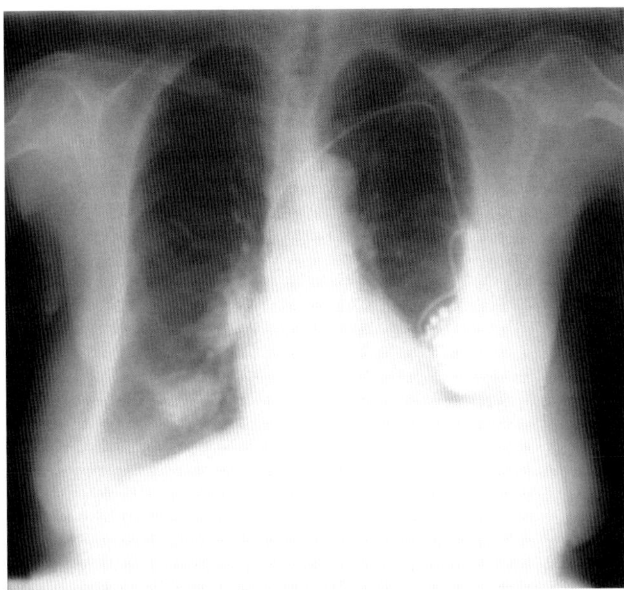

Fig. 98 Chest radiograph from a patient admitted for insertion of a permanent pacing system. An incidental lesion was noted at the right base and subsequently found to be a hydatid cyst.

• Serology: a significant number of false negatives occur, especially with solitary, intact cysts at sites other than the liver
• Direct diagnosis by microscopy if aspiration or surgery is performed.

Disease syndromes and complications

• Most infections are found incidentally on radiological examination. Cysts can affect any organ, but liver and lung are the most common sites.
• Local pressure symptoms.
• Cyst rupture may result in an allergic reaction to parasite antigens.
• Secondary bacterial infection of a cyst.

Therapy

• Specialist advice is needed regarding treatment of symptomatic disease [2]
• Surgical resection
• Fine needle aspiration and installation of a cysticidal agent
• Medical therapy (e.g. albendazole) may be useful adjunctive therapy but has a low cure rate.

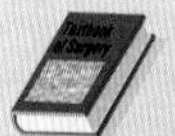

1 Clarkson MJ. Hydatid disease. *J Med Microbiol* 1997; 46: 28.
2 Khuroo MS, Wani NA, Javid G *et al.* Percutaneous drainage compared with surgery for hepatic hydatid cysts. *N Engl J Med* 1997; 337: 881.

Investigations and practical procedures

3.1 Getting the best from the laboratory

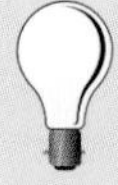

- Are the specimen and form correctly labelled?
- Are you sure what samples to take? If not call the laboratory.
- Where possible, try to obtain cultures before antibiotics.
- Is the specimen from the infected site?
- Does the specimen need to be transported urgently?

Although there are few practical procedures that are unique to clinical infectious diseases, the accurate diagnosis and management of infection requires the correct use and interpretation of diagnostic microbiology services [1,2]. It is essential that the laboratory staff are aware of the following:

- What pathogens are suspected
- What specimens may be available
- Patient details, including recent antimicrobial therapy, travel and underlying immunocompromise.

For example, in routine practice blood cultures are discarded after 7 days' incubation and this will fail to isolate *Brucella* sp. which takes 10–14 days to grow.

Microbiology specimens

When trying to diagnose any infection, it is vital that the correct specimens are sent to the laboratory. Tables 70, 71 and 72 detail what samples are needed and how to take them.

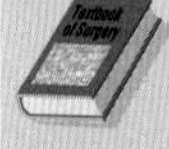

1 Andremont A. The past, present and future of the clinical microbiology laboratory. In: Armstrong D, Cohen J (eds) *Infectious Diseases*. London: Mosby, 1999: 3.1–3.8.
2 Koneman EW, Allen SD, Janda WM *et al. Color Atlas and Textbook of Diagnostic Microbiology*, 5th edn. New York: Lippincott Williams & Wilkins, 1997.

Table 70 Common samples used for the diagnosis of respiratory tract infections.

Sample	How to take	Potential pathogens
Throat swab	If exudate visible try to swab that area. Swab gently between uvula and tonsils	β-Haemolytic streptococci Diphtheria
Sputum	Give sputum pot to the patient. Try to send purulent specimens rather than saliva. Ask physiotherapy to help	Bacteria and TB: microscopy and culture Not suitable for viruses or PCP
Induced sputum	3% saline is inhaled using an ultrasonic nebulizer. Droplets penetrate to alveoli. Use trained staff	Increased yield for diagnosis of TB Sensitivity of 70% for PCP
Bronchoalveolar lavage	Procedure of choice for immunocompromised host Saline aspirated through a bronchoscope wedged in terminal bronchi Samples should be sent to microbiology, virology and cytology.	Bacteria/mycobacteria: microscopy and culture Viruses: IF, culture PCP: IF, cytology Fungi: cytology, culture Parasites: cytology
Gastric washings	After an overnight fast drink 250–500 mL sterile water and then aspirate via a nasogastric tube	Detection of TB where patient is not producing sputum Centrifuge, stain and culture for TB
Nasopharyngeal aspirate	Saline gargled and then spat or aspirated into a sterile container	Respiratory viruses: IF, culture
Nasopharyngeal swab	Special swab passed through nose until reaches pharynx	*Bordetella pertussis*
Pleural aspirate	Best transported fresh in sterile containers to both microbiology and cytology	Bacteria and mycobacteria: microscopy and culture, PCR

PCP, *Pneumocystis carinii* pneumonia; IF, immunofluorescence; PCR, polymerase chain reaction; TB, tuberculosis.

Table 71 Samples used for the diagnosis of genitourinary infections.

Sample	How to take	Potential pathogens
Midstream urine (MSU)	Clean penis/vulval area	Microscopy and culture for bacteria
	Use sterile collecting bowl, catch midstream urine	DNA-based tests for *Chlamydia*
Early morning urine	All of the first voided urine collected on three mornings	TB: low yield on microscopy, higher with culture
Terminal urine	Best early morning, last 20–30 mL	Schistosomiasis
Genitourinary specimens	Essential to take correct samples on appropriate media	Bacteria, viruses and *Chlamydia*

Table 72 Other samples used for the diagnosis of infections

Sample	How to take	Potential pathogens
Stool	No point in sending formed stool unless looking for parasites In dysentery stool should be transported quickly (hot)	Culture for bacteria Microscopy for parasites Electron microscopy and ELISA for viruses ELISA for *Clostridium difficile* toxin
Blood	Inoculate into culture bottles (see below)	Aerobic/anaerobic bacteria, mycobacteria and fungi (increased with specific media)
Bone marrow	See *Haematology*, Section 3.2.	*Brucella*, *Salmonella* and mycobacteria
Serum	Timed serology	Many organisms
Wounds	If pus is present collect and send to laboratory If not then use bacterial swabs	Bacteria, fungi
Pus	Aspirates of pus should be placed into a sterile container and transported rapidly to the laboratory	Bacteria, mycobacteria, fungi
Ascites	Transport fresh to lab in sterile tube Consider inoculating into blood culture bottles	Bacteria, mycobacteria and fungi readily cultured on appropriate media
CSF	Lumbar puncture (see *Emergency medicine*, Section 3.5).	Bacteria: microscopy, culture, antigen detection, PCR Mycobacteria: culture, PCR Viruses: culture and PCR Syphilis: serology Fungi: culture, antigen detection
Vesicles	If intact aspirate fluid with insulin syringe and transport to lab Scrape base on to a microscope slide	Vesicle fluid can be used for electron microscopy and culture Scrapings for IF
Tissue	Separated for histology and microbiology Must not dry out, transport to lab immediately	Bacteria, mycobacteria, viruses and fungi Immunohistochemisty can be applied to tissue
Skin scrapings	Superficial scrapings with glass slide of blunt blade collected in Petri dish or envelope Nail clippings for onychomycosis	Dermatophytes and other fungi

ELISA, enzyme-linked immunosorbent assay; IF, immunofluorescence; PCR, polymerase chain reaction.

3.2 Specific investigations

Blood cultures

Preparation is important to reduce contamination.

1 Have the blood culture bottles ready and clean the tops liberally with alcohol.

2 Venepuncture site should be free from visible contamination or superficial infection. Liberally swab the site with alcohol or iodine and allow to dry for 1–2 min.

3 Enter the vein using a 'no touch' technique.

4 Directly inoculate into the prepared blood culture bottles without delay. Always inoculate blood culture bottles before other samples are filled to minimize contamination.

5 Fill the bottles up to their capacity (generally 10 mL/bottle) because insufficient blood volume reduces the yield.

Do not change needles between blood culture bottles. This does not reduce contamination, but does increase the risk of needlestick injury.

Always take a minimum of two sets of blood cultures (where one set = 1 aerobic + 1 anaerobic bottle). Taking only one set makes interpretation of possible contaminants very difficult.

Malaria films

Correctly taken blood films are essential in the management of malaria (see Section 1.20, p. 53). Two types of films are used:

1 Thin film: this enables the level of parasitaemia to be measured and the species identified. The film is prepared in the same way as for a regular blood film. (See *Haematology*, Section 3.1.)

2 Thick film: this concentrates the parasites and increases sensitivity. One or two drops of blood are allowed to dry on a glass slide and are treated with an osmotic agent to lyse the red blood cells. The slide is stained with Giemsa stain and viewed under the microscope.

Skin snips

These are used to diagnose filariasis resulting from *Onchocerca volvulus*. (See Section 2.14.4, p. 147.) In onchocerciasis, microfilaria are found in the most superficial skin layers.

1 Skin is lifted up with a needle and a disposable blade used to shave off a tiny skin fragment without drawing blood.

2 Typically four to five specimens are taken from different sites.

3 The skin fragments are placed in a drop of water or saline and viewed under a microscope.

4 The microfilaria will emerge 30 min to several hours later.

Tuberculin testing

There are a number of methods described to test for skin reactivity to mycobacterial antigens. The two most widely used are:

1 Mantoux test

2 Heaf test.

Both tests aim to inoculate tuberculin purified protein derivative (PPD) into the dermis. Intradermal injection is critical, because the procedure is likely to fail if the PPD is injected subcutaneously. The forearm is the preferred site for both tests.

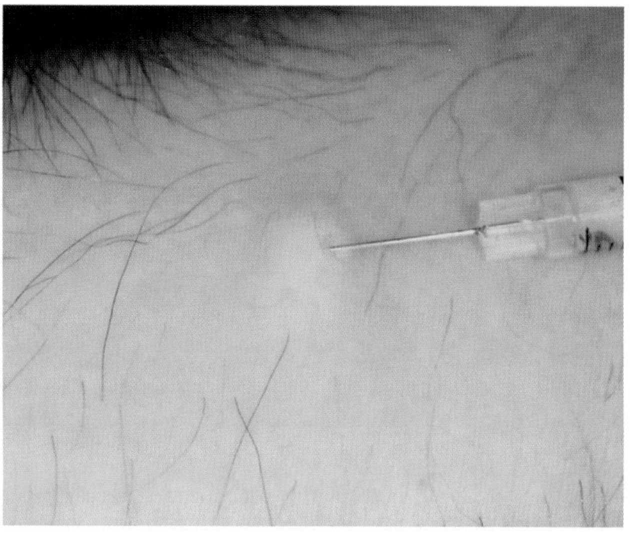

(a)

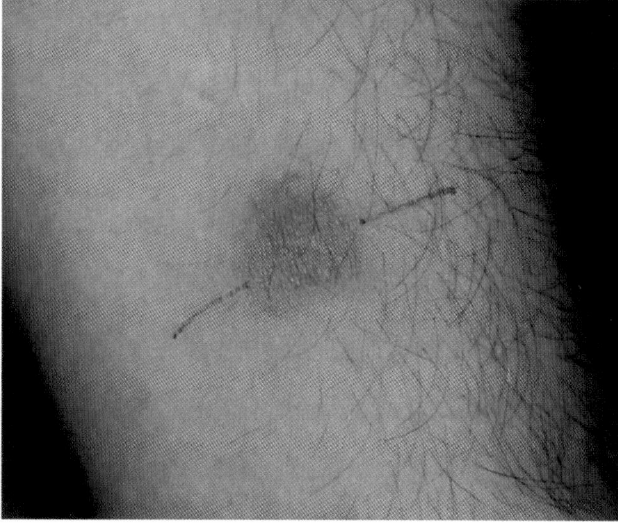

(b)

Fig. 99 Mantoux test: (a) injection of purified protein derivative (PPD). A 25-g needle is used to enter the dermis and PPD slowly injected. If the needle is in the correct site, a 'bleb' will be raised as shown. (b) Positive Mantoux reaction.

Mantoux test

1 0.1 mL PPD is injected into the dermis (Fig. 99) with a fine needle.

2 Mantoux reaction is read at 48–72 h.

3 Measured by the area of induration rather than erythema.

PPD for use in the Mantoux test comes in the strengths 10, 100 and 1000 IU/mL:

- If TB is suspected, start with the 10 IU/mL strength (i.e. 1 IU injected) and if negative move up to the next strength.
- When screening for exposure, most people generally use the 100 IU/mL strength.

Interpretation of the area of induration:

- <5 mm—negative
- 5–10 mm—intermediate
- >10 mm—positive.

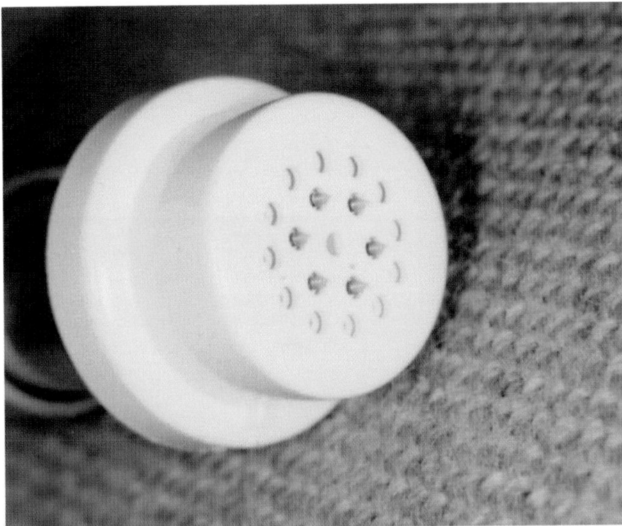

(a)

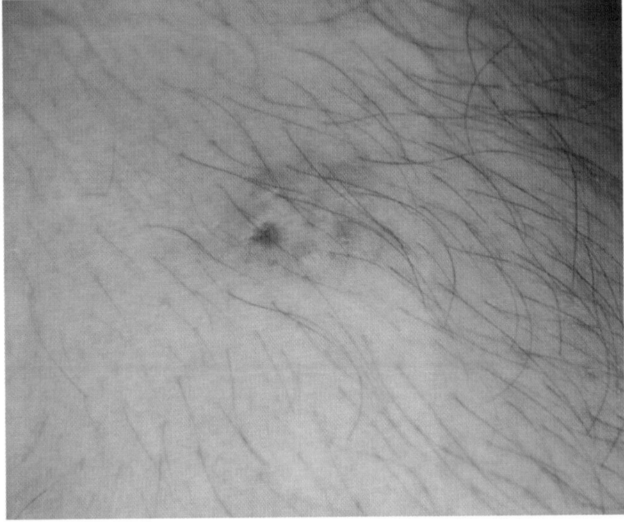

(b)

Fig. 100 (a) Heaf gun after use showing the six needles that penetrate the skin. (b) Grade 2 positive Heaf test.

Table 73 Grading of Heaf reaction.

Grade	Reaction
0	No reaction at site
1	Discrete induration at least four puncture points
2	Induration of puncture sites merge to form a ring but leave centre clear
3	Confluent induration of 5–10 mm
4	Confluent induration of >10 mm

Heaf test

The Heaf test uses a spring-loaded device to fire six tiny needles 1 mm into the skin (Fig. 100). This reduces the likelihood of a false result as a result of operator error.

1 A drop of 100 000 IU/mL strength tuberculin is placed on the skin and the Heaf gun applied.

2 The gun is triggered by firm downward pressure and the six needles inoculate the PPD into the dermis.

3 The head of the gun is then discarded in a sharps bin.

4 The Heaf test is read at 5–7 days and is graded (Table 73).

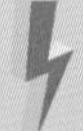

Always check that you are using the correct strength tuberculin:

- Injection of 0.1 mL of the 100 000 IU/mL solution used for Heaf testing is likely to cause a severe reaction
- Conversely, using the Mantoux strength solutions for the Heaf test will lead to a negative result.

Acknowledgement

The senior editor would like to thank Dr A Robinson for helpful advice in the preparation of this section.

4 Self-assessment

Answers are on pp. 223–227.

Question 1

Figure 101 shows a swelling that developed 4 weeks after starting combination anti-retroviral therapy in an AIDS patient with a CD4 count of 20 cells/microlitre. Incision and drainage of an abscess was performed. What is the likely cause?

A mycobacterium avium intracellulare
B mycobacterium tuberculosis
C staphylococcus albus
D staphylococcus aureus
E lymphoma

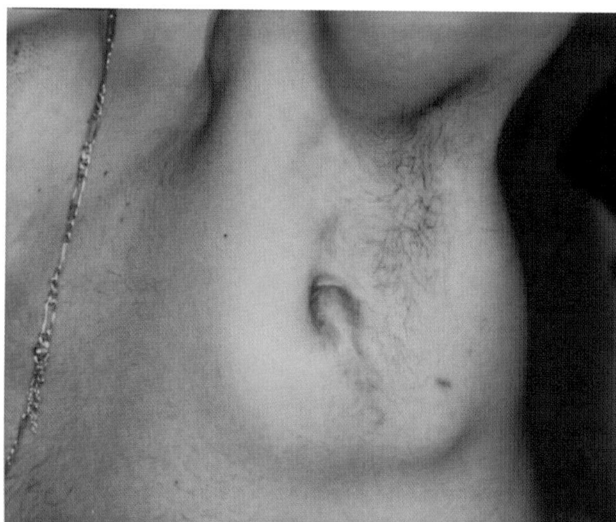

Fig. 101 Question 1.

Question 2

A 40-year-old woman with chronic renal failure due to IgA nephropathy presents 3 years after a renal transplant with spots on her hands (see Figure 102). These have gradually increased in number over a period of 6 months. What is the cause?

A chicken pox
B papilloma virus
C cytomegalovirus
D Epstein Barr virus
E molluscum contagiosum

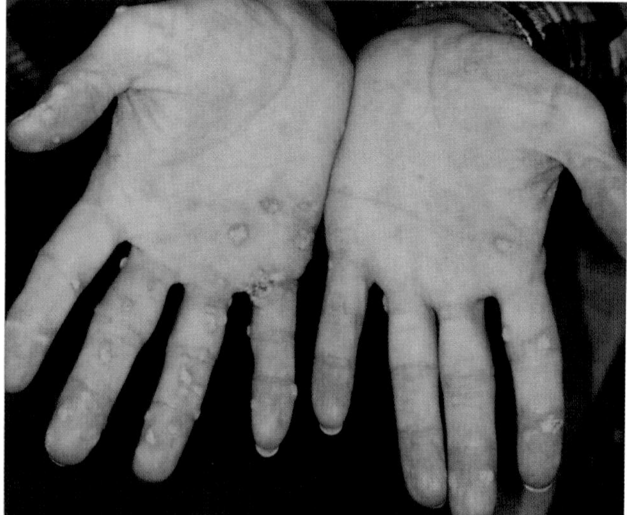

Fig. 102 Question 2.

Question 3

A 33-year-old man presents with abdominal pain 3 months after returning from a trip to India. Figure 103 shows a CT scan of his abdomen. What is the most likely cause of the abscess in his liver?

A tuberculosis
B pyogenic bacteria
C amoebiasis
D brucellosis
E hydatid

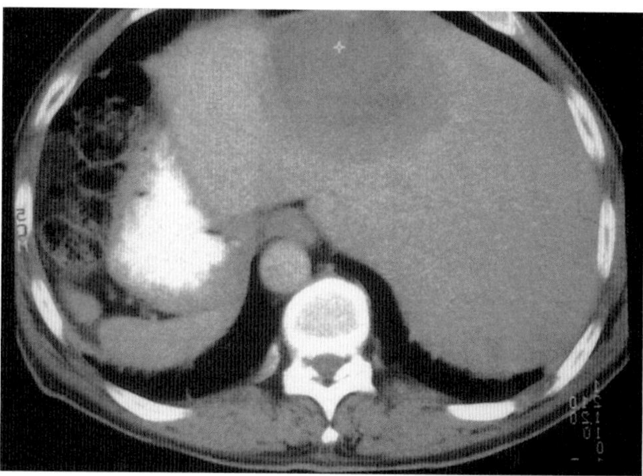

Fig. 103 Question 3.

Question 4

A 20-year-old student becomes acutely unwell and is admitted on medical take with headache and fever. On examination he is hypotensive, but there are no focal signs. A year ago he went on a trekking holiday in southern Africa, but there is no more recent travel history.

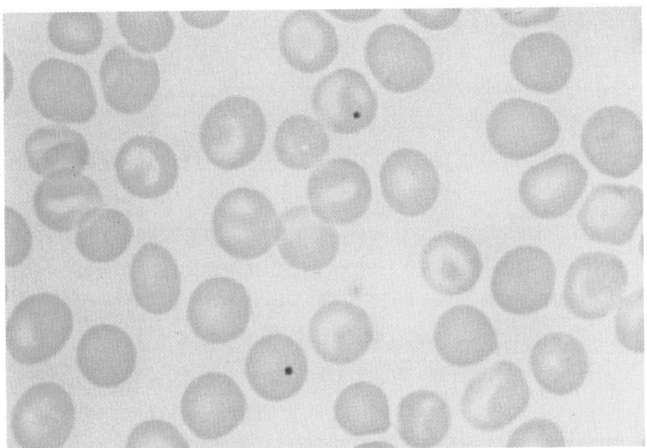

Fig. 104 Question 4.

Figure 104 shows his blood film. What is the likely diagnosis?

A falciparum malaria
B vivax malaria
C meningococcal septicaemia
D pneumococcal septicaemia
E dengue

Question 5

Figure 105 shows a serum sample from a 33-year-old woman presenting with arthritis and ankle swelling who is found to have proteinuria and abnormal liver function. What is the most likely diagnosis?

A rheumatoid arthritis
B systemic lupus erythematosus
C parvovirus infection
D hepatitis B infection
E hepatitis C infection

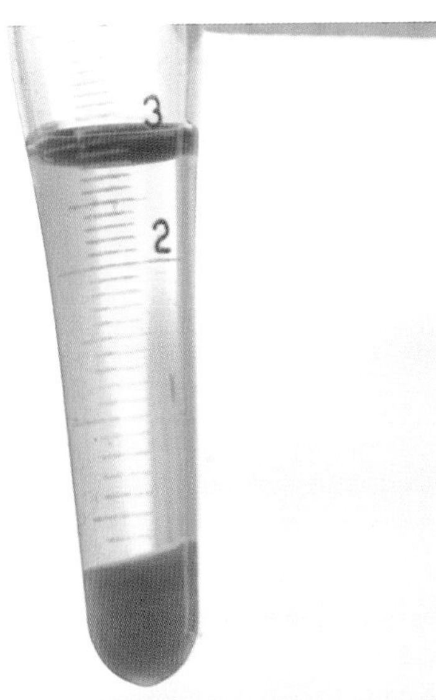

Fig. 105 Question 5.

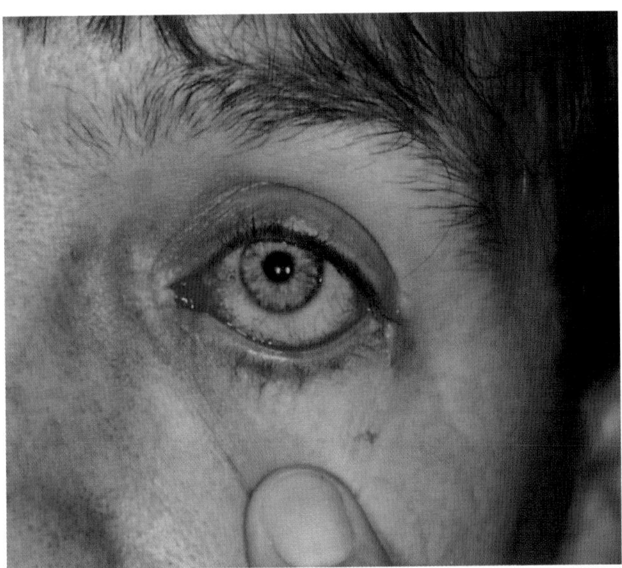

Fig. 106 Question 6.

Question 6

Figure 106 shows the eye of a 40-year-old woman presenting with a runny nose, fever and myalgia. What is the most likely diagnosis?

A streptococcal infection
B staphylococcal infection
C haemophilus infection
D varicella zoster infection
E adenovirus infection

Question 7

A 58-year-old man presents with fever and malaise. He is very unwell, with severe hypotension. He has an abscess on his foot. Figure 107 shows a Gram stain of material aspirated from this. What is the diagnosis?

A streptococcal infection
B staphylococcal infection
C infection with *Clostridium tetani*
D infection with *Clostridium perfringens*
E infection with *Neisseria meningitidis*

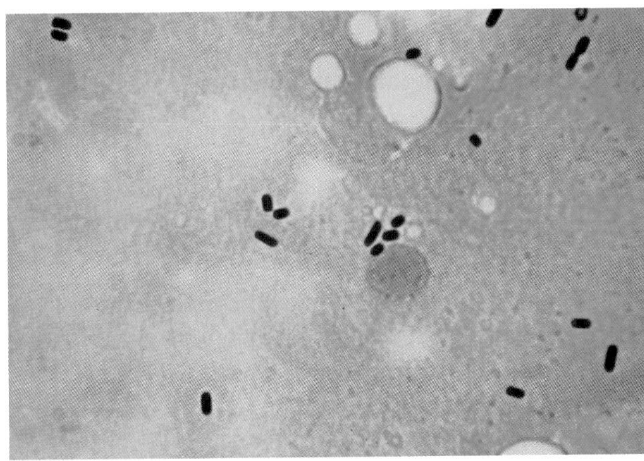

Fig. 107 Question 7.

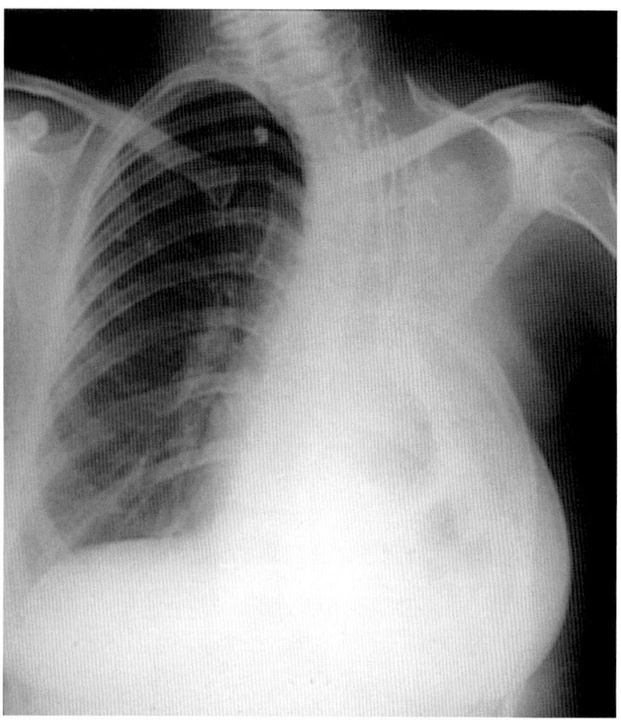

Fig. 108 Question 8.

Question 8

A 74-year-old woman has developed a large inguinal hernia that is causing her distress. It has not proved possible to restrain this with a truss and she would like to have it corrected surgically. Her chest radiograph is shown (see Figure 108). What is the explanation?

A congenital kyphoscoliosis
B congenital kyphoscoliosis with left sided pleural effusion
C tuberculosis treated with thoracoplasty
D tuberculosis treated with plombage
E left sided pleural effusion

Question 9

A 65-year-old man with a history of controlled chronic myeloid leukaemia presents confused and unwell with a high fever but no other localizing signs of infection. Which combination of drugs would be the most appropriate treatment pending CSF analysis and blood culture results? (Select 2 options from this list)

A third generation cephalosporin
B high dose intravenous ampicillin
C high dose intravenous benzyl penicillin
D intravenous metronidazole
E oral aciclovir
F intravenous ciprofloxacin
G high dose intravenous flucloxacillin
H oral metronidazole
I intravenous vancomycin
J oral rifampicin

Question 10

You are called to see a 79-year-old man on the urology ward who has become unwell. He had a transurethral prostatectomy 6 hours ago and is now afebrile, vomiting, hypotensive and hypoxic. Preoperative investigations included a chest radiograph consistent with chronic obstructive airway disease, a CSU showing profuse growth of mixed coliforms and routine screening for methicillin-resistant *staphylococcus aureus* (MRSA) was positive. Blood tests showed mild renal impairment. Which two of the following are LEAST appropriate steps for immediate management?

A oxygen administration via a facemask
B fluid resuscitation
C commencement of oral ciprofloxacin 500 mg b.d.
D commencement of intravenous cefuroxime 1.5 g t.d.s. with addition of 500 mg t.d.s. metronidazole
E commencement of intravenous cefuroxime 1.5 g t.d.s. with addition of vancomycin 750 mg b.d.
F taking an ECG
G repeating a chest radiograph
H taking blood cultures
I placement on regular observations
J taking blood gases

Question 11

A 32-year-old woman who might be pregnant has recently returned from Africa. She is febrile and drowsy with a *Plasmodium falciparum* malaria parasite count of 1%, haemoglobin of 9.8 g/dl, platelets of 20×10^9/l, creatinine of 200 μmol/l and mild jaundice. Which two of the following are essential parts of her management?

A CT of her head
B platelet transfusion
C blood glucose monitoring
D exchange transfusion
E dialysis
F liver ultrasound
G prophylactic phenobarbitone
H steroids
I antimalarial treatment given intravenously
J antibiotic cover

Question 12

A 48-year-old man presents with a 5-day history of fever and cough. He has no significant past medical history but is very unwell. His chest radiograph shows patchy shadowing, mainly in the right lower lobe. What two antibiotic regimen from the list below would it be most appropriate to give him?

A co-trimoxazole 120 mg/kg daily in 2–4 divided doses
B ciprofloxacin 400 mg 12-hourly intravenously
C erythromycin 1 g 6-hourly intravenously
D clarithromycin 250 mg 8-hourly orally
E ciprofloxacin 500 mg 12-hourly orally

F erythromycin 500 mg 6-hourly intravenously
G benzylpenicillin 1.2–2.4 g 6-hourly intravenously
H rifampicin 600 mg 12-hourly intravenously
I amoxicillin 250 mg 8-hourly orally
J cefotaxime 1 g 8-hourly intravenously

Question 13

A 49-year-old factory worker presents unwell with fever and confusion. He is hypotensive and hypoxic. The most notable finding on clinical examination is a necrotic skin lesion on his back. He is transferred to intensive care, given supportive management and broad-spectrum antibiotics, and the surgical team consulted. The next day blood cultures flag positive with Gram-positive rods. Which two organisms should you be concerned about?

A Group A Streptococcus
B *Staphylococcus aureus*
C *Clostridium tetani*
D *Listeria monocytogenes*
E *Bacteroides fragilis*
F *Pseudomonas aeruginosa*
G *Bacillus anthracis*
H *Clostridium perfringens*
I diptheroids
J *Escherichia coli*

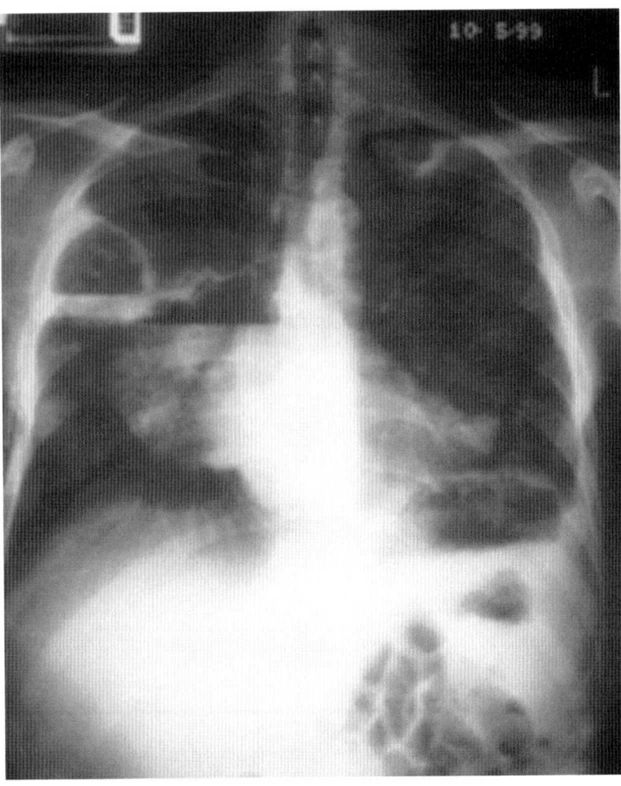

Fig. 109 Question 14.

Question 14

This chest radiograph (Figure 109) is from a 25-year-old intravenous drug user who presented with a 10-day history of fever and a cough productive of copious amounts of green sputum. What are the two most likely aetiological agents?

A *Streptococcus pneumoniae*
B *Staphylococcus epidermidis*
C *Haemophilus influenzae*
D *Mycoplasma pneumoniae*
E *Staphylococcus aureus*
F *Legionella pneumophila*
G *Klebsiella pneumoniae*
H *Mycobacterium avium intracellulare*
I *Escherichia coli*
J *Salmonella typhi*

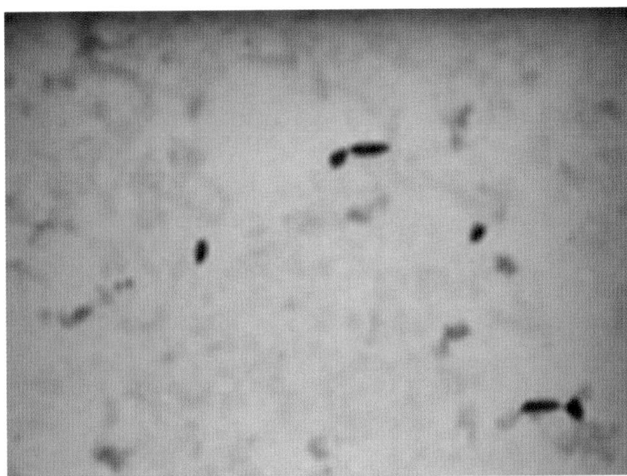

Fig. 110 Question 15.

Question 15

A 34-year-old intravenous drug abuser presents with a persistent fever and shortness of breath. His chest radiograph shows bilateral discrete lesions. Blood cultures taken on admission flag positive after 24 hours. The Gram stain is shown (Figure 110). What is the organism (select one of options A–E) and what is the most likely underlying diagnosis (select one of options F–J)?

A *Staphylococcus aureus*
B *Streptococcus bovis*
C *Candida albicans*
D *Pneumocystis carinii*
E *Mycobacterium tuberculosis*
F HIV infection
G left-sided endocarditis
H right-sided endocarditis
I miliary tuberculosis
J pneumonia

Question 16

A 42-year-old woman has recently been diagnosed HIV positive and has a CD4 count of 180 and HIV viral load of 200 000 copies/ml. She presents with behavioural change. She is alert but withdrawn, uncommunicative, not eating and at times appears to be mute. CT brain with contrast and MRI brain show a moderate degree of cerebral atrophy but are otherwise normal. CSF analysis reveals 20 lymphocytes, protein 0.74 g/l and glucose 3.5 mmol/l (plasma 5.6 mmol/l). Which two of the following are most likely?

A CMV encephalitis
B new variant Creutzfeldt–Jacob disease
C cryptococcal meningitis
D cerebral lymphoma
E depression
F neurosyphilis
G progressive multifocal leucoencephalopathy
H cerebral toxoplasmosis
I HIV encephalopathy
J tuberculous meningitis

Question 17

A 17-year-old gay man has recently become sexually active. He presents with a 1-week history of fever, myalgia, sore throat and a macular rash. A blood film shows a reactive lymphocytosis and liver function tests are abnormal. HIV-1 antibody is negative. Which two of the following tests are most likely to provide a diagnosis?

A hepatitis C antibody
B throat, urine and stool cultures for viruses
C measurement of anti-CMV IgG
D Paul–Bunnell test
E HIV p24 antigen
F coxsackie virus serology
G HIV-2 antibody test
H blood cultures
I parvovirus B 19 IgM
J serum VDRL/TPHA

Question 18

A 48-year-old man who had been referred with deranged liver function tests attends for a follow up outpatient appointment to discuss the results of his recent tests. He is told that he has chronic hepatitis B (HBV). Which one of the following statements is correct?

A cirrhosis develops in about 20% of people with chronic hepatitis B
B all persistent HBV infection is symptomatic
C most primary infections in adults lead to persistent HBV infection
D all primary HBV infection is symptomatic
E all asymptomatic chronic HBV carriers have grossly abnormal findings on liver biopsy

Question 19

You are called to see a 78-year-old woman on an orthopaedic ward. She fell and sustained a fractured left humerus 2 weeks previously. On admission she was noted to have an infected right venous leg ulcer and had been started on antibiotics for associated cellulitis 6 days previously. The nursing staff are concerned at a significant deterioration in her condition: she is now confused and pyrexial, and the leg ulcer has increased in size with some central necrosis and adjacent blistering. On examination some crepitus is felt. You wonder if this could be necrotising fascitiis. Which one of the following statements is correct?

A it is unlikely to be necrotising fasciitis as she is already on antibiotics
B an MRI scan maybe useful in confirming the diagnosis
C necrotising fasciitis is always caused by infection with Group A Streptococci
D crepitus does not occur in necrotising fasciitis
E bullae are unsusual in necrotising fasciitis

Question 20

A 40-year-old woman, recently returned from a 2-month trip to India, presents with a week's history of fever, malaise, myalgia and headache. There are no abnormal findings on examination. A full blood count shows Hb 13.6 g/dl, WCC 14.2×10^9/l (neutrophils 12.4×10^9/l), platelets 148×10^9/l. A malaria film is negative. Which one of the following would be UNLIKELY?

A rickettsial disease
B amoebic liver abscess
C leptospirosis
D urinary tract infection
E sepsis from pyodermic insect bites

Question 21

A 30-year-old man, recently returned from trekking in Nepal, presents with a 6-day history of bloody diarrhoea with abdominal cramps but no fevers. He has taken some antibiotics, obtained in Nepal, with little effect. Which one of the following would be an UNLIKELY cause?

A *Entamoeba histolytica*
B *Trichuris*
C acute schistosomiasis
D ulcerative colitis
E *Clostridium difficile* colitis

Question 22

A 78-year-old man has been ventilated on the Intensive Care Unit for 10 days following surgical repair of a ruptured abdominal aortic aneurysm. His respiratory function is deteriorating and it is thought that he has developed a ventilator-associated pneumonia. Which one of the following drugs might be most suitable for treatment?

A benzylpenicillin

B cefuroxime
C augmentin
D vancomycin
E piperacillin/tazobactam (Tazocin)

Question 23
A 67-year-old man with chronic renal failure (cause unknown) for which he receives regular haemodialysis treatment has been admitted to the renal ward on many occasions with access difficulties. He is now admitted with fever and malaise. Blood cultures grow a vancomycin-resistant enterococcus (VRE). Which one of the following drugs would be most suitable treatment?
A meropenem
B linezolid
C gentamicin
D tobramycin
E co-trimoxazole (Septrin)

Question 24
A 74-year-old woman with chronic leg ulceration for which she has been admitted to hospital many times is admitted once again with fever and malaise thought to be due to infection of these ulcers. Swabs of the ulcer grow Methicillin-resistant *Staphylococcus aureus* (MRSA). Which one of the drugs listed can be used to treat this condition?
A flucloxacillin
B augmentin
C vancomycin
D cefuroxime
E meropenem

Question 25
A renal transplant patient develops fever and haematuria. Which viral infection should be considered most likely?
A polyoma virus (BK)
B Epstein-Barr virus (EBV)
C herpes simplex virus (HSV)
D varicella zoster (VZV)
E human herpes virus6 (HHV-6).

Question 26
A woman who is 36 weeks pregnant presents with chickenpox. How should she be treated?
A varicella-zoster immune globulin
B steroids
C aciclovir
D painkillers only
E immediate delivery of the child

Question 27
An intubated patient on the Intensive Care Unit for 8 days following a road traffic accident has a persistent fever and some lung shadowing. Which of the following organisms is most likely to be involved?
A *Streptococcus pneumoniae*
B *Staphylococcus epidermidis*
C *Staphylococcus aureus*
D *Pseudomonas aeruginosa*
E *Legionella pneumophila*

Question 28
A 28-year-old woman has noticed this blistering eruption appear over her body every 2–3 months for the last year (see Figure 111). On each occasion she has had symptoms of genital soreness and has taken some potassium citrate and cranberry juice. What is the most likely diagnosis?
A fixed drug eruption
B erythema multiforme
C disseminated gonococcal disease
D bullous pemphigus
E urticaria

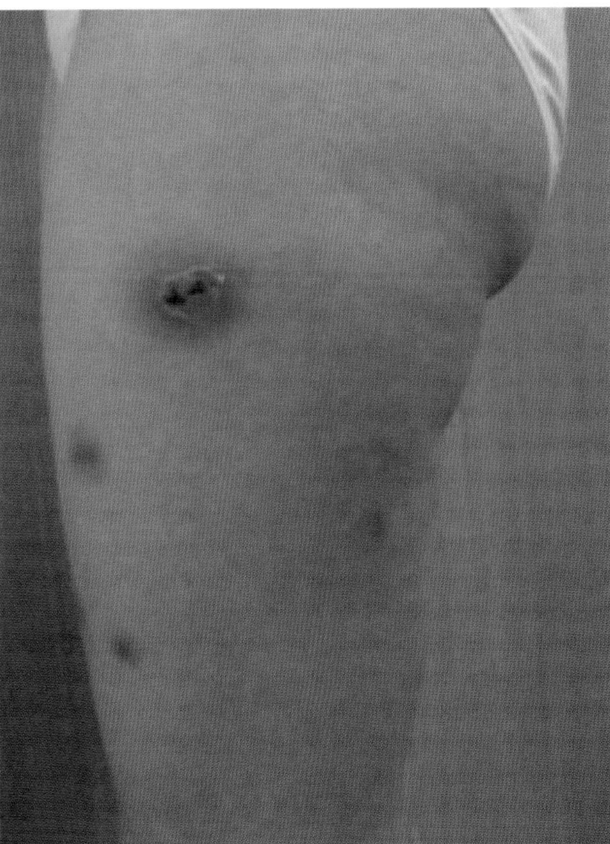

Fig. 111 Question 28.

Question 29
A 25-year-old woman complains of an increasing offensive vaginal discharge over the last 2 weeks. She is feeling feverish and has lower abdominal pains. She is not sexually active and has had a sexual health screen after she finished her last relationship some 3 months ago when a cervical erosion was noted. She has never had a sexually

transmitted infection. She is on no medication and her last normal menstrual period was 17 days ago. She discontinued her oral contraceptive some 4 weeks ago. What is the most likely diagnosis?
A candidal infection
B *Neisseria gonorrhoeae* infection
C cervical malignancy
D retained foreign body in the vagina
E pregnancy

Question 30

A patient reports that he is allergic to erythromycin. Which one of the following would you NOT usually accept as being compatible with an allergic reaction?
A fever
B widespread rash
C shortness of breath
D diarrhoea
E localized skin eruption

Question 31

An 89-year-old man presents to casualty with a fever and a several week history of headache. On examination he is confused, has neck stiffness and a right seventh cranial nerve palsy. He has no visible rash. A lumbar puncture reveals CSF Protein 4.0 g/l, Glucose 1.2 mmol/l (plasma glucose 4.6 mmol/l), and on microscopy 300 white cells/μl, predominantly lymphocytes. Serum VDRL is positive and TPHA is negative. The most likely diagnosis is:
A viral meningitis
B neurosyphilis
C herpes simplex encephalitis
D tuberculous meningitis
E *Listeria* meningitis

Question 32

A 32-year-old woman presents with community-acquired pneumonia. She is very unwell, but reports that she is 'allergic to penicillin', having had an anaphylactic reaction after treatment of a urinary tract infection several years ago. You would give her:
A cefotaxime 2 g six-hourly and erythromycin 1 g six-hourly, both intravenously
B erythromicin 500 mg six-hourly orally
C amoxicillin 250 mg eight-hourly and clarithromycin 250 mg twice daily, both orally
D erythromycin 1 g six-hourly intravenously
E ciprofloxacin 500 mg twice daily orally

Question 33

A 77-year-old man presents with sudden onset of weakness of his right arm on a background of a 3-week history of thoracolumbar backpain, weight loss, fever and night sweats. Blood tests show haemoglobin 9.8 g/dL, white cell count (WCC) 12.0 × 10^9/l, platelets 450 × 10^9/l, erythrocyte sedimentation rate (ESR) 110 mm/hr, creatinine 180 μmol/L. Stick testing of his urine reveals microscopic haematuria. What is the most likely diagnosis?
A spinal osteomyelitis
B myeloma
C infective endocarditis
D mycobacterium tuberculosis infection
E tertiary syphilis

Question 34

A 48-year-old man presents on the medical take with right lower lobe pneumonia. In the acute assessment of an adult with community-acquired pneumonia which one of the following is NOT of prognostic importance?
A urea > 7 mmol/l
B confusional state
C PaO_2 < 10 kPa
D respiratory rate > 30/min
E diastolic BP < 60 mmHg

Question 35

A 57-year-old woman develops a fever 7 days post bone marrow transplantation. She is placed empirically on broad-spectrum antibiotics but remains febrile. On the 11th day she develops a few painless, red, papular lesions on her trunk and lower limbs. What is the likely cause of these lesions?
A candidal infection
B staphylococcal infection
C aspergillus infection
D graft versus host disease
E recurrence of her haematological disease.

Question 36

A 26-year-old woman presents with a short history of confusion, diarrhoea and breathlessness. On examination she is pyrexial at 38.5°C, pulse 120/min, BP 80/60 mmHg and respiratory rate 26/min. She has a faint blanching macular rash across the trunk. She is disorientated without meningism. Which of the following diagnoses is most likely?
A *Salmonella enteritidis* infection
B pneumococcal meningitis
C anaphylaxis
D N-methyl-3,4-methylenedioxymethamphetamine ('Ecstasy') overdose
E toxic shock syndrome

Question 37

A 30-year-old man presents with diplopia, dysphagia and dysarthria. After 12 hours he has weakness of his arms but remains afebrile and is not confused. Over the next 12 hours he develops respiratory failure and requires artificial ventilation. What is the likely diagnosis?

A tetanus
B diphtheria
C botulism
D strychnine poisoning
E rabies

Question 38

A 38-year-old man presents with breathlessness and cough. He is unwell, with high fever, and has signs of consolidation in his right lower lobe. The most likely pathogen is:

A legionella
B *Neisseria meningitidis*
C *Streptococcus pneumoniae*
D HIV
E *Staphylococcus aureus*

Question 39

An HIV-positive patient presents with abdominal bloating and discomfort. He is afebrile, with blood pressure 110/60 mmHg, pulse 98/min, respiratory rate 24/min. The chest is clear, heart sounds normal, but palpation reveals some right upper quadrant tenderness. Blood tests show Na 141 mmol/L, K 3.9 mmol/L, urea 7.2 mmol/L, creatinine 111 µmol/L, bilirubin 48 µmol/L, alkaline phosphatase 500 IU/L, gamma-glutamyl transpeptidase (GGT) 220 IU/L, alanine aminotransferase (ALT) 80 IU/L. Arterial blood gases (breathing air) are pH 7.28, PaO_2 12.0 kPa, PCO_2 3.2 kPa, base excess –11.9. A chest radiograph is normal. The CD4 count is 180 cells/mL and HIV viral load is undetectable. What is the most likely diagnosis?

A *Pneumocystis carinii* pneumonia
B myocardial infarction
C *Mycobacterium avium* infection
D lactic acidosis
E hepatitis C infection

Question 40

Two days after returning from a 1-week trip around Thailand, a 25-year-old woman presents with sudden onset of fever, headache and severe myalgia. Three days after her symptoms started she develops a generalized erythematous rash. Her Hb is 12g/dl, WCC $2.1 \times 10^9/l$ and platelets $65 \times 10^9/l$. What is the most likely diagnosis?

A *Plasmodium vivax* malaria
B typhoid fever
C paratyphoid fever
D dengue fever
E tick-borne encephalitis

Dermatology

AUTHORS:
K. Harman, G. Ogg, N. Stone

EDITOR:
K. Harman

EDITOR-IN-CHIEF:
J.D. Firth

1 Clinical presentations

1.1 Blistering disorders

Case history

A 70-year-old man presents with blisters on his arms and legs.

Clinical approach

The brief history gives little away, but a careful history and examination will narrow down the diagnostic possibilities (Table 1). Your immediate priority is to recognize and treat diseases that may become life threatening, in particular toxic epidermal necrolysis (TEN), pemphigus vulgaris (PV), eczema herpeticum and varicella zoster in the immunosuppressed.

Widespread erosion of the skin as a result of blistering is potentially life-threatening due to the consequences of fluid, electrolyte and protein loss and in particular, secondary infection causing septicaemia.

History of the presenting problem

The history alone may point to a particular diagnosis if key questions are asked:

Table 1 Skin disorders presenting with blisters or erosions.

Immunobullous disorders	Bullous pemphigoid and pemphigoid gestationis Pemphigus vulgaris Dermatitis herpetiformis Cicatricial pemphigoid
'Reactive'	Bullous erythema multiforme Toxic epidermal necrolysis Staphylococcal scalded skin syndrome Bullous drug eruptions Bullous insect bites Acute contact dermatitis
Infections	Herpes simplex Varicella zoster (chicken pox) Herpes zoster (shingles) Bullous impetigo Cellulitis (occasionally, if severe)
Miscellaneous	Porphrias (cutanea tarda and variegate) Pompholyx (dyshidrotic eczema) Diabetic bullae Burns

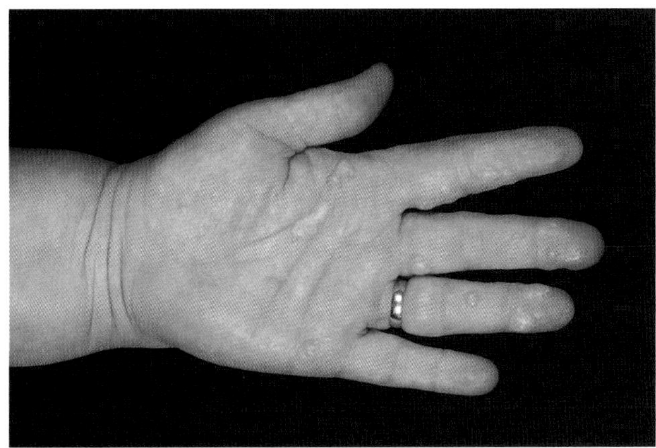

Fig. 1 Pompholyx (Dyshidrotic eczema). Multiple itchy vesicles on the palms and lateral borders of the digits. The thick epidermis results in deep-seated blisters which resemble tapioca grains when the blisters are small.

- How old is the patient? This is an important consideration: this man is 70. PV, porphyria cutanea tarda, bullous pemphigoid (BP) and cicatricial pemphigoid (CP) usually present in the middle aged/elderly. By contrast, dermatitis herpetiformis (DH), chicken pox, pemphigoid gestationis (PG), bullous impetigo and staphylococcal scalded skin syndrome (SSSS) usually present in children/young adults, and the latter two almost exclusively in children.
- How long? Infections and reactive conditions will have a short history over hours/days whilst blisters occurring over several weeks/months are typical of immunobullous disorders and porphyrias.
- Do you itch? Pruritus is a very useful symptom to elicit and here suggests DH, pemphigoid (BP and PG), contact dermatitis, chicken pox, pompholyx (Fig. 1) or insect bites.
- Is it painful? Pain is prominent in herpes zoster, eczema herpeticum and cellulitis. Tenderness or burning of the skin occurs in TEN and SSSS. The skin will also be sore if there are widespread erosions, regardless of cause, especially if secondarily infected.
- Which drugs? A history of all medications taken in the month prior to the onset of blisters is crucial. Erythema multiforme (EM), TEN and bullous drug eruptions may all be drug triggered (see Section 2.6, p. 195).
- Are you pregnant? Clearly not applicable in this man, but if so consider PG, a specific dermatosis of pregnancy.
- What were you doing before the blisters appeared? Particularly relevant in acute contact dermatitis. Ask about occupation and hobbies, e.g. a gardener with an itchy rash on his hands may be allergic to a plant. Ask about application of any creams to the affected area.

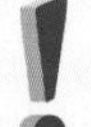

When you assess a patient with blisters or ulcers of the skin, always ask about soreness or ulceration of the mucous membranes, particularly the eyes, mouth and genitalia. Patients may be too embarrassed to tell you about genital ulcers and often fail to realize they are linked to their skin problems.

Relevant past history

Immunobullous disorders may be associated with other autoimmune diseases and DH with gluten-sensitive enteropathy. Some patients with porphyria cutanea tarda have hepatitis C or alcohol-induced liver disease. Immunosuppressed patients are more susceptible to infections, in which they are more serious.

Examination

Skin

Site and distribution

Many bullous disorders show a predilection for certain sites (Table 2). If very localized or asymmetrical, think of an exogenous cause such as infections (Fig. 2) or contact dermatitis (see Figs 22, p. 178 and 47, p. 198). Watch out for the dermatomal distribution of herpes zoster (Fig. 3).

Morphology

Close attention to the appearance of individual lesions may provide the diagnosis:

Table 2 Blistering diseases in which the distribution may help make a diagnosis.

Site which is commonly affected	Diagnosis
Mucous membranes	Pemphigus vulgaris EM and TEN (lips too) CP
Limbs	DH (extensor surfaces, especially knees and elbows) EM (particularly hands/feet) Bullous insect bites (often clustered) Pompholyx (palms, soles and sides of digits) Diabetic bullae (lower legs)
Centripetal	Chicken pox PG (often begins on the abdomen)
Photosensitive distribution	Variegate and porphyria cutanea tarda Photosensitive drug eruptions
Dermatomal	Herpes zoster
Localized and asymmetrical	Herpes simplex (usually clustered) Bullous impetigo Cellulitis Acute contact dermatitis

CP, cicatricial pemphigoid; DH, dermatitis herpetiformis; EM, erythema multiforme; PG, pemphigoid gestationis; TEN, toxic epidermal necrolysis.

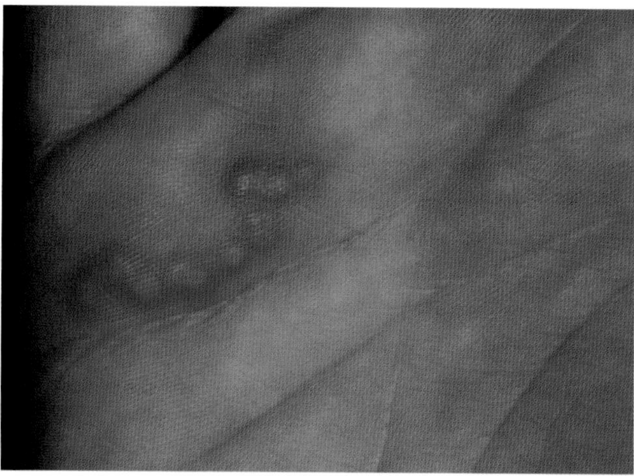

(a)

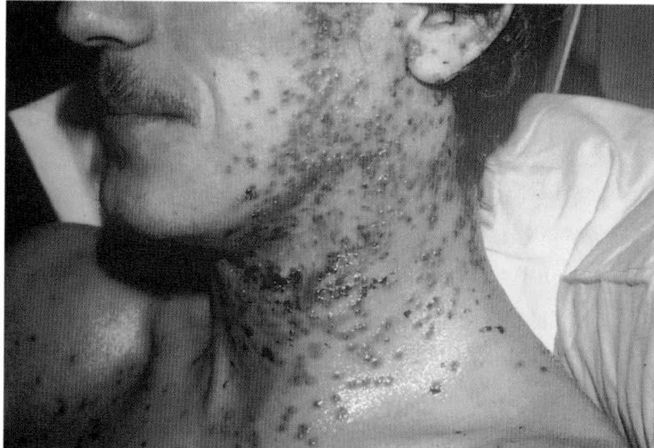

(b)

Fig. 2 (a) Herpes simplex. A localized cluster of small vesicles and pustules on an erythematous base which will become eroded then crust over. (b) Eczema herpeticum. The herpes simplex virus spreads easily through abnormal, eczematous skin and can become widespread. The clue to the diagnosis is the presence of multiple vesicles, papules and punched-out erosions which are monomorphic, i.e. the same size and shape. They are best seen peripherally rather than centrally where they often become confluent. It is a painful and serious condition.

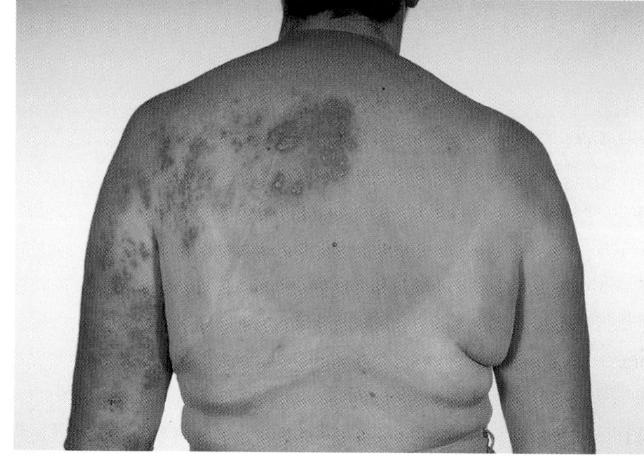

Fig. 3 Herpes zoster. Pain preceded the appearance of this eruption in the left T2 dermatome. There are erythematous papules with clusters of overlying blisters and pustules visible on the back. These will subsequently crust before healing.

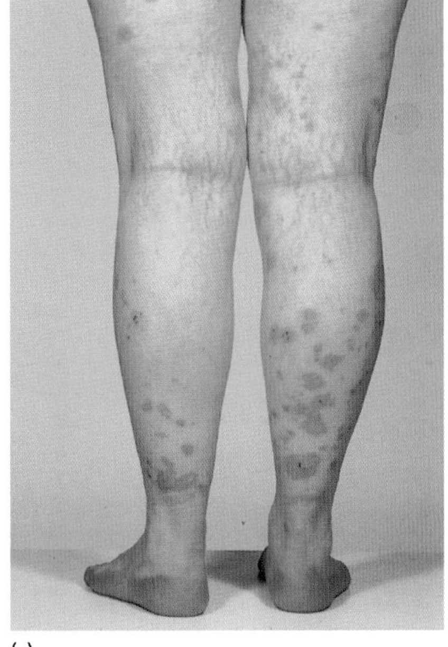

(a)

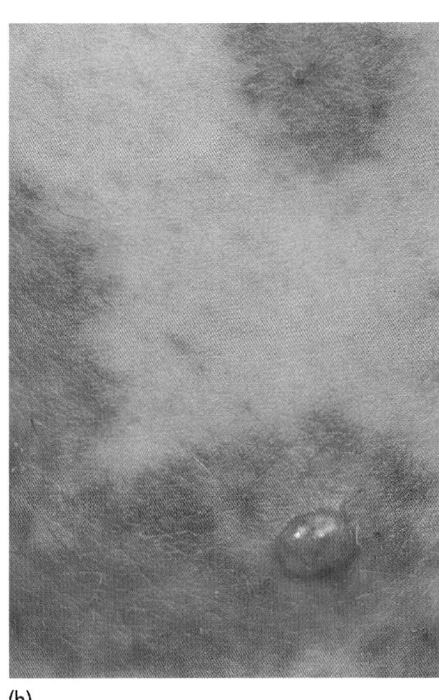

(b)

Fig. 4 Pemphigoid gestationis. This pregnant woman presented with an itchy eruption which had been treated as scabies. There were erythematous papules and plaques (a), but on careful inspection, one tense blister was found (b). Bullous pemphigoid has a similar appearance.

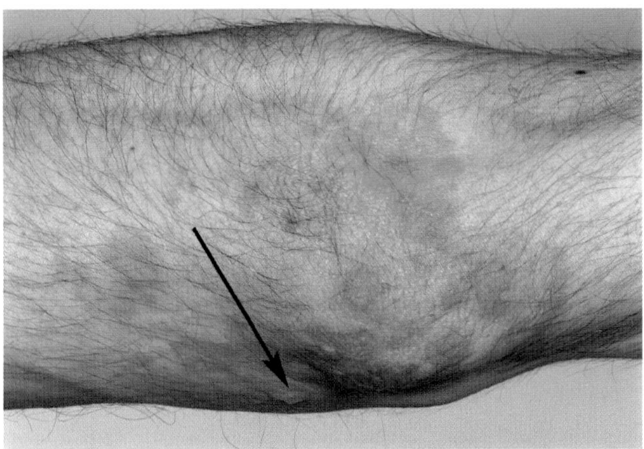

Fig. 5 Dermatitis herpetiformis. This patient with gluten-sensitive enteropathy complained of intense pruritus prior to the appearance of erythematous papules and plaques on the elbows (shown), buttocks and knees. One blister is visible (arrowed).

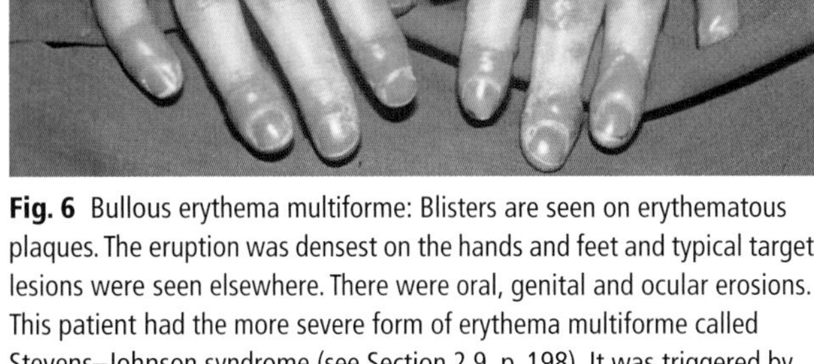

Fig. 6 Bullous erythema multiforme: Blisters are seen on erythematous plaques. The eruption was densest on the hands and feet and typical target lesions were seen elsewhere. There were oral, genital and ocular erosions. This patient had the more severe form of erythema multiforme called Stevens–Johnson syndrome (see Section 2.9, p. 198). It was triggered by mycoplasma pneumonia in this case.

- in herpes simplex virus (HSV) infection, a cluster of small vesicles or punched-out erosions is typical (Fig. 2a).
- multiple, monomorphic erosions on a background of eczema should make you think of eczema herpeticum (Fig. 2b).
- target-like lesions may be seen in EM (see Section 1.2, p. 169 and Fig. 11a, p. 171).
- lesions of variable age are typical in chicken pox (see Section 1.2 and Table 3).
- Blisters on a background of erythema and oedema are typical in herpes zoster, BP, PG, EM, DH, acute contact dermatitis and insect bites (Figs 3–6).
- Underlying and surrounding inflammation and erythema is minimal in porphyria, PV and diabetic bullae (Figs 7–9).
- In TEN and SSSS there is diffuse, widespread erythema and the epidermis tends to shear off in sheets rather than form discrete blisters (see Fig. 13).

The blisters of BP are more resilient than those of PV because they are sited deeper (at the dermoepidermal junction compared to within the epidermis). Therefore, BP blisters are often tense with fluid (Fig. 4b) and may be up to several cm in size before bursting, whilst PV blisters are easily ruptured to leave erosions (Fig. 7a).

Nikolsky's sign

This is positive if a shearing force applied to apparently normal, perilesional skin results in epidermal detachment. It is traditionally a sign of PV but may also be positive in TEN and SSSS.

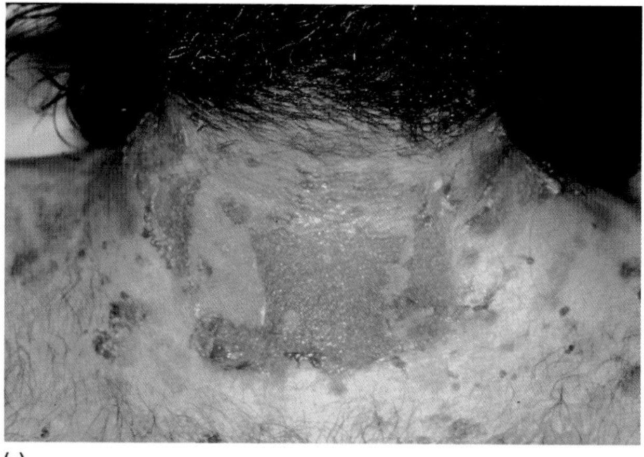

(a)

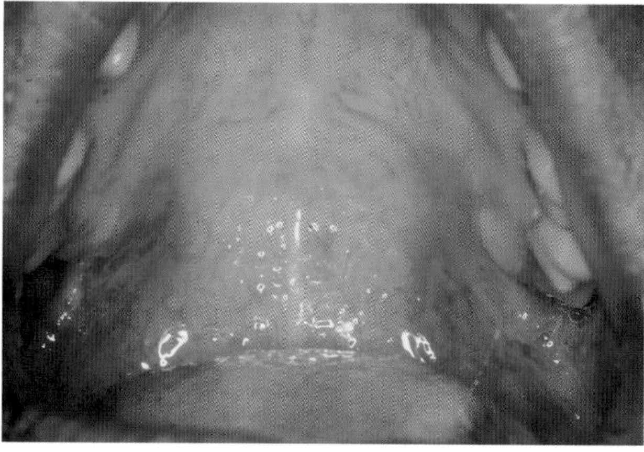

(b)

Fig. 7 Pemphigus vulgaris. The fragile blisters in pemphigus rarely remain intact so erosions are more commonly seen (a). In almost all cases, there will be erosions in the oral cavity, seen here on the soft palate (b).

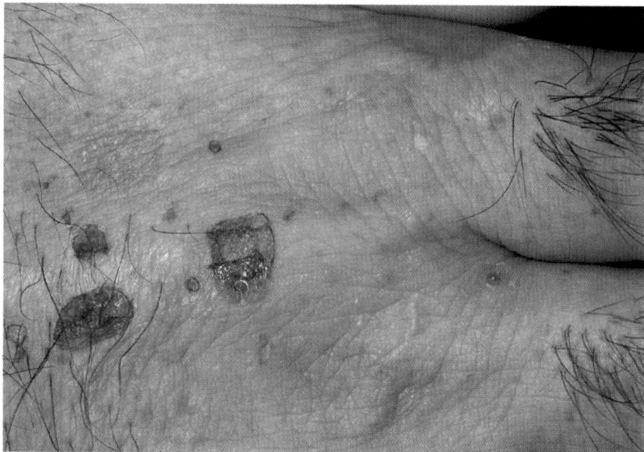

Fig. 8 Porphyria cutanea tarda. Blisters preceded these erosions seen on the dorsum of the hand of a patient who complained of skin fragility and increased hair growth (note the hypertrichosis). There is minimal inflammation of the skin (unlike Figs 2–6) and atrophic scars are also visible.

Other features

The skin is fragile in variegate and porphyria cutanea tarda and there may be scarring, hypertrichosis, hyperpigmentation and milia. Scarring is also a feature of CP.

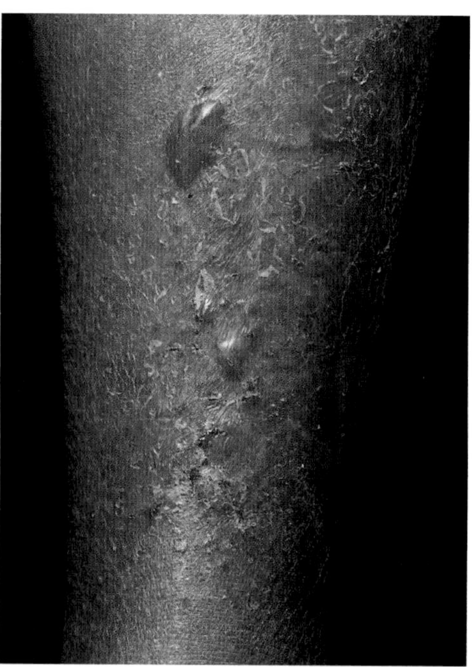

Fig. 9 Diabetes: large bullae on a non-inflamed base on the lower legs of a diabetic male.

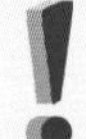

Blisters easily rupture to produce erosions. Therefore, always consider a blistering disorder if there are skin or mucous membrane erosions. Don't forget to send skin for direct immunofluorescence in these cases—histology alone is insufficient to clinch the diagnosis of an immunobullous disorder.

Approach to investigation and management

Investigations

The choice of investigations will be guided by your clinical findings:

- skin swabs for bacterial and viral culture (don't forget to use viral transport medium)
- vesicle fluid for electron microscopy—for urgent confirmation of suspected viral infections
- blood cultures
- blood tests—indirect immunofluorescence may be positive in immunobullous disorders (see Section 3.2, p. 212); antiendomysial, reticulin, gliadin or tissue transglutaminase antibodies if DH suspected; HSV and mycoplasma serology in EM; blood count may show eosinophilia in BP or drug eruptions, neutrophilia in cellulitis
- porphyrin screen—blood, urine, stool
- skin biopsy for histology and direct immunofluorescence
- patch tests.

Management

- Immunobullous diseases—see Sections 2.2 (p. 192), 2.5 (p. 195) and 2.12 (p. 202).

• Bullous EM and TEN—see Section 2.9 (p. 198).
• Contact dermatitis—see Section 2.8 (p. 197).
• Herpes simplex, chicken pox and herpes zoster—see *Infectious diseases*, Section 2.10, but eczema herpeticum must be treated with systemic aciclovir.
• Cellulitis, bullous impetigo and SSSS—see *Infectious diseases*, Sections 1.3 and 2.5.1.
• Porphyrias—see *Biochemistry and metabolism*, Section 6.
• Bullous drug eruptions. Stop the suspected drug—see Section 2.6 (p. 195).

If there is widespread erosion of the skin, general management is as outlined for TEN, regardless of diagnosis—see Section 2.9 (p. 198).

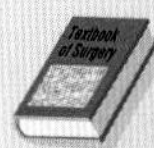

Fitzpatrick TB, Johnson RA, Wolff K *et al. Color Atlas and Synopsis of Clinical Dermatology: Common and Serious Diseases* (3rd edn). New York: McGraw-Hill, 1997.
Habif TP. *Clinical Dermatology: A Colour Guide to Diagnosis and Therapy* (2nd edn). St Louis: CV Mosby, 1990.

1.2 Acute generalized rashes

Case history

A 20-year-old woman presents with a 12-h history of fever and a generalized rash.

Several life-threatening disorders present with a rash and fever. The cutaneous findings alone may be diagnostic and allow life-saving treatment to be started without delay.

Clinical approach

Many disorders present acutely with a generalized rash: diagnostic confusion is common. Table 3 lists these disorders along with key clinical features to help differentiate them. Your main priority is to be able to recognize and treat those that are life-threatening.

History of the presenting problem

There are several key questions to ask when assessing patients with acute rashes:
• How old is the patient. This woman is 20. Many disorders present in certain age groups and so some diagnoses, e.g. Kawasaki's disease and SSSS, can be discounted here simply on the basis of age (see Table 3).
• Have you been unwell recently? A prodromal illness is common in viral exanthems and symptoms associated with a triggering infection may be present in erythema multiforme (EM), Stevens–Johnson syndrome (SJS), toxic epidermal necrolysis (TEN), staphylococcal scalded skin syndrome (SSSS), toxic shock syndrome (TSS), scarlet fever, vasculitic rashes and acute urticaria.
• Has anyone else been unwell recently? Find out about any infectious contacts.
• Are you itchy? Is the skin sore? Pruritus is characteristic of urticaria and is common in chicken pox and pityriasis rosea. It may accompany drug eruptions. If the skin is tender or burning, think of TEN, SSSS and generalized pustular psoriasis.
• Do lesions come and go? Urticarial weals last a few hours only, a characteristic feature.
• Tongue swelling, dyspnoea or wheeze? Angioedema or anaphylaxis may accompany urticaria but are unlikely to be relevant here because the history is usually very acute.
• Where did the rash start? May be very helpful, e.g. measles and rubella typically start on the face and spread to the trunk and limbs, unlike maculopapular drug eruptions, the main differential diagnosis otherwise (Fig. 10).
• Are you menstruating? Relevant in toxic shock syndrome.

Drug history

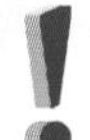

An accurate drug history is vital when assessing skin problems. Patients may fail to tell you about over-the-counter and 'alternative' therapies so specifically ask about these in addition to prescribed drugs. Include all drugs taken in the preceding month. See Section 2.6 (p. 195).

Relevant past history

Unlikely to be relevant here with the exception of generalized pustular or guttate psoriasis in which there may be a preceding history. You may also obtain a history of drug allergy.

Examination

General

• General impression: Is the patient well, unwell or very unwell?
• A full physical examination is required.
• Don't forget to check for fever, lymphadenopathy and sources of infection that may liberate toxins, e.g. pharyngitis, wounds, retained tampons.

Skin

Distribution

Compare the head and neck vs trunk vs limbs and don't forget the palms, soles and flexural areas. The distribution may provide diagnostic clues, e.g. EM has a predilection

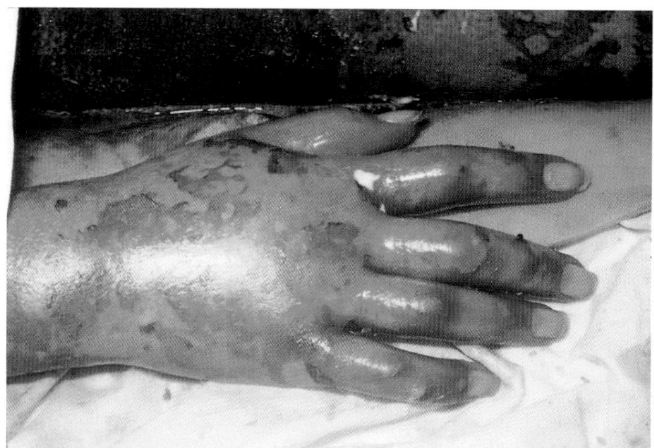

Fig. 13 Toxic epidermal necrolysis. The epidermis has sloughed off in places to reveal the raw, glazed surface of the underlying dermis. Friction on 'normal' skin may slough off the epidermis (Nikolsky's sign) so skin handling should be minimized. The appearance of staphylococcal scalded skin syndrome is similar.

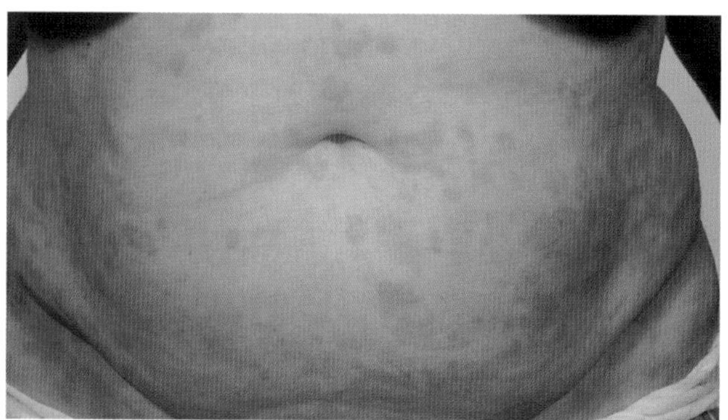

Fig. 14 Urticaria. Erythematous, oedematous papules and plaques which are itchy. The skin surface is normal. The key feature, which distinguishes urticaria from other dermatoses, is the transient nature of lesions which last for only a few hours and leave no mark.

WEALS

Characteristic of urticaria (Fig. 14) (see Section 2.16, p. 206).

PUSTULES

- Multiple tiny pustules on a background of diffuse erythema suggests a drug eruption or pustular psoriasis (Fig. 15) (see Section 1.3, p. 173).
- Scanty pustules can occur in bacteraemia, particularly gonococcaemia or *S. aureus* endocarditis.

SCALE

If lesions have a scaly surface, think of guttate psoriasis, pityriasis rosea and secondary syphilis (Fig. 16). Only the latter will affect the palms/soles.

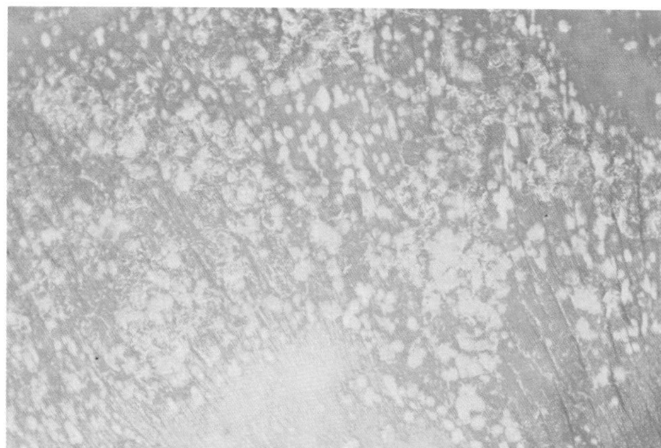

Fig. 15 Pustules: small, superficial, discrete collections of pus are sheeted across erythematous skin. The differential diagnosis is a drug eruption or pustular psoriasis.

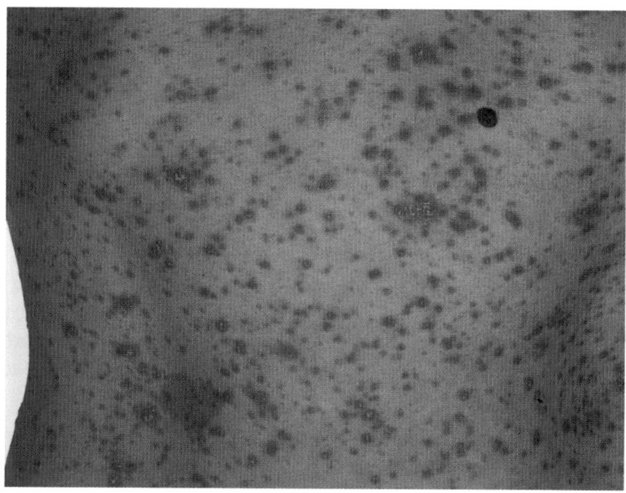

Fig. 16 Guttate psoriasis. This young woman developed an acute papular eruption on her trunk and proximal limbs. On close inspection, the surface of these deep red papules was scaly. In this case guttate psoriasis was triggered by a sore throat one week previously and the ASO titre was raised.

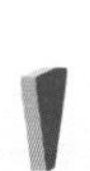

Don't forget the mucosal surfaces! Always check the mouth, eyes and genitalia. If affected, the differential diagnosis narrows (see Table 3).

Approach to investigation and management

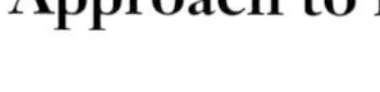

Investigations

- Blood tests—A blood count may show an eosinophilia in drug eruptions or thrombocytopaenia in TSS, some cases of purpura and sometimes in varicella. Thrombocytosis may occur in Kawasaki's disease and neutrophilia is a feature of pustular psoriasis or underlying bacterial infection. Do a coagulation screen if purpura is present. Check renal and liver function tests. Take acute and convalescent blood for serology in viral exanthems. Check mycoplasma and HSV serology in EM/SJS/TEN and an anti-streptolysin O (ASO) titre in scarlet fever and vasculitis. Check treponema serology if secondary syphilis is suspected.

- Blood cultures.
- Swab skin pustules, which will be sterile in drug eruptions and pustular psoriasis, and positive if due to bacteraemia or secondary infection.
- Swab suspected sources of infection in toxin-mediated diseases, e.g. throat, umbilical stump, skin wounds, nose, vagina.
- Chest X-ray—Look for evidence of mycoplasma pneumonia in EM/SJS/TEN, and pneumonitis in chicken pox or SJS/TEN.
- Examination of blister fluid or scrapings from blister base (Tzanck smear)—these tests should be performed for urgent confirmation of suspected viral infections. Light microscopy will identify virally infected cells and electron microscopy will identify virus particles. Otherwise, send swabs for viral culture.
- Skin biopsy—In many cases a skin biopsy will not be necessary, but proceed if the diagnosis is uncertain, particularly to distinguish SSSS and TEN.
- ECG and echocardiogram—If Kawasaki's disease is suspected.

Management

- Toxin-mediated disorders—treat the underlying bacterial infection (see *Infectious diseases*, Section 2.5). TSS may lead to multiorgan failure and ITU support may be needed. SSSS is treated similarly to TEN (see Section 2.9, p. 198) but it is far less severe as epidermal detachment is very superficial and re-epithelialization occurs within a few days.
- EM/SJS/TEN—see Section 2.9 (p. 198).
- Kawasaki's disease—aspirin and intravenous immunoglobulin reduce the long-term cardiac complications [1].
- Chicken pox or disseminated HSV: intravenous aciclovir —see *Infectious diseases*, Section 2.10.2.
- Urticaria—antihistamines and treat any infectious triggers. See Section 2.16 (p. 206).
- Drug eruptions—stop the suspected drug! See Section 2.6 (p. 195).
- Viral exanthems—symptomatic treatment in most cases. See *Infectious diseases*, Section 2.11.
- Pityrisis rosea—reassure. Symptomatic treatment only but warn patient that resolution takes 6–8 weeks.
- Guttate and pustular psoriasis—see Sections 1.3 and 2.14 (p. 203).

If unable to make a diagnosis, consider other infectious exanthems, e.g. adenoviruses, enteroviruses, CMV, EBV, toxoplasmosis, leptospirosis, Legionnaire's disease, HIV seroconversion and listeria, or acute rheumatic fever or connective tissue diseases such as systemic lupus erythematosis and Still's disease (see *Rheumatology and clinical immunology*, Sections 1.10 and 1.11).

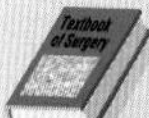

Du Vivier A. *Atlas of Clinical Dermatology* (2nd edn). London: Gower Medical Publishing, 1993.

Fitzpatrick TB, Johnson RA, Wolff K *et al. Color Atlas and Synopsis of Clinical Dermatology. Common and Serious Disease.* (3rd edn). New York: McGraw-Hill, 1997.

Newburger JW, Takahashi M, Beiser AS *et al.* A single infusion of gamma globulin as compared with four infusions in the treatment of acute Kawasaki syndrome. *N Engl J Med* 1991; 324: 1633–1639.

1.3 Erythroderma

Case history

A 50-year-old man is red all over.

Clinical approach

Widespread, confluent erythema involving more than 90% of the skin surface is termed erythroderma: there are several causes (Table 4). Psoriasis and eczema are the commonest. Your first priority is to resuscitate the patient, who may be extremely unwell. The cause of erythroderma can then be established and specific treatment instituted.

Erythroderma is life threatening because of the complications of widespread cutaneous vasodilatation, increased catabolism and loss of the normal homeostatic functions of the skin.

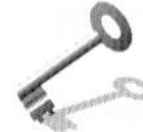

Complications of erythroderma

- Fluid loss, hypovolaemia, prerenal failure.
- Hypoalbuminaemia
- Excess heat convection, loss of thermoregulation, hypothermia
- High-output cardiac failure.

Table 4 The differential diagnosis of erythroderma.

Endogenous diseases	Psoriasis (pustular and non-pustular) Eczema Sézary syndrome Pityriasis rubra pilaris (PRP) Paraneoplastic
'Reactive'	Drug eruptions Allergic contact dermatitis Toxic epidermal necrolysis (TEN) Infectious exanthems, e.g. toxic shock syndrome, staphylococcal scalded skin syndrome (SSSS)

History of the presenting problem

• How long has the skin been red? An acute history with no pre-existing dermatoses is suggestive of a drug reaction, TEN or an infectious exanthem. Although eczema and psoriasis can sometimes progress very rapidly, there will usually be a past history. Sézary syndrome and pityriasis rubra pilaris (PRP) are slower to evolve, and in PRP, there is typically cranio-caudal migration.
• Take a very careful drug history! What drugs have been taken in the last month? Anything from 'over-the-counter'? Are you absolutely sure? Not one tablet? If you think of anything, please let me know.
• Does the skin itch or burn? Itching is severe in eczema and Sézary syndrome. Skin tenderness or burning occurs in generalized pustular psoriasis, TEN and SSSS.
• Have you been unwell recently? Infections may trigger exacerbations of psoriasis. There may be an underlying infection or prodromal illness in infectious exanthems (see Section 1.2, p. 169).
• Check for symptoms that suggest malignancy. Erythroderma can occasionally be paraneoplastic.

Relevant past history

Enquire about drug reactions and allergies. There may be a history of psoriasis or eczema.

Examination

General

Initial assessment of the patient:
• General impression—well, unwell, very unwell or nearly dead? If nearly dead, call for help from ICU.
• Check vital signs—temperature, pulse, respiration, blood pressure.
• Is the patient's intravascular volume depleted? The only reliable signs in this context are a low jugular venous pressure (JVP) and postural hypotension. Where is the JVP? What is the blood pressure, lying and sitting, since standing will probably not be prudent? It can be difficult to establish these in someone who is erythrodermic and unwell: but the worse they are, the more important it is to know. If volume depleted, obtain venous access and start resuscitation immediately, whilst you complete the history and examination.
• A full general physical examination is required.

Skin

When there is diffuse erythema, ascertaining a cause from the morphology of individual skin lesions is difficult (Fig. 17a). Other clues need to be sought:

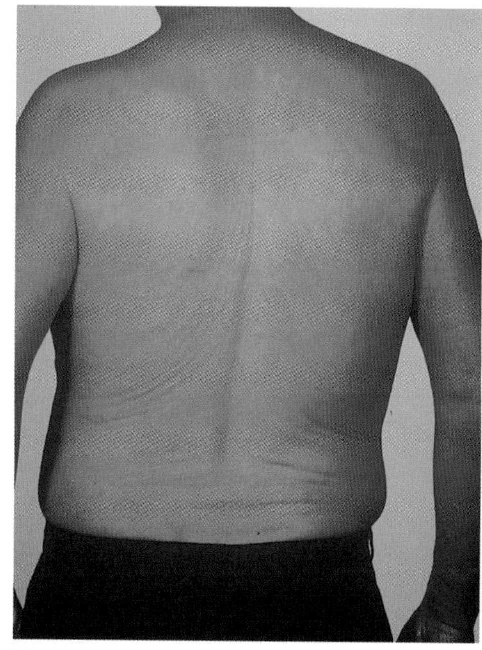

(a)

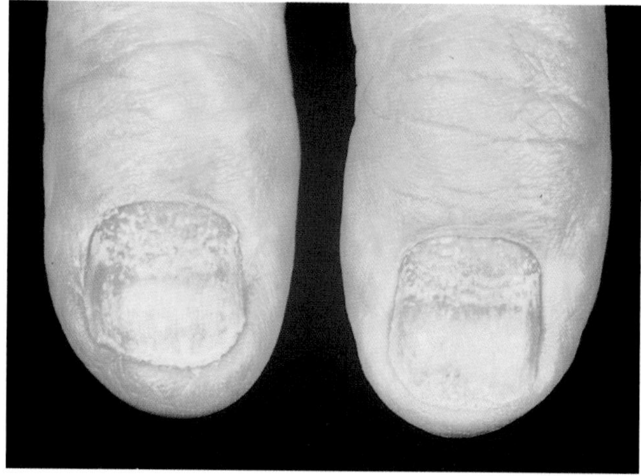

(b)

Fig. 17 Erythrodermic psoriasis (a) and psoriatic nails (b). The skin was scaly on close inspection but ascertaining the cause of erythroderma is difficult if the skin is examined in isolation. However, in this case there was a past history of plaque psoriasis and the nails were thickened and dystrophic with subungual hyperkeratosis and surface pits.

• Look for pustules—Sheets of superficial pustules can occur in drug reactions and generalized acute pustular psoriasis (Figs 15 and 18). The distinction can be difficult, but patients with a drug reaction tend to be less toxic and there may be a past history of plaque psoriasis in pustular psoriasis.
• Blisters, erosions or Nikolsky's sign positive—If present, think of TEN or SSSS (see Section 1.1, p. 167) (see Fig. 13).
• Scaling—Scaling is common in all long-standing cases of erythroderma (Fig. 19) and may be thick in psoriasis. In very acute cases scaling may not be seen, but if present it is more suggestive of psoriasis, eczema and drug eruptions rather than infectious exanthems.

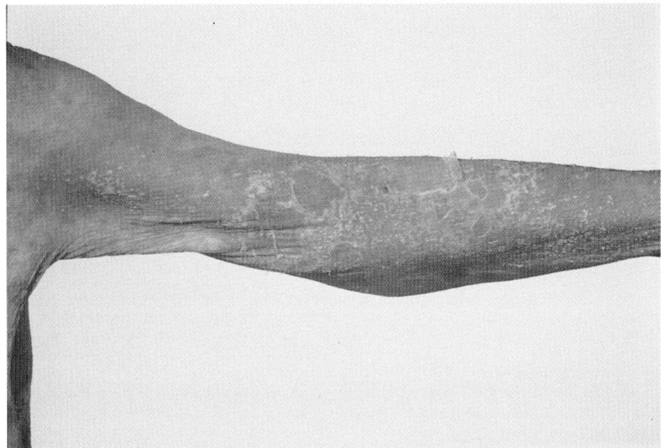

Fig. 18 Generalized pustular psoriasis: There are multiple superficial pustules studded on a background of diffuse erythema and scaling in a patient with a history of plaque psoriasis.

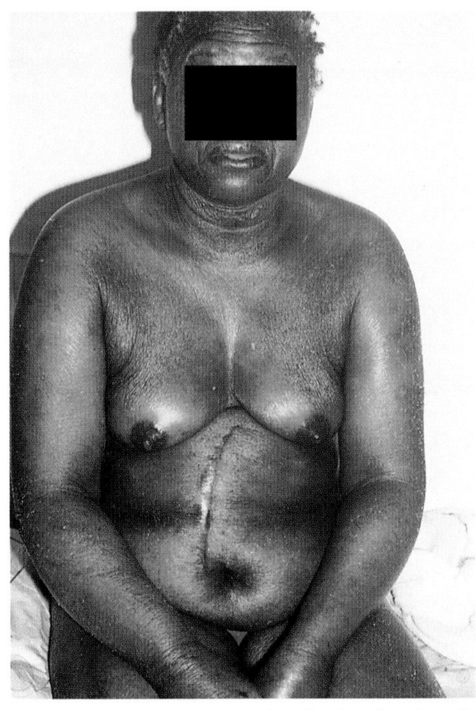

Fig. 19 An erythrodermic drug eruption. The offending drug (zopiclone) was continued for several weeks and over this time the eruption became erythrodermic and scaly. It can be difficult to appreciate erythema in black skin but the skin was hot to touch and the patient was unwell, shivering and dehydrated.

Mucous membranes

Ulceration occurs in TEN; erythema of the mouth and eyes occurs in TSS. (Table 3a).

Lymphadenopathy

Reactive hyperplasia of regional nodes occurs in erythroderma, regardless of cause, so it is probable that small nodes will be palpable. Large nodes suggest a diagnosis of Sézary syndrome or a drug hypersensitivity syndrome.

Palms and soles

Thickening of the skin is prominent in psoriasis, Sézary syndrome and PRP.

Alopecia

A telogen effluvium (see Section 1.6, p. 183) may occur in erythroderma regardless of cause. However, total alopecia suggests Sézary syndrome.

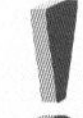

Always check the nails when assessing any patient with a skin disorder. Nail abnormalities will provide diagnostic clues. In this case psoriasis would be suggested by pitting, onycholysis, ridging and thickening of the nails (Fig. 17b) (see Fig. 51, p. 204). Nail thickening is also seen in Sézary syndrome and PRP.

Approach to investigation and management

Investigations

- Full blood count: eosinophilia—atopic eczema, drug reactions; neutrophilia—generalized pustular psoriasis or a triggering bacterial infection; lymphocytosis—Sézary syndrome.
- Blood film—Sézary cells are present in Sézary syndrome.
- IgE—Raised in atopic eczema.
- Swabs for M, C & S—Swab possible sources of *S. aureus* infection that may have triggered TSS or SSSS, e.g. wounds, retained tampons.
- Lymph node biopsy—If nodes are enlarged and Sézary syndrome is suspected.
- Skin biopsy.

For further investigations relevant to TSS/SSSS/TEN, see Sections 1.2 (p. 169) and 2.9 (p. 198).

Management

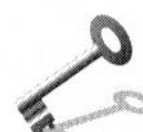

Supportive general management of the erythrodermic patient

- Fluid replacement if volume depleted—if the JVP is down and there is postural hypotension, give colloid or 0.9% saline rapidly until the JVP has risen into the normal range and there is no postural drop in blood pressure. Then give fluid at a rate equal to measured output plus a large allowance (often 2–3 L per day) for greatly increased insensible losses, adjusted in the light of clinical examination of volume status repeated at least twice daily
- Keep careful fluid balance charts and weigh the patient daily (if possible)
- Monitor electrolytes and renal function daily whilst the patient remains acutely ill.
- Nurse in a warm environment
- Bed rest
- Nutritional supplementation—nutritional supplements, nasogastric feeding or parenteral nutrition will be required
- Treat the skin with bland emollients

Specific treatment

- Psoriasis—When erythrodermic, systemic treatment is usually required. Generalized pustular psoriasis is particularly serious. See Section 2.14 (p. 203).
- Eczema—See Sections 2.7 (p. 196) and 2.8 (p. 197).
- Erythrodermic drug eruptions—Stop any suspected drug triggers. Symptomatic treatment ± systemic steroids. See Section 2.6 (p. 196).
- Sézary syndrome—See Section 2.4 (pp. 193).
- TEN, SSSS and TSS—See Sections 1.2 (p. 173) and 2.9 (p. 198).
- Pityrisis rubra pilaris is a rare, idiopathic disorder. It is difficult to treat and resolves spontaneously in most cases. Retinoids, cyclosporin and methotrexate have been used.
- Paraneoplastic—Treat the underlying neoplasm.

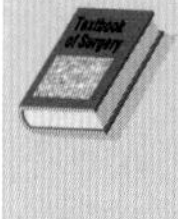

Fitzpatrick TB, Johnson RA, Wolff K *et al. Color Atlas and Synopsis of Clinical Dermatology. Common and Serious Diseases* (3rd edn). New York: McGraw-Hill, 1997.
Habif TP. *Clinical dermatology: A Colour Guide to Diagnosis and Therapy* (2nd edn). St Louis: CV Mosby, 1990.

1.4 A chronic, red facial rash

Case history

A 25-year-old woman presents with a 2-month history of a red facial rash.

Clinical approach

This is an extremely common dermatological presentation. A common skin disease is the most likely diagnosis, but some systemic disorders can present with an eruption that preferentially affects the face. The diagnosis can often be made from a good history and examination alone (Tables 5 and 6).

History of the presenting problem

- Does your face itch? If yes, you are likely to be dealing with eczema. Other facial dermatoses are not especially itchy.
- Have you had this problem before? Atopic eczema might have been present on and off since childhood. Seborrhoeic dermatitis also tends to wax and wane. A fungal infection (tinea) or the rash of systemic lupus erythematosus (SLE) would have a shorter history.
- Is it worse in the summer or after sun exposure? SLE, discoid lupus erythematosus (DLE), photosensitive eczemas and dermatomyositis can all be photoaggravated.

Table 5 Differential diagnosis of a chronic red facial rash.

Common	Atopic eczema Contact dermatitis Seborrhoeic dermatitis Acne Rosacea *Tinea faciei*
Less common	Discoid lupus erythematosus Systemic lupus erythematosus Dermatomyositis Sarcoidosis Photosensitive eczema (endogenous or exogenous)

- Is the rash present elsewhere on your body?
- Any new cosmetics or creams? These may be the trigger in contact dermatitis. In addition, nail-varnish allergy may present with facial eczema from touching the skin.
- Do you have any pets? A history of contact with animals may be present with *Tinea faciei* (ringworm).

Associated symptoms

Check for:

- symptoms of proximal muscle weakness or an underlying carcinoma that would suggest dermatomyositis
- joint pains, indicating psoriatic arthropathy or lupus
- shortness of breath, indicating active pulmonary sarcoid
- easy flushing, associated with rosacea
- Raynaud's phenomenon, occurring with both SLE and DLE, and sometimes dermatomyositis.

Relevant past history

- Is there a personal or family history of atopy (eczema, asthma or hayfever)?
- There may be a history of lupus or sarcoidosis.

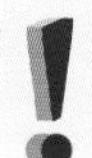

Always enquire about a personal or family history of atopy (asthma, eczema, hay-fever) when assessing a patient with skin problems. Atopic eczema could be the primary diagnosis or a contributory factor, e.g. atopy complicated by contact dermatitis.

Examination

Skin

Morphology of the rash

Consider Table 6, and ask:

- Is the rash eczematous, i.e. red, scaly and macular? (Figs 20–23).

Table 6 Causes of a chronic red facial rash: clinical findings.

Diagnosis	Morphology, distribution	Other findings
Atopic eczema	Red, scaly, macular. Poorly defined. Lichenification. Eyelids commonly involved	Atopy. Generalized dry skin (xerosis) and active flexural eczema
Contact dermatitis	Red, scaly, macular. Distribution may be odd, suggesting an exogenous cause	Absence of atopic features
Seborrhoeic dermatitis	Red, scaly, macular. Nasolabial folds, eyebrows, hairline	Look for a similar rash over sternum, flexures, behind ears plus a scaly scalp
Acne	Comedones, papules, pustules. Nodules and scarring when severe. Forehead, nose, chin, jawline	Look for upper chest and back involvement
Rosacea	Erythema, papules, pustules, telangiectasia. Forehead, nose, cheeks, chin.	Easy flushing. May be an associated rhinophyma. No rash on body
Tinea faciei	Often annular. Red, scaly, advancing margin	Usually a solitary lesion
SLE	Macular erythema across cheeks—'Butterfly rash'. Erythematous papules and plaques over light-exposed areas	Nail-fold telangiectasia, Raynaud's phenomenon, livedo reticularis, fingerpulp vasculitic lesions
DLE	Scaly round/oval plaques with prominent follicles within. Well defined. Heal with scarring	Scarring alopecia. Unusual to find lesions on body cf. psoriasis
Dermatomyositis	Peri-orbital oedema and heliotrope rash (i.e. purplish colour). Macular erythema cheeks and forehead	Gottron's papules on dorsum of hands. Nail-fold telangiectasia and ragged cuticles
Sarcoidosis	Bluish/red papules and plaques infiltrating the nose, cheeks and earlobes (lupus pernio variant). Red/brown papules, plaques or nodules.	Lupus pernio variant may be associated with upper respiratory tract involvement. Check for systemic disease
Photosensitive eczema	Features of eczema as above	Sparing of covered sites with a cut-off on the neck or upper chest/back

DLE, discoid lupus erythematosus; SLE, systemic lupus erythematosus.

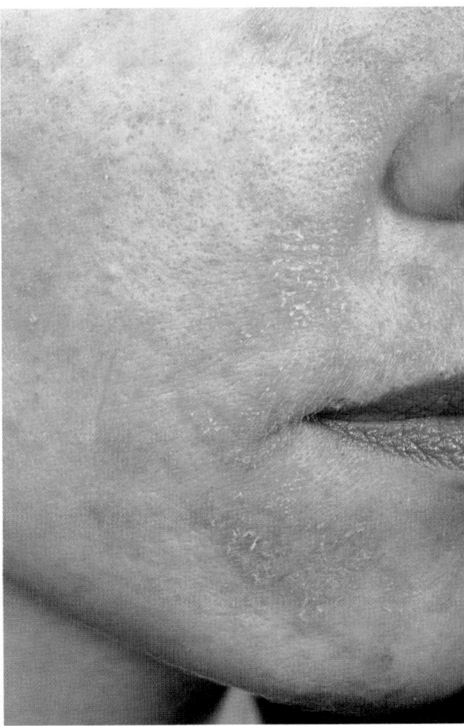

Fig. 20 Seborrhoeic dermatitis. Poorly defined, erythematous, scaly macules and patches. Seborrhoeic dermatitis has a predilection for the nasolabial folds, eyebrows and scalp, allowing it to be differentiated from atopic eczema.

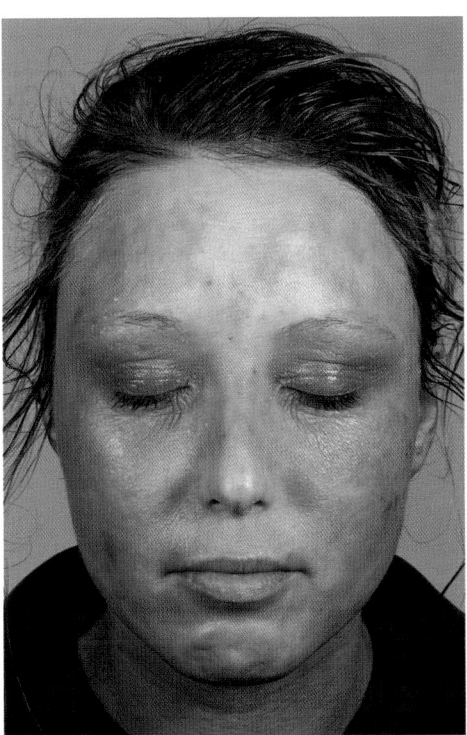

Fig. 21 Atopic eczema. Poorly defined, erythematous, scaly macules and patches. Note the additional eyelid lichenification and excoriations that are common features of atopic eczema due to rubbing and scratching. There was involvement of the limb flexures, intense itching and a history of atopy.

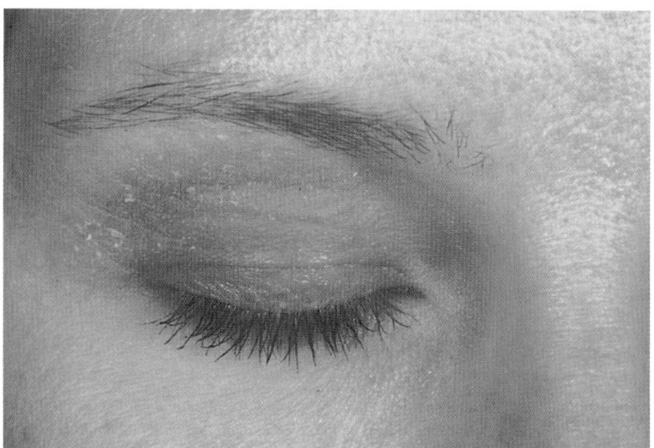

Fig. 22 Contact dermatitis. Erythematous, scaly, lichenified eyelids as in Fig. 21, but the patient was not atopic and the skin was clear elsewhere on the body. She was allergic to the eye make-up she had been using.

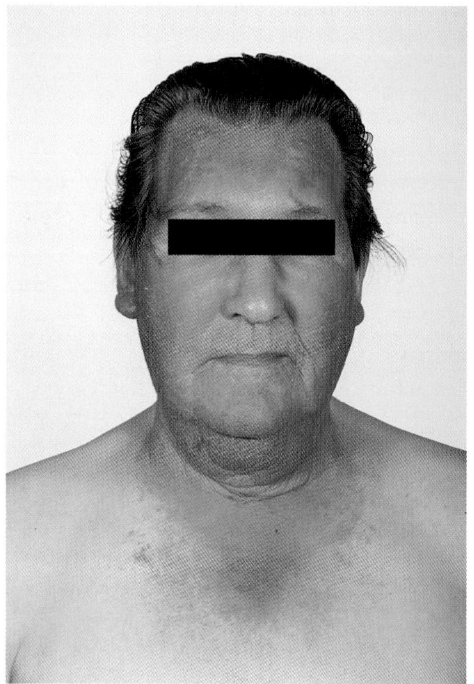

Fig. 23 Photosensitive eczema: This man complained of a scaly, itchy eruption on his face and hands. The V-shaped cut-off at the neck indicates it is photo-induced. The patient had been given a thiazide diuretic in the autumn but the rash had not appeared until spring when he began spending time outdoors gardening.

- Is it papular or pustular? (Figs 24 and 25).
- Are there comedones? (Fig. 25).
- Are there scaly plaques that might indicate psoriasis? However, if there is additional plugging of the hair follicles or scarring, it could be DLE (Fig. 26).

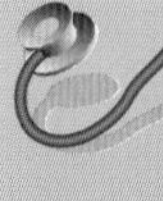

The presence of scaling is a helpful physical sign. It indicates a disease process that involves the epidermis. In this case, it would be present in eczema, tinea and DLE and absent in acne, rosacea and sarcoidosis. Mild scaling may be seen in dermatomyositis and SLE.

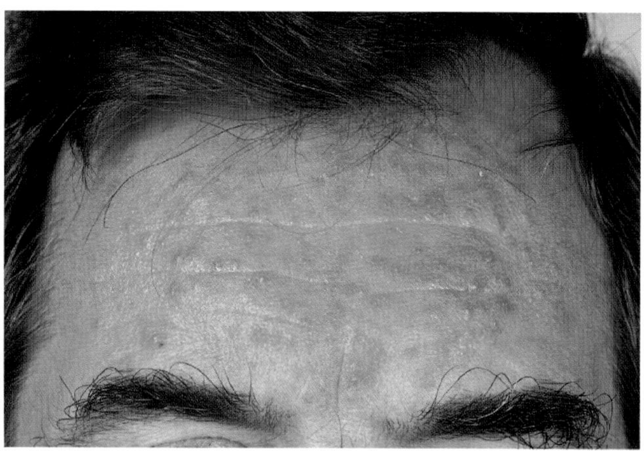

(a)

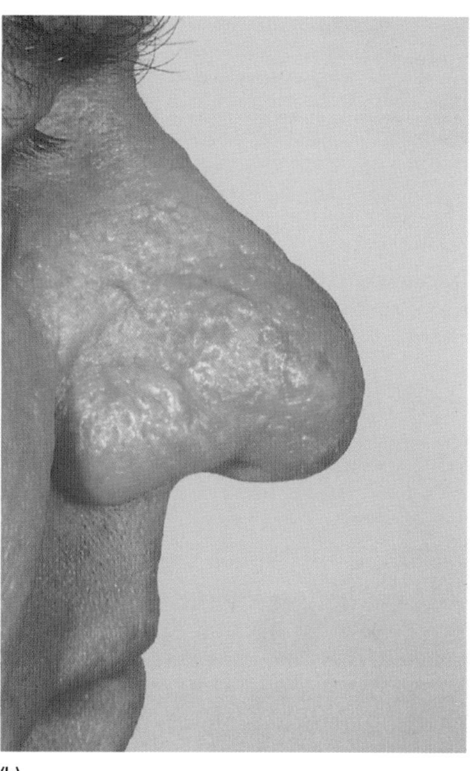

(b)

Fig. 24 Rosacea. (a) Erythema, papules and scattered pustules which typically affect the convex surfaces of the face, including the forehead as shown here. Telangiectasiae are also a common feature. By contrast with acne, comedones are absent. (b) In long-standing cases, a rhinophyma may be the end result.

Rash distribution

Seborrhoeic dermatitis classically affects the eyebrows and nasolabial folds. Check if the distribution is photosensitive—there will be sparing behind the ears, under the chin and nose, in the upper eyelid fold, and a cut-off at the neck. Is the rash asymmetrical, as often seen with fungal infections? (Table 6).

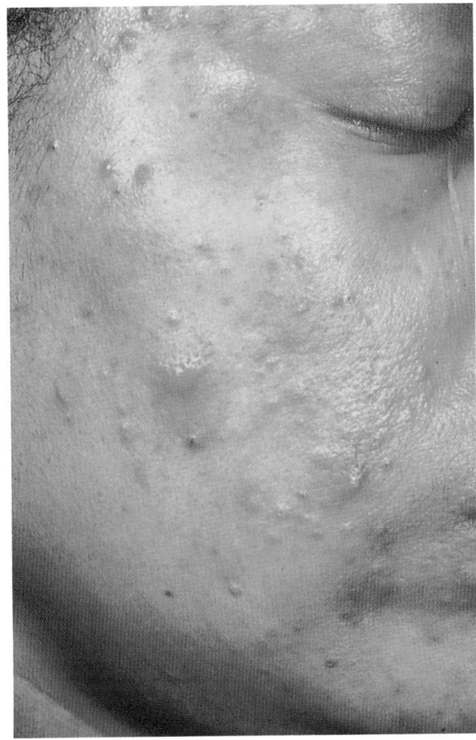

Fig. 25 Acne: comedones, the earliest feature of acne, are very prominent in this case. Erythematous papules and a pustule are also visible.

Looking beyond the face

• Facial atopic eczema will be associated with generally dry skin (xerosis) and flexural eczema.
• Remember to look for a scaly scalp in seborrhoeic dermatitis and for scarring alopecia with DLE.
• Examination of the dorsum of the hands and nail folds is vital if dermatomyositis is suspected (Fig. 27).

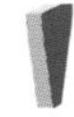

When assessing a patient who complains of a localized skin problem, as in this case, it is vital to examine the whole skin including the scalp. There will often be hidden diagnostic clues!

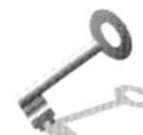

Acne and rosacea are very common and both are characterized by erythematous papules and pustules. Look for comedones ('white heads' and 'black heads'), nodules and scarring, which do not occur in rosacea. In addition, rosacea affects the infra-orbital portion of the cheeks, which tend to be spared by acne.

Approach to investigation and management

Investigations

• Skin scrapings in suspected tinea. See Section 2.13, p. 203.
• Skin biopsy for histology and direct immunofluorescence—Important for the diagnosis of the less common conditions, DLE, dermatomyositis and sarcoidosis. See Sections 3.1 (p. 211) and 3.2 (p. 212).
• Patch testing—To diagnose or exclude allergic contact dermatitis. See Section 3.3 (p. 213).
• Blood tests—Check serum angiotensin-converting enzyme if sarcoidosis is suspected (Fig. 28) and creatine phosphokinase in dermatomyositis. Check antinuclear antibodies, which are positive in the majority of cases of SLE (Fig. 29) but only 35% of cases of DLE. Antibodies to the nuclear antigen Jo-1 are detectable in some cases of dermatomyositis.
• Chest X-ray if sarcoidosis suspected.

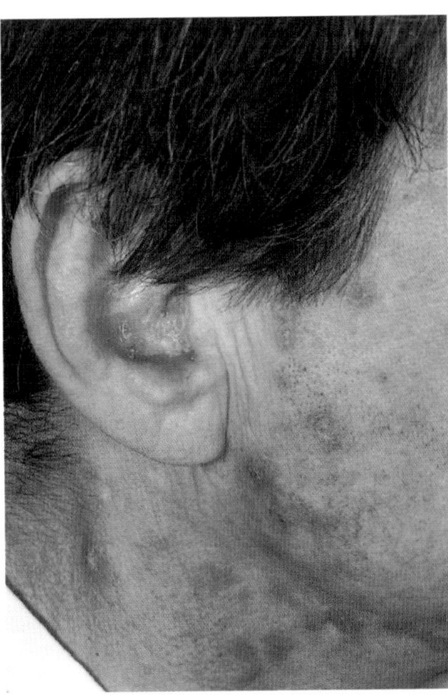

(a)

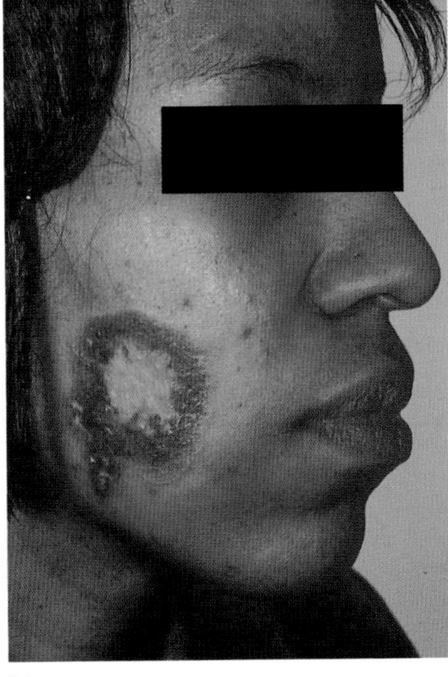

(b)

Fig. 26 Discoid lupus erythematosus: Well defined, scaly erythematous plaques (a). Dilated, plugged follicles may be seen on close inspection, particularly in the ears. Chronic DLE results in scarring which is often atrophic with postinflammatory hypopigmentation or hyperpigmentation as shown (b). Hyperpigmentation is commoner in racially pigmented skin.

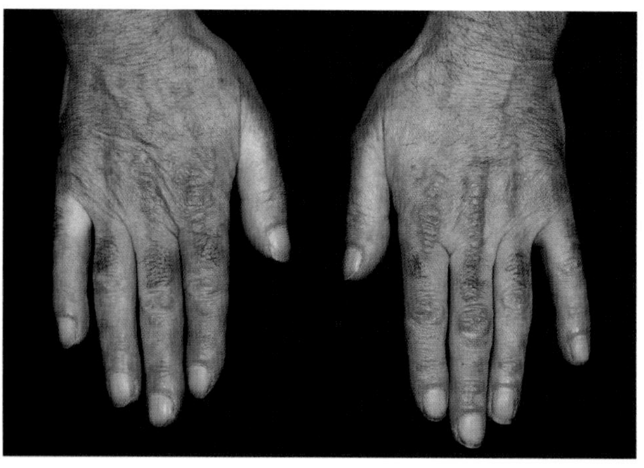
(a)

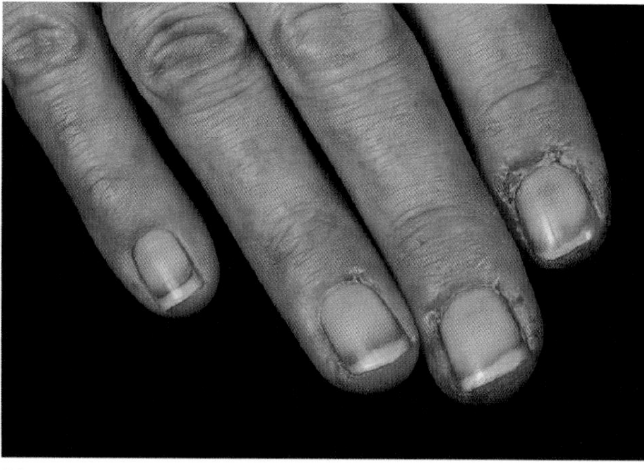
(b)

Fig. 27 Dermatomyositis. (a) Flat topped purple papules and plaques running along the extensor surfaces of the fingers and onto the hands. They are referred to as Gottren's papules over the knuckles. Note the nicotine-stained fingers. This patient had an underlying bronchial carcinoma. (b) Ragged cuticles with erythema and telangiectasiae of the nailfolds are typical of dermatomyositis but can also occur in lupus and other connective tissue diseases.

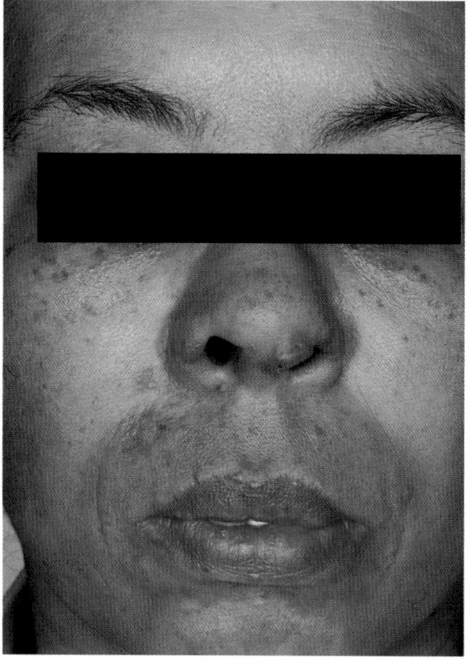

Fig. 28 Sarcoidosis: Red-brown papules and nodules around the nostrils and lips.

Management

- Atopic eczema—see Section 2.7 (p. 196).
- Contact dermatitis—see Section 2.8 (p. 197).
- Tinea—see Section 2.13 (p. 203).
- Dermatomyositis—see Section 2.3 (p. 192); see *Rheumatology and clinical immunology*, Section 2.3.5.
- Sarcoidosis—see *Respiratory medicine*, Section 2.8.2.
- Lupus erythematosus—see *Rheumatology and clinical immunology*, Section 2.4.1.
- Photosensitive eczema can be exogenous or endogenous.

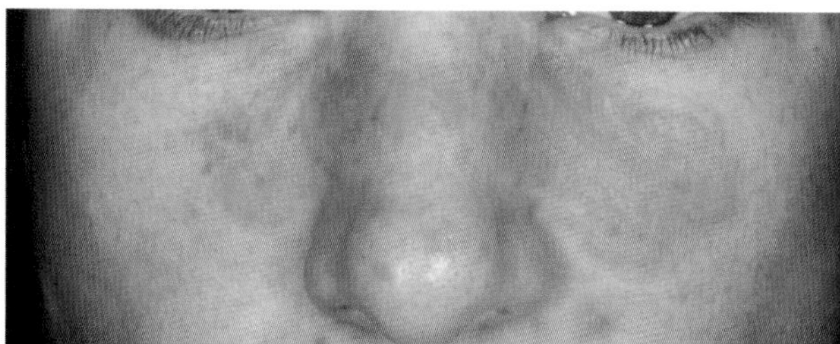

Fig. 29 Systemic lupus erythematosus: Erythematous plaques over the cheeks and bridge of the nose—a typical butterfly rash.

Exogenous cases are typically drug triggered so the drug should be stopped.

Fitzpatrick TB, Johnson RA, Wolff K *et al. Color Atlas and Synopsis of Clinical Dermatology. Common and Serious Diseases* (3rd edn). New York: McGraw-Hill, 1997.

Habif TP. *Clinical Dermatology: A Colour Guide to Diagnosis and Therapy* (2nd edn). St Louis: CV Mosby, 1990.

1.5 Pruritus

Case history

A 30-year-old man complains of a 6-month history of generalized pruritus.

Clinical approach

The first issue is to decide whether or not there is a co-existing rash. The differential diagnoses then fall into two

Table 7 Causes of pruritus.

Pruritus without a rash	Obstructive liver disease Hyper/hypothyroidism Chronic renal failure Iron deficiency Polycythaemia rubra vera Haematological malignancy esp. lymphoma Dry skin Drugs Idiopathic or psychological (non-organic)
Pruritus with a rash	Eczema Lichen planus Urticaria Scabies and other infestations Drug eruptions Bullous pemphigoid Dermatitis herpetiformis Pityriasis rosea Sézary syndrome Insect bites

groups (Table 7), which can be dissected on the basis of further history, examination and investigation.

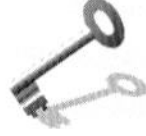

Pruritus in the absence of a rash can be an indication of an underlying systemic disease, including malignancy. You must search carefully for an underlying cause: non-organic pruritus is a diagnosis of exclusion and only to be made after proper consideration of all recognized causes.

History of the presenting problem

• For how long? Is there a temporal association with other events, e.g. drug ingestion, foreign travel.
• Have you noticed a rash? Is it there all the time? If there is an intermittent rash that is temporally related to itching, the diagnosis is likely to be urticaria.
• Do you itch all the time? Any provoking factors? The itching associated with urticaria may be intermittent: some types are provoked, e.g. cholinergic urticaria by exercise. Pruritus often seems worse at night, but particularly so in scabies.
• Do you feel well? A full functional enquiry should follow with particular emphasis on features that might suggest anaemia, hyper- or hypothyroidism, renal or liver impairment or malignancy.
• How's your appetite? Are you sleeping well? Are you tearful? Pruritus can reflect psychiatric problems, including depression, so try to elicit symptoms that might point to a psychiatric diagnosis. Beware, however, that pruritus of any cause may disturb sleep and concentration.

Relevant past history

There may be a documented history of anaemia, thyroid, liver or renal problems. Ask about drug and alcohol intake. Further clues may be available in the family history, e.g. an atopic tendency. A psychiatric history is also relevant here.

Examination

Skin

Is there a visible rash or generalized xerosis (dryness)? Examine the whole skin. The diagnosis revolves around whether the skin is normal.

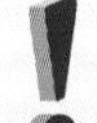

Scratching and rubbing of normal skin can lead to secondary changes that may mislead the unwary into diagnosing a primary skin disease. Look particularly for linear erosions and nodules that spare inaccessible areas, e.g. the central back (Fig. 30). This indicates scratching.

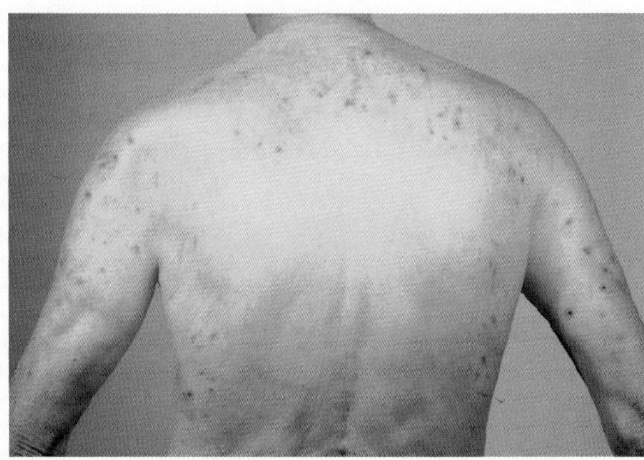

Fig. 30 Skin changes secondary to scratching: There are linear scratch marks and excoriated papules, but the upper, central back is spared.

Distribution

If there is a rash, the distribution may be characteristic:
• atopic eczema (flexures)
• scabies (interdigital web spaces, genitals)
• dermatitis herpetiformis (extensor surfaces, especially buttocks and limbs)
• lichen planus (wrists and mucosae)
• pityriasis rosea (trunk).

Morphology of lesions

In particular, look for:
• track formation, linear burrows (e.g. scabies, larva migrans)
• blisters or vesicles (e.g. autoimmune bullous disorders, acute dermatitis)
• flat-topped violaceous papules (e.g. lichen planus)
• grouped excoriated papules (e.g. dermatitis herpetiformis)
• weals which indicate urticaria.

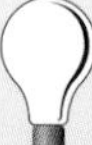

In an itchy patient, always look very closely for signs of scabies. It is commonly missed! Look for burrows and nodules in the typical sites (Fig. 31) (see Section 2.15, p. 205).

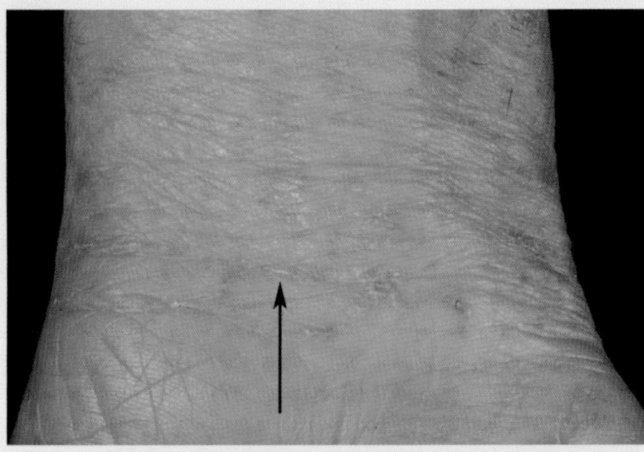

(a)

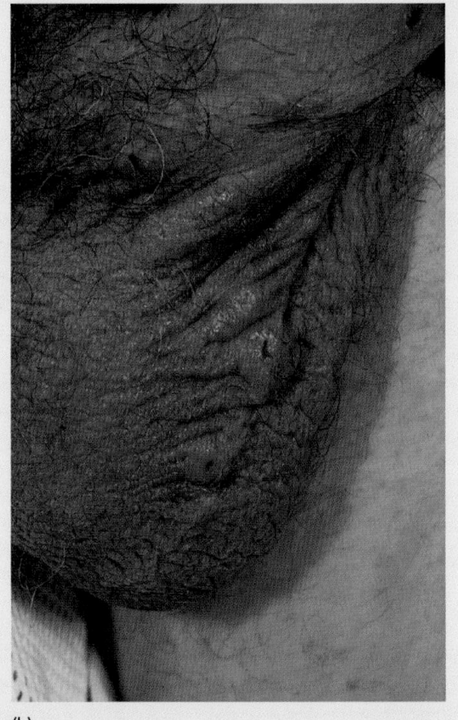

(b)

Fig. 31 Scabies. Linear burrows, seen here on the flexor surface of the wrist and indicated with an arrow (a), and nodules on the male genitalia (b) are characteristic signs.

General

A full general examination is vital, particularly if there is no evidence of skin disease. Emphasis should be placed on signs of anaemia, hyper- or hypothyroidism, renal or liver impairment and malignancy. Don't forget to check for lymphadenopathy and do a pelvic and rectal examination.

Approach to investigation and management

Investigation

If the skin is normal

• Blood tests—Check blood count and blood film, ferritin, renal, liver and thyroid function, and erythrocyte sedimentation rate (ESR).
• Chest X-ray.
• Further tests will depend on your clinical suspicions and blood test results. However, if the blood tests indicated above and a chest radiograph are normal and there are no symptoms or signs to suggest malignancy, further tests are probably not justified. However, testing for faecal occult blood and a cervical smear are non-invasive and simple.

If the skin is abnormal

Your battery of tests will depend on the suspected diagnosis (see relevant sections of this module).

Management

Treat any underlying dermatological or systemic disease. If the ferritin is normal but at the low end of the normal range, it is worth giving iron supplements.

For symptomatic treatment, start with bath oils and emollients, particularly if the skin looks dry. Dry skin resulting in pruritus is common, particularly in the elderly. Anti-histamines may be helpful but if these fail, tricyclic antidepressants or phototherapy are sometimes used. Formal psychiatric assessment is appropriate if there is any indication of an underlying or associated psychiatric disorder.

• Eczema—See Sections 2.7 (p. 198) and 2.8 (p. 199).
• Urticaria—See Section 2.16 (p. 207).
• Lichen planus—See Section 2.11 (p. 202).
• Scabies—See Section 2.15 (p. 206).
• Bullous pemphigoid—See Section 2.2 (p. 192).
• Dermatitis herpetiformis—See Section 2.5 (p. 195).
• Drug eruptions—Stop suspected drug.
• Sézary syndrome/cutaneous T-cell lymphoma—See Section 2.4 (p. 194).

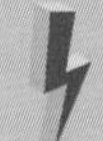

When pruritus persists with no identifiable cause, re-evaluate periodically with repeated tests because pruritus can precede the development of detectable malignancy.

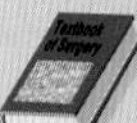

Fitzpatrick TB, Johnson RA, Wolff K *et al. Color Atlas and Synopsis of Clinical Dermatology. Common and Serious Diseases* (3rd edn). New York: McGraw-Hill, 1997.

Greaves MW. Pruritus. In: Champion R, Burton J, Burns A, Breathnach S (eds) *Textbook of Dermatology* (6th edn). Oxford: Blackwell Science, 1998.

Greaves MW, Wall PD. Pathophysiology of itching. *Lancet* 1996; 348: 938–940.

1.6 Alopecia

Case history

A 30-year-old woman complains of recent hair loss.

- Loss of hair or hair shedding is termed effluvium.
- Reduced hair density, the result of an effluvium, is termed alopecia.

Clinical approach

Hair loss and alopecia cause great distress and should be dealt with sympathetically.

In determining the cause of alopecia, determine whether:
- it is generalized or patchy
- there is inflammation or scarring of the underlying skin
- it is sudden or gradual in onset.

History of the presenting problem

- How long? Gradual or sudden hair loss? Sudden hair shedding suggests either an anagen or telogen effluvium or alopecia areata.
- Relationship to life events, illness, crash diets and drugs? The temporal relationship to drugs, stressful events, childbirth, surgery and illness is important, particularly in anagen (the phase of hair growth) and telogen (resting phase) effluvium (see later in this case description). An anagen effluvium occurs shortly after the precipitating event, e.g. chemotherapy, whilst a telogen effluvium occurs 1–4 months later.
- Do you tie back or braid your hair? Tension on the hair shafts can cause damage and eventually scarring of the follicles. This is most common in black women from tight braiding of the hair.
- Does the scalp itch? Have you noticed a rash? Do you have skin problems elsewhere? If alopecia is associated with skin abnormalities, the differential is very different to cases where the skin is normal (Table 8).

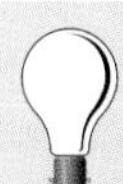

Causes of a telogen effluvium
- Parturition or abortion
- Major surgery
- Serious illness
- Fever
- Crash dieting
- Emotional stress
- Drugs.

Causes of an anagen effluvium
- Cytotoxic drugs
- Poisoning, e.g. heavy metals.

Table 8 Causes of alopecia.

Scarring (usually patchy)	Discoid lupus erythematosus Lichen planus Cicatricial pemphigoid Sarcoidosis Tumours, e.g. basal cell carcinoma Burns Radiation Infections including fungal kerion Traction (late stages)
Non-scarring and patchy	Androgenetic alopecia Alopecia areata Tinea capitis Traction (in early stages) Secondary syphilis
Non-scarring and generalized	Iron deficiency Telogen effluvium Anagen effluvium Drugs Alopecia totalis Endocrine, e.g. thyroid disease, hypopituitarism Malnutrition Systemic lupus erythematosus Chronic disease

Relevant past history

A history of systemic disease may be relevant. A full functional enquiry is necessary with emphasis on features that might suggest anaemia or thyroid disease. Ask about alopecia in male and female relatives—often present in both males and females with androgenetic alopecia. The psychiatric history is sometimes relevant.

Examination

Scalp

Distribution

The distribution will provide diagnostic clues. It may be generalized or patchy and there may be preferential loss in certain areas. For example:
- loss from the temples and crown in androgenetic alopecia
- traction alopecia (due to tying back or braiding of hair) can be patchy but is usually most marked along the fronto-temporal hairline.

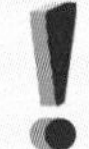

Approximately 85% of hairs are in the anagen phase (actively growing) and 15% are in telogen (the resting phase). Anagen effluvium therefore results in sudden loss of almost all the hair. By contrast, patients are alarmed by dramatic hair shedding in a telogen effluvium, but in most cases the majority of hair remains.

The other diagnosis to consider in sudden, extensive hair loss is alopecia totalis and universalis, which are severe forms of alopecia areata.

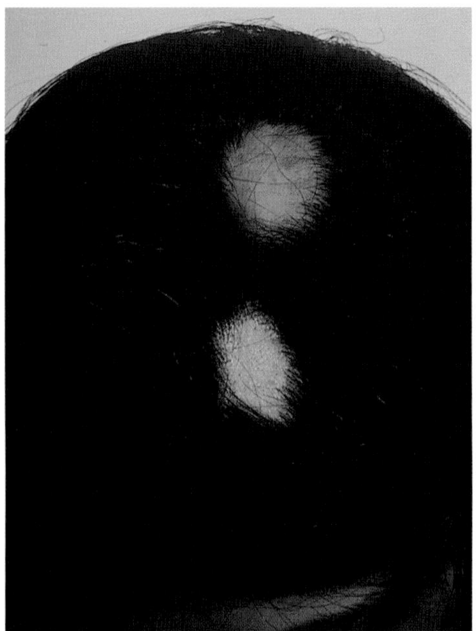

Fig. 32 Alopecia areata. Round/oval, discrete patches of complete hair loss (white hairs may be preferentially spared). Exclamation mark hairs are just visible at the periphery of the upper patch. The skin is entirely normal and follicles would be clearly visible on close inspection.

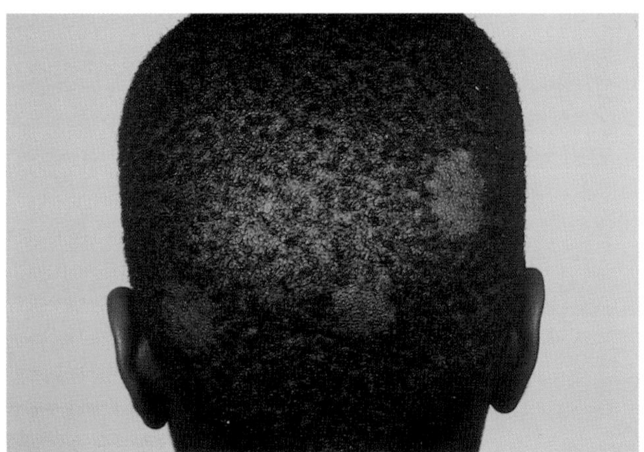

Fig. 33 Tinea capitis. Discrete patches of alopecia with a scaly skin surface that could be accentuated with gentle abrasion. Tinea capitis is commonest in children, especially among black and asian populations. Skin scrapings and plucked hairs should be sent for direct microscopy and culture.

Morphology of lesions

Look closely at the areas of hair loss (Figs 32–36). Is the skin normal? Look for inflammation or scaling. Is the colour normal? Hyper- or hypopigmentation may be the after-effect of inflammation and is common in DLE. Look for scarring—smooth, shiny skin with invisible hair follicles. Exclamation-mark hairs are diagnostic of alopecia areata and are often seen at the periphery of lesions (see Section 2.1, p. 191).

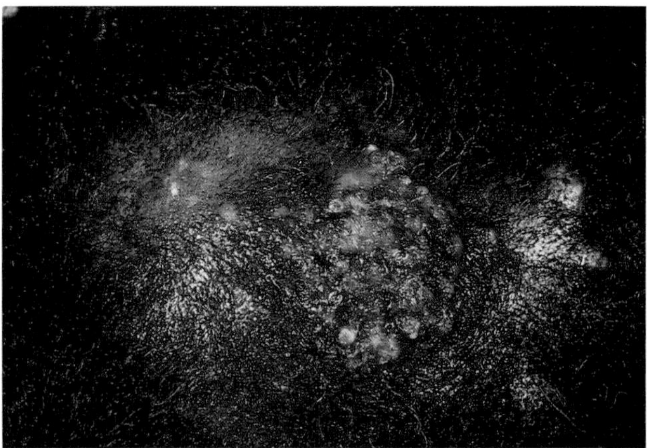

Fig. 34 Fungal kerion. An inflammatory, boggy mass associated with alopecia. This is due to an inflammatory response to the fungus and does not reflect secondary bacterial infection. It will respond to systemic antifungal agents alone and does not require incision and drainage.

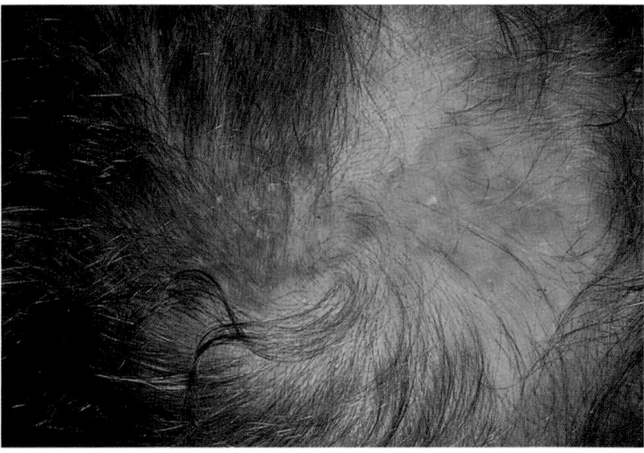

(a)

(b)

Fig. 35 (a) Discoid lupus erythematosus: Scaly, erythematous plaques in the scalp of an adult patient who had similar lesions on the face. (b) Scarring alopecia following discoid lupus erythematosus: The scalp is shiny and atrophic and no follicular openings can be seen, indicating scarring in this patient who had discoid lupus. The hair will not regrow.

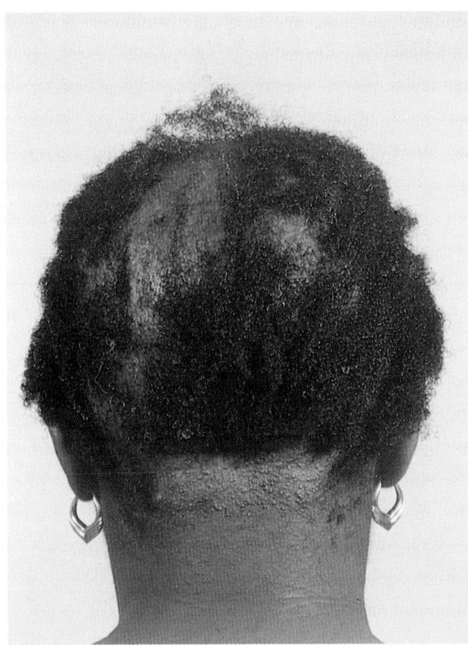

Fig. 36 Traction alopecia: Patchy hair loss in a patient who had braided her hair over many years.

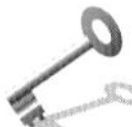

Androgenetic alopecia is the commonest cause of alopecia, most often recognized in men, presenting with thinning over the vertex and fronto-temporal recession. It is also common in women, but is usually very mild, with thinning over the vertex and (usually) preservation of the frontal hairline. It rarely signifies underlying endocrine disease.

General

A full cutaneous and general examination may throw light on the underlying aetiology.

• Look for hair loss on the body and signs of anaemia, thyroid disease, autoimmune or skin disease.

• Check for features of androgen excess in females with androgenetic alopecia, e.g. acne, hirsuitism, virilization.

• Don't forget to look at the nails too—they may be abnormal in lichen planus or alopecia areata, and may show a Beau's line in telogen effluvium.

Approach to investigation and management

Investigations

• Microscopy and culture of skin scrapings and plucked hairs—This is to exclude tinea capitis in any patient with patchy alopecia. (Wood's light is a quick screening investigation. Green fluorescence may be seen in some cases of tinea capitis, but a negative result does not exclude the diagnosis.)

• Skin biopsy for histology and direct immunofluorescence—To ascertain the diagnosis in cases of scarring alopecia.

• Blood tests—If generalized alopecia is present, check blood count and haematinics, particularly ferritin, thyroid function and antinuclear antibodies. An underlying endocrine abnormality is unusual in females with androgenetic alopecia alone but it is worth checking, particularly if severe and of recent onset in a young woman with no family history. Endocrine investigation is essential if there is virilization (see *Endocrinology*, Section 1.6).

Iron deficiency is a common cause of generalized alopecia in women. It may also be a compounding factor in other types of alopecia. Check the ferritin even if the haemoglobin is normal. For optimal hair growth, aim to boost the ferritin above 70 μg/L.

Management

• Alopecia areata—See Section 2.1 (p. 191).

• Lupus erythematosus—See *Rheumatology and clinical immunology*, Section 2.4.1.

• Lichen planus—See Section 2.11 (p. 201).

• Tinea capitis—See Section 2.13 (p. 203).

• Telogen and anagen effluvium—Recovery can be expected.

• Androgenetic alopecia—No satisfactory treatment. Topical minoxidil can partially restore hair loss as does systemic finasteride, a type-2 5-α reductase inhibitor, but the latter is not licensed for this indication in the UK. Anti-androgens can be used in females.

• Cicatricial pemphigoid—As for bullous periphigoid see Section 2.2 (p. 192).

• Sarcoidosis—See *Respiratory medicine*, Section 2.8.2.

• Traction alopecia—Advise the patient to wear a loose hairstyle.

Treatment of scarring alopecia should be aggressive to prevent further damage. In cases where alopecia is severe in the patient's eyes but is not apparent to the physician, there may be an underlying psychological or psychiatric problem.

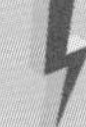

Fungal kerions are boggy, inflammatory masses which most commonly occur on the scalp of Asian and Black children. They may be mistaken for bacterial abscesses. Samples should be taken to confirm/exclude the presence of dermatophytes and to avoid unecessary incision and drainage.

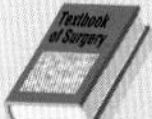

Fitzpatrick TB, Johnson RA, Wolff K *et al. Color Atlas and Synopsis of Clinical Dermatology. Common and Serious Diseases* (3rd edn). New York: McGraw-Hill, 1997.

Habif TP. *Clinical Dermatology: A Colour Guide to Diagnosis and Therapy.* (2nd edn). St Louis: CV Mosby, 1990.

Du Vivier A. *Atlas of Clinical Dermatology* (2nd edn). London: Gower Medical Publishing, 1993.

1.7 Abnormal skin pigmentation

Case history

A 40-year-old woman presents with a 2-year history of a change in skin colour.

Clinical approach

Pigmentary abnormalities are common. Although distressing for the patient, they are usually harmless, but you should recognize when a change in skin colour indicates an underlying systemic disease.

Pigmentary changes are usually due to an increase or decrease in melanin. Other substances, such as bilirubin and drug metabolites, can cause hyperpigmentation when present in excess. There can be very specific colour changes, such as the yellow/orange colour of carotenaemia.

History of the presenting problem

• When did you notice the colour change? This patient was 38 years old when the problem began so genetic conditions can be discounted, e.g. albinism, Ashleaf macules in tuberous sclerosis, or *café au lait* macules in neurofibromatosis (see *Neurology*, Sections 2.8.2 and 2.8.3). Most pigmentary problems are acquired, as in this case.

• Has your skin become darker or lighter? Is the change all over or just in some areas? The answer to these two questions will divide the possible diagnoses into four groups (Tables 9–12).

Table 9 Differential diagnosis of acquired, localized hypopigmentation.

Diagnosis	Clinical features
Vitiligo	Completely depigmented macules. Not scaly. Well defined edge. Often symmetrical
Postinflammatory hypopigmentation	Incomplete pigment loss. Poorly defined edge. Look elsewhere for active lesions
Pityriasis versicolor	Pale, scaly, well defined macules usually on upper central back and chest
Leprosy	Incomplete pigment loss, sometimes scaly. Anaesthetic. Feel for enlarged nerves near patches
Halo naevi	As for vitiligo, but occurring around a melanocytic naevus (mole). Usually on trunk of children/young adults
Chemicals	Occupational or therapeutic use, e.g. *p*-tertiary butyl phenol, hydroquinone

Table 10 Differential diagnosis of acquired, generalized hypopigmentation.

Diagnosis	Clinical features
Hypopituitarism	Due to lack of MSH
Generalized vitiligo	Look for islands of normal skin

MSH, melanocyte-stimulating hormone.

Table 11 Differential diagnosis of acquired, localized hyperpigmentation.

Diagnosis	Clinical features
Freckles (ephelides)	Small (<3 mm) macules usually on sun exposed sites. Look for other signs of photoageing and skin tumours. If severe, think of xeroderma pigmentosa
Chloasma (melasma)	Patchy pigmentation on facial skin. Often symmetrical. Cheeks, chin, forehead, upper lip. Almost always females. Worsens with sun exposure
Acanthosis nigricans	Thickened, velvety areas of skin, usually in flexures. Patient often obese unless associated with underlying malignancy
Postinflammatory hyperpigmentation	Patchy and poorly defined. More common in racially pigmented skin. Look for remaining areas of the rash that caused the inflammation
Haemosiderosis	Poorly defined, macular, red/brown pigmentation. Usually on lower legs in association with varicose veins or venous ulceration
Drugs	For example, minocycline–blue/black, chlorpromazine (hydroxy)chloroquin and amiodarone—blue/grey on sun-exposed sites, gold (chrysiasis)—blue/grey pigmentation on sun-exposed
Alkaptonuria (ochronosis)	Blue-grey pigmentation is generalized but often only visible over the pinnae, tip of nose and extensor tendons of the hand

Table 12 Differential diagnosis of acquired, generalized hyperpigmentation.

Diagnosis	Clinical features
Addison's disease, Nelson's syndrome	Diffuse hyperpigmentation, particularly of the flexures, palmar creases and oral mucosa
Ectopic ACTH/MSH	E.g. oat-cell tumours. Addison-like pigmentation
Acromegaly, hyperthyroidism, phaeochromocytoma	Occasionally associated with Addison-like pigmentation
Malnutrition, malabsorbption, chronic infections and cachectic states	Diffuse brown or grey pigmentation
Chronic renal failure	Diffuse brown pigmentation
Systemic sclerosis	Diffuse brown/grey pigmentation
Haemochromatosis (Bronzed diabetes)	Bronzed or grey pigmentation, particularly of exposed sites
Hyperbilirubinaemia	Yellow pigmentation of skin and sclera (bilirubin has a high affinity for elastin)
Hepatic cirrhosis	Particularly primary biliary cirrhosis. Diffuse, brown pigmentation.
Drugs	E.g. mepacrine—diffuse yellow pigmentation (sclera normal). Busulphan, bleomycin, cyclophosphamide—brown pigmentation
Carotenaemia	Yellow pigmentation of skin, particularly the palms, with normal sclera. Associated with hypothyroidism or diabetes but most commonly due to dietary excess, particularly carrots.

• Was there a skin problem or rash present before the colour change?
• What drugs are you taking? As ever, an accurate drug history is crucial. Many cytotoxic agents can cause pigmentation so don't just dwell on medications taken on a regular, daily basis.

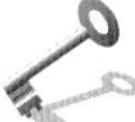

Inflammation of the skin frequently resolves to leave hyper- or hypopigmentation, particularly in racially pigmented skin. It is particularly common with some conditions, such as lichen planus or fixed drug eruptions, and takes many months to disappear (Fig. 37).

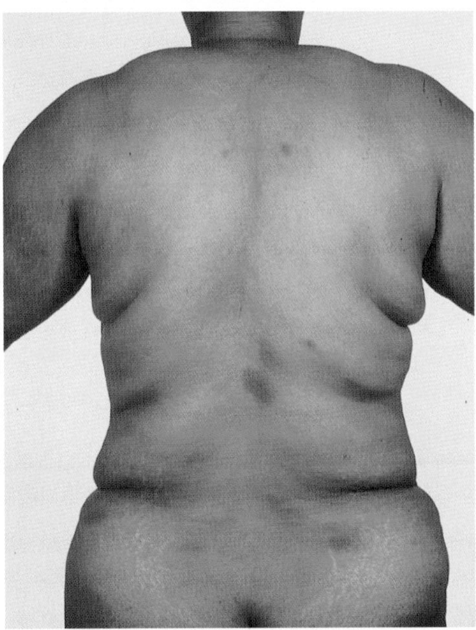

Fig. 37 Post-inflammatory hyperpigmentation. There are several oval hyperpigmented patches. The patient complained of an intermittent red rash which always occurred at these sites. The history and physical signs are typical of a fixed drug eruption. The trigger was ibuprofen which was taken occasionally for dysmenorrhoea.

Relevant past history

• Autoimmune diseases, particularly thyroid disease, pernicious anaemia and diabetes are associated with vitiligo (Fig. 38a). Autoimmunity is also associated with halo naevi (Fig. 38b) and Addison's disease.
• Hypertension may be associated with Cushing's disease, acromegaly, phaeochromocytoma or hyperthyroidism, which can all occasionally cause Addison's-like diffuse hyperpigmentation.
• Hepatic cirrhosis of any aetiology can cause a diffuse hypermelanosis, which is particularly associated with haemochromatosis and primary biliary cirrhosis.

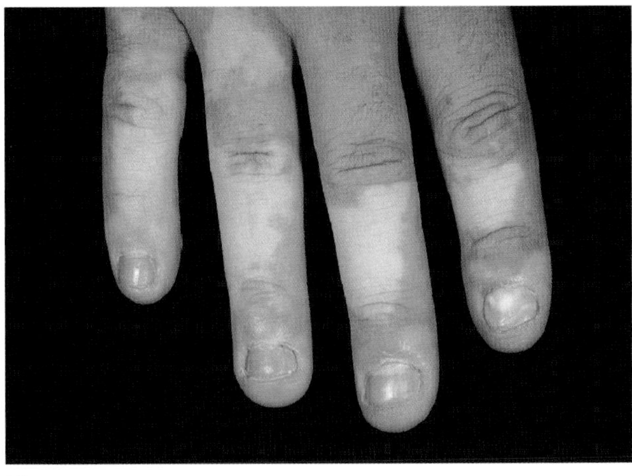

(a)

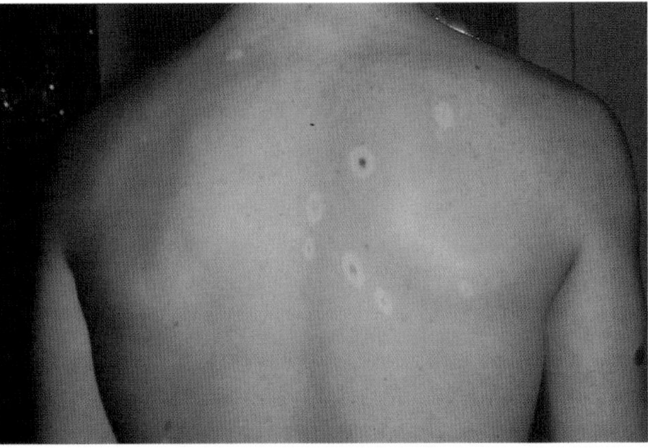

(b)

Fig. 38 (a) Vitiligo: well-defined patches of complete depigmention with a normal skin surface. This contrasts with postinflammatory hypopigmentation in which pigment loss is usually partial. (b) Halo naevi: well-defined, oval patches of completely depigmented skin which are identical to vitiligo. However, in the centre of each patch is a melanocytic naevus (benign mole) which in some cases has completely depigmented. Halo naevi are most commonly seen in teenagers and young adults, who should be reassured. The skin may repigment eventually.

• Diabetes could be associated with vitiligo, haemochromatosis, acanthosis nigricans or carotenaemia.
• A previous history of skin tumours or photosensitivity in a patient with multiple freckles should suggest a possible diagnosis of xeroderma pigmentosum.

Examination

Skin

• Is there increased or decreased pigmentation? If there is hyperpigmentation, what colour? If there is hypopigmentation, is it complete (depigmentation) or partial (hypopigmentation) pigment loss? Complete depigmentation suggests vitiligo (Fig. 38a).
• Localized or generalized? If localized, are the edges well defined, e.g. pityriasis versicolor, vitiligo, or patchy

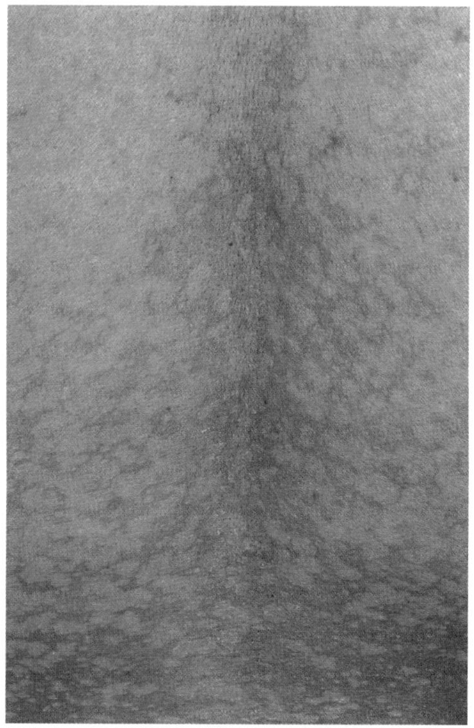

Fig. 39 Pityriasis versicolor: the abnormal areas are the well-defined, hypopigmented macules which were covered in a fine scale that can be accentuated with gentle abrasion. Skin scrapings were stained with Parker's stain which demonstrated *Malassezia furfur.*

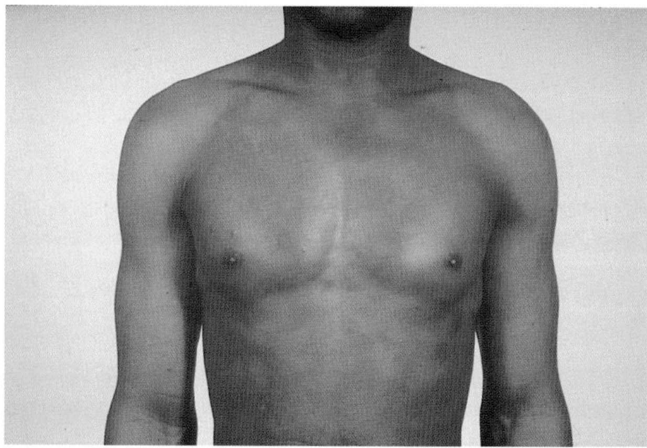

Fig. 40 Leprosy: hypopigmented patches in which sensation was reduced. The patient had lived in Africa.

and poorly defined, e.g. post-inflammatory pigmentary change?

• Is the skin surface normal? Does the skin feel normal? In most cases, apart from a colour change, the skin will look and feel normal. However, pityriasis versicolor is scaly (Fig. 39), although you may need to gently scrape the skin surface to see this clearly. Areas of leprosy may feel thickened and may be scaly (Fig. 40). The skin is thickened with a velvety surface in acanthosis nigricans (Fig. 41). The skin will be tight and sclerotic in systemic sclerosis.

• Abnormal sensation? If there is reduced sensation within a hypopigmented area, think of leprosy.

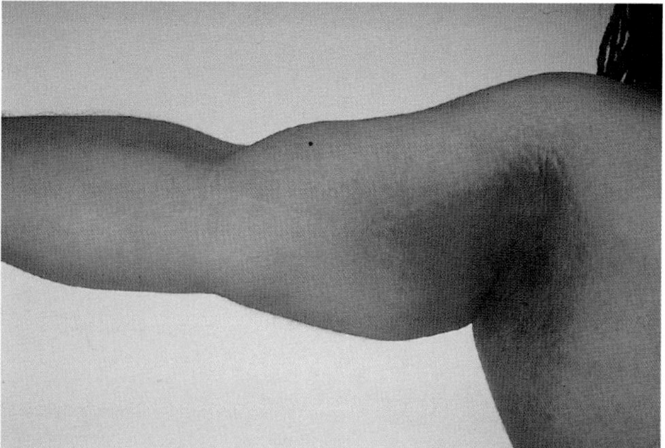

Fig. 41 Acanthosis nigricans: thickened, warty, hyperpigmented skin which most commonly occurs in the flexures, including the axillae as shown.

General

In most cases, extra-cutaneous findings are unlikely. However:

• look for signs of malignancy in acanthosis nigricans

• if there is diffuse hyperpigmentation, look for hepatomegaly and stigmata of liver disease, signs of Addison's disease, acromegaly, hyperthyroidism, phaeochromocytoma or pituitary tumours

• there may be signs of hypothyroidism in carotenaemia or signs of hypopituitarism in diffuse hypopigmentation.

Approach to investigation and management

Investigations

In the majority of cases, it is possible to make a diagnosis based on the history and examination alone. The following investigations may be helpful:

• Wood's light—A hand-held source of filtered UV light which causes areas of epidermal hypopigmentation to fluoresce, making them more prominent in subtle cases, e.g. vitiligo, Ash leaf macules.

• Skin scrapings for mycological examination—Pityriasis versicolor is caused by the yeast *Malassezia furfur*. The hyphae are best exhibited with Parker's stain (Parker's ink/KOH).

• Skin biopsy—Histology is necessary to confirm suspected leprosy and is needed if there is diagnostic doubt.

• Blood tests—An autoimmune screen in vitiligo or Addison's disease to screen for associated autoimmune diseases. Also check liver and renal function, glucose, insulin level (if acanthosis nigricans suspected), full blood count, ferritin and perform endocrine work-up in suspected Addison's disease, ectopic adrenocorticotrophic hormone (ACTH)/melanocyte-stimulating hormone (MSH) secretion, acromegaly, hyper/hypothyroidism, phaeochromocytoma, hypopituitarism.

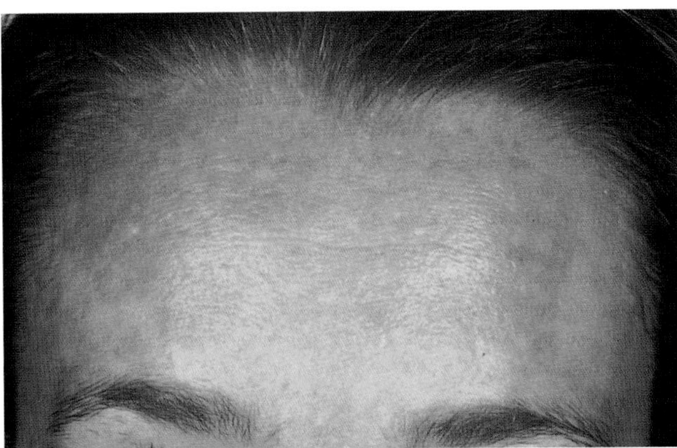

Fig. 42 Melasma: hyperpigmented patches on the forehead with a normal skin surface. There was similar pigmentation on the cheeks and upper lip which became more prominent after sun exposure. The patient was taking an oral contraceptive pill.

Management

- Vitiligo—See Section 2.17 (p. 207).
- Leprosy—See *Infectious diseases*, Section 2.6.2.
- Haemochromatosis, Addison's disease and other endocrine diseases—See *Endocrinology*, Sections 2.2.2 and 2.5.3.
- Acanthosis nigricans—See Section 2.20 (p. 210).
- Post-inflammatory pigmentary change—No treatment required.
- Pityriasis versicolor—Topical azoles usually. Systemic in extensive cases.
- Melasma (Fig. 42)—Stop the oral contraceptive pill. Use sunblocks and camouflage.

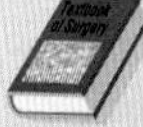

Bleehan SS. Disorders of skin colour. In: Champion R, Burton J, Burns A, Breathnach S (eds) *Textbook of Dermatology* (6th edn). Oxford: Blackwell Science, 1998.

Du Vivier A. *Atlas of Clinical Dermatology* (2nd edn). London: Gower Medical Publishing, 1993.

1.8 Patches and plaques on the lower legs

Case history

A 40-year-old woman presents with a 6-month history of an enlarging lesion on her lower leg.

Clinical approach

The differential diagnosis is wide given the brief history, but the first priority is to consider skin cancer, particularly malignant melanoma, which is the most serious sort and commonly presents on the legs in women. In addition, there are a number of other skin diseases that preferentially affect the leg and may be linked with systemic diseases (Table 13).

Table 13 Likely causes of a patch or plaque on the lower leg.

Category	Diagnosis
Tumours	Basal cell carcinoma Bowen's disease Squamous cell carcinoma Malignant melanoma Kaposi's sarcoma
Inflammatory	Discoid eczema Venous eczema Hypertrophic lichen planus
Endocrine	Necrobiosis lipoidica Pre-tibial myxoedema
Infection	Cellulitis Tinea Erythema chronicum migrans
Others	Granuloma annulare Morphea Erythema nodosum

Malignancy should be suspected in any patient who gives a history of a solitary, enlarging skin lesion. It is an increasing problem in the UK, with a rising incidence of both melanoma and non-melanoma skin cancers.

History of the presenting problem

- How did it start? How long ago? Has it changed? This information may be crucial. A lesion arising at the site of a pre-existing melanocytic naevus ('mole') suggests melanoma. In erythema chronicum migrans (Lyme disease) there will be a history of a papule that evolves into an enlarging ring. Tinea also enlarges in an annular fashion. Erythema nodosum and cellulitis usually present acutely, so are unlikely here.
- Is it painful? Does it itch? If itch is a prominent symptom, you may be dealing with a patch of eczema. Pain is a very prominent feature in pyoderma gangrenosum, erythema nodosum and cellulitis.
- Do you feel well? Patients with erythema nodosum, cellulitis, pyoderma gangrenosum and Lyme disease often feel unwell with 'flu-like symptoms.

Relevant past history

Past medical history and family history are relevant in many conditions that preferentially affect the legs:

- pretibial myxoedema is associated with Graves' disease
- necrobiosis lipoidica is associated with diabetes mellitus

Table 14 Causes of leg ulceration.

Category	Disease
Tumours	Basal cell carcinoma Sqamous cell carcinoma Malignant melanoma Kaposi's sarcoma
Large vessel disease	Venous ulceration Atherosclerosis Polyarteritis nodosa Systemic sclerosis
Small vessel disease	Diabetes Systemic lupus erythematosus Rheumatoid arthritis Systemic sclerosis Cutaneous vasculitis
Blood abnormalities	Immune complex disease Sickle cell anaemia Cryoglobulinaemia
Neuropathy	Diabetes Leprosy Syphilis
Infection	Mycobacterium Fungal
Trauma	
Others	Pyoderma gangrenosum Necrobiosis lipoidica

• a history of varicose veins or venous thrombosis would be expected in venous eczema
• erythema nodosum has many associations (see Section 2.10, p. 200) but although the lower leg is the commonest site, the history here does not fit this diagnosis.

A history of UV exposure is relevant in the case of the commonest skin tumours. Ask about sunbathing, severe sunburn, use of sunbeds, an outdoor occupation and whether they have lived in a hot climate.

Examination

Skin

Distribution

The exact location of the lesion may provide diagnostic clues:
• venous eczema or ulcers affect the lower legs and ankles, particularly the medial aspect.
• necrobiosis lipoidica and pretibial myxoedema usually affect the shins
• tender subcutaneous lumps on the lower legs would be in keeping with erythema nodosum
• sun-induced skin tumours are also commoner on the lower legs than thighs.

Morphology of lesions

Look carefully. Many of the likely diagnoses here have a characteristic morphology (see Sections 2.10, p. 200 and 2.11, p. 201). The presence of primary ulceration should alert the clinician to other diagnoses (Table 14) and this should be reflected in the subsequent general examination.

General examination

A full cutaneous and systemic general examination is important as this may shed light on the underlying aetiology. Particular emphasis should be placed on signs of arterial/venous disease, diabetes, thyroid disease or skin disease elsewhere.

Approach to investigation and management

Investigation

Unless there is a clear-cut clinical diagnosis, the most important investigation of a solitary skin lesion is a skin biopsy to confirm/exclude a skin tumour.

Skin scrapings should be sent for mycology if fungal infection is suspected. Blood sugar, thyroid function tests and thyroid autoantibodies may also be necessary depending on the clinical features and dermatopathological assessment.

Management

• Tumours—See *Oncology*, Section 2.7.
• Lichen planus—See Section 2.11 (p. 201).
• Eczema—See Sections 2.7 (p. 196) and 2.8 (p. 197).
• Tinea—See Section 2.13 (p. 203); see *Infectious diseases*, Section 2.9.
• Erythema nodosum—See Section 2.10 (p. 200).
• Pyoderma gangrenosum—See Section 2.18 (p. 208).

Fitzpatrick TB, Johnson RA, Wolff K *et al. Color Atlas and Synopsis of Clinical Dermatology. Common and Serious Diseases* (3rd edn). New York. McGraw-Hill, 1997.
Habif TP. *Clinical Dermatology: A Colour Guide to Diagnosis and Therapy* (2nd edn). St Louis: CV Mosby, 1990.

2 Diseases and treatments

2.1 Alopecia areata

Aetiology/pathophysiology/pathology

Alopecia areata (AA) is thought to be an organ-specific autoimmune disease and shows a familial tendency. Biopsies show a perifollicular T-cell infiltrate.

Epidemiology

Alopecia areata is common (2% of dermatology referrals in the UK and USA). The peak onset is in young adults but AA can affect children. Males and females are equally affected.

Clinical presentation

Common

• Uninflamed, non-scaly, non-scarring, round/oval patch of complete alopecia.
• Exclamation mark hairs at the margins are pathognomonic (broken hairs 3–4 mm in length, narrower and less pigmented proximally).

The scalp is the commonest site, but any hair-bearing areas can be affected. Hair loss within patches is rapid. See Figs 32 (p. 184) and 43.

Uncommon

• Nail pitting.
• Diffuse scalp or whole-body hair loss (alopecia totalis and universalis).

Investigation

Autoimmune screen to exclude associated disease.

Differential diagnosis

Consider other causes of patchy, non-scarring alopecia (see Table 8, p. 183), e.g. androgenetic alopecia, ringworm and traction alopecia, but the diagnosis is usually straightforward.

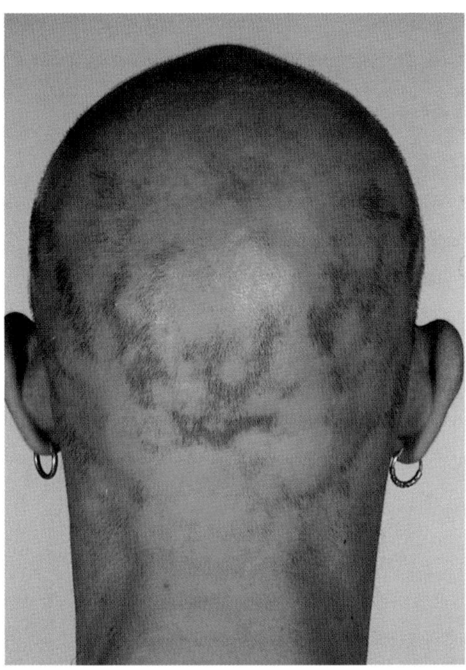

Fig. 43 Alopecia areata: it can be appreciated that multiple oval/round patches have resulted in extensive alopecia in this case. The skin surface appears entirely normal and hair follicles would be visible on close inspection.

Treatment

• Topical or intralesional steroids, contact irritants or allergens, PUVA, minoxidil.
• Systemic treatment is usually avoided.
• Relapse is common after stopping treatment.

Prognosis

The prognosis is variable. Spontaneous regrowth of individual patches may occur after a few months but relapse is common. Poor prognostic indicators include prepubertal onset, atopy, Down's syndrome, widespread disease, or scalp margin involvement.

Disease associations

Diseases associated with AA: Atopy, Down's syndrome and autoimmune diseases, particularly thyroid disease, pernicious anaemia, vitiligo and systemic lupus erythematosus.

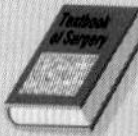

Dawber RPR, De Berker D, Wojnarowska F. Alopecia areata. In: Champion R, Burton J, Burns A, Breathnach S (eds) *Textbook of Dermatology* (6th edn). Oxford: Blackwell Science, 1998.
Du Vivier A. *Atlas of Clinical Dermatology.* 2nd edn. London: Gower Medical Publishing, 1993.

2.2 Bullous pemphigoid and pemphigoid gestationis

Aetiology/pathophysiology/pathology

Pemphigoid gestationis (PG) (syn. herpes gestationis) and bullous pemphigoid (BP) are autoimmune diseases in which IgG binds to the dermo-epidermal junction (DEJ) of skin/mucous membranes leading to dermo-epidermal separation and blister formation. The target antigen in most cases is type XVII collagen (BP180), a component of hemidesmosomes. BP is occasionally drug induced.

Epidemiology

BP can occur at any age, even childhood, but is most common in the elderly. PG is associated with pregnancy.

Clinical presentation

Pruritus and a rash.

Physical signs

Common

- Initially erythematous, urticaria-like plaques on which tense blisters then form (cf. pemphigus vulgaris) and which may be up to several centimetres in diameter (see Fig. 4).
- Generalized distribution but BP particularly affects the flexural surfaces, and PG the abdomen.

Uncommon

- Oral erosions, itchy nodules.
- Neonatal PG due to transplacental passage of pathogenic IgG.

Investigation/staging

- Skin biopsy—Will show a blister at the DEJ and direct immunofluorescence shows IgG along DEJ (see Section 3.2, p. 212).
- Serum for indirect immunofluorescence—serum IgG binds to the DEJ of normal skin.
- Blood count may show an eosinophilia.

Differential diagnosis

- BP: Bullous drug eruptions, other immunobullous diseases, urticaria, erythema multiforme (EM).
- PG: Polymorphic eruption of pregnancy, urticaria.

Treatment

- BP: Systemic corticosteroids ± adjuvant drug (commonly azathioprine).
- PG: Topical corticosteroids if possible ± systemic corticosteroids.

Complications

The commonest complications are treatment related. Infection of skin erosions may lead to septicaemia.

Prognosis

- In BP there is significant treatment-related morbidity/mortality, but ultimately BP may remit.
- PG resolves after delivery but may recur in subsequent pregnancies. The prognosis for the infant is good.

Disease associations

Other autoimmune diseases.

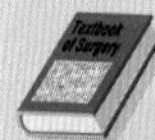

Fitzpatrick TB, Johnson RA, Wolff K *et al. Color Atlas and Synopsis of Clinical Dermatology. Common and Serious Diseases* (3rd edn). New York: McGraw-Hill, 1997.
Nousari HC, Anhalt GJ. Pemphigus and bullous pemphigoid. *Lancet* 1999; 354: 667–672.

2.3 Dermatomyositis

Aetiology

Dermatomyositis (DM) is an inflammatory disease of skin and striated muscle that is likely to be immunologically based.

Epidemiology

It affects all races, is twice as common in women and has a weak familial tendency. Adults aged 40–60 years are predominantly affected, in whom there is an association with underlying carcinoma and lymphoma. Children are sometimes affected (juvenile DM).

Clinical presentation

Common

- Rash, particularly of sun-exposed sites.
- Proximal muscle weakness and pain causing difficulty climbing stairs or brushing hair.
- General malaise, fever.

Uncommon

- Difficulties with speech and swallowing.
- Raynaud's phenomenon.
- Joint pains and swellings.
- Dyspnoea.

Physical signs

Common

- Purple/red (heliotrope), oedematous facial rash particularly affecting the eyelids, cheeks and forehead. May be scaly.
- Purple/red papules over knuckles (Gottron's papules). Streaking erythema along the dorsum of the fingers (see Fig. 27a, p. 180).
- Prominent, dilated nail-fold capillaries with ragged cuticles (see Fig. 27b, p. 180).
- Proximal muscle weakness.

Uncommon

- Rash can occur on any area, particularly on the back/chest/scalp.
- Diffuse alopecia.
- Weakness can affect any muscle group.
- Calcification of muscles/skin (particularly in childhood cases).
- Arthritis, pulmonary fibrosis, cardiac failure.

Investigation

- Blood tests: Creatine phosphokinase is often increased. ANA/DNA binding is often negative in DM (cf. Lupus), but Jo-1 antibodies may be detected.
- Electromyography (distinguishes neuropathic from myopathic weakness).
- Muscle biopsy (may show inflammation and oedema).
- Skin biopsy (may resemble subacute lupus).
- Tests to investigate possible underlying malignancy.

Differential diagnosis

Systemic lupus erythematosus, polymyositis, systemic sclerosis, muscular dystrophies.

Treatment

- Treat any underlying malignancy.
- High-dose oral steroids, in a reducing regime.
- Additional immunosuppression may be needed, e.g. azathioprine, cyclosporin.
- Physiotherapy to prevent contractures.

Complications

- Respiratory failure, bulbar palsy.
- Muscle contractures and subcutaneous calcification, especially in children.
- Complications of treatment (common).

Prognosis

The overall mortality rate is 25%, the majority of deaths being due to underlying malignancy. Poor prognostic factors are old age, pulmonary involvement, skin necrosis and dysphagia. Calcinosis may be a good prognostic sign. The course of the disease is highly variable.

Disease associations

- Carcinoma and lymphoma in adults.
- Penicillamine treatment.

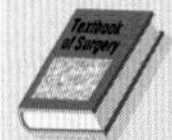

Rowell NR, Goodfield MJD. Connective tissue diseases. In: Champion R, Burton J, Burns A, Breathnach S (eds) *Textbook of Dermatology* (6th edn). Oxford: Blackwell Science, 1998.

2.4 Mycosis fungoides and Sézary syndrome

Aetiology/pathophysiology/pathology

These are primary T-cell lymphomas of the skin due to clonal proliferation of skin-homing T-cells (CLA+ and usually CD4+). In Sézary syndrome (SS), there is haematogenous dissemination. Biopsies show atypical lymphocytes in the dermis which exhibit epidermotropism (cells tend to abut and invade the epidermis).

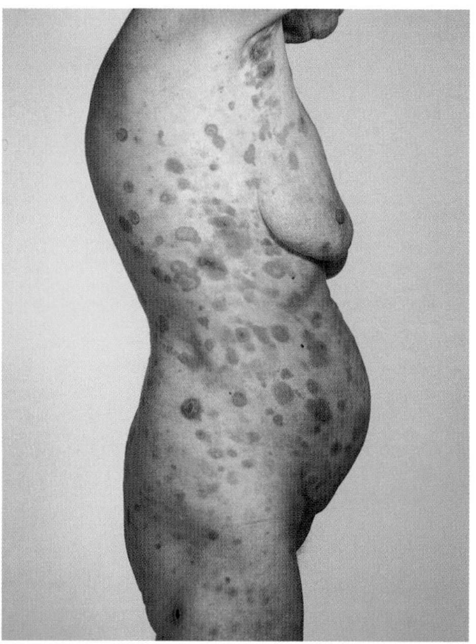

Fig. 44 Mycosis fungoides. Erythematous patches and plaques in a patient who was thought to have psoriasis. However, note the wide variety in colour, size and shape of individual lesions in contrast to those of psoriasis in Fig. 50.

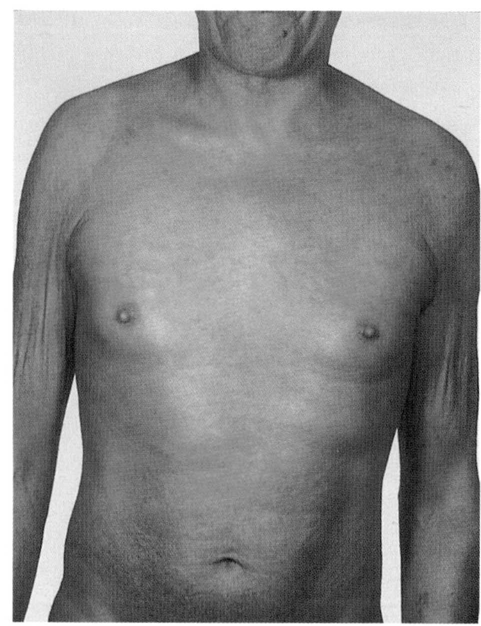

Fig. 45 Sézary syndrome (SS). A scaly erythroderma that may be indistinguishable from other causes such as psoriasis or eczema (see Section 1.3, p. 173). However, in SS the lymph nodes are enlarged and Sézary cells are seen on a blood film.

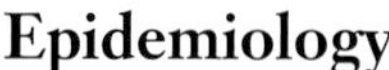

Epidemiology

Primary cutaneous lymphomas are rare with an annual incidence of 1 per 100 000.

• Mycosis fungoides (MF) is the commonest subtype, accounting for 43% of cases.
• SS accounts for 5% of cases.

Clinical presentation

Mycosis fungoides

• In patch-stage disease there are scaly, erythematous patches that may be bizarre in shape and heterogeneous in size and colour. They show a random, asymmetrical distribution but with a predilection for the pelvic girdle and breasts (Fig. 44). They may be itchy. Patches are occasionally hypopigmented.
• The appearance of erythematous, scaly plaques heralds plaque-stage disease.
• Nodules are seen in tumour-stage disease.
• All three stages may be present concurrently ± lymphadenopathy, hepatosplenomegaly, erythroderma.

Sézary syndrome

• Pruritus ++
• Erythroderma (scaly) (Fig. 45)
• Thickening of palms, soles, nails
• Lymphadenopathy
• ± Alopecia, ectropion.

Investigation/staging

• Skin biopsy
• FBC and blood film—lymphocytosis, Sézary cells (large, atypical lymphocytes with cerebriform nuclei)
• Serum LDH
• Chest X-ray
• CT chest, abdomen, pelvis
• Lymph node biopsy if node enlargement
• Bone marrow examination
• T-cell receptor gene rearrangement studies on skin, lymph node, blood to demonstrate clonality (specialist centres only).

Differential diagnosis

• Patch- and plaque-stage cutaneous T cell lymphoma—eczema, psoriasis or tinea.
• Sézary syndrome—Other causes of erythroderma (see Section 1.3, p. 173).

Treatment

The aim is control not cure. Treatment is stage dependant, but options include topical corticosteroids, PUVA, topical chemotherapy e.g. nitrogen mustard, systemic chemotherapy, radiotherapy, interferon, retinoids, photopheresis.

Prognosis

The natural history is variable. Patch/plaque-stage disease may persist for many years. Once there are tumours or extra-cutaneous disease, as in Sézary syndrome, the prognosis is poor (median survival 3 years).

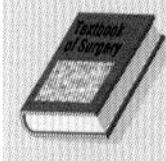

Fitzpatrick TB, Johnson RA, Wolff K *et al. Color Atlas and Synopsis of Clinical Dermatology. Common and Serious Diseases* (3rd edn). New York: McGraw-Hill, 1997.

Du Vivier A. *Atlas of Clinical Dermatology.* (2nd edn). London: Gower Medical Publishing, 1993.

2.5 Dermatitis herpetiformis

Aetiology/pathophysiology/pathology

Dermatitis herpetiformis (DH) is characterized by IgA deposits in the tips of dermal papillae (see Section 3.2, p. 212) which are believed to be pathogenic but, the antigen is not known. Biopsies show neutrophil micro-abscesses in the dermal papillae or frank blister formation at the dermo-epidermal junction. DH is associated with gluten-sensitive enteropathy (90%) and HLA-DRB1*0301, DQA1*0501/DQB1*02.

Epidemiology

Commonest in Europe, particularly Ireland, and rare in the Black, Asian and Oriental populations. The onset can be at any age, but typically in young adults (15–40 years).

Clinical presentation

Common

- Intense pruritus, burning or stinging of skin
- An eruption of small blisters on erythematous papules is classical. More commonly, excoriated papules are seen. Typically affects the extensor surfaces, especially elbows, knees, buttocks, sacrum, neck and scapulae (see Fig. 5, p. 167).

Uncommon

- Oral ulcers
- Pruritus/burning without rash in early stages.

Investigation/staging

- Skin biopsy (histology and direct immunofluorescence)
- Serum autoantibodies: anti-reticulin, gliadin, endomysial or tissue transglutaminase antibodies
- Jejunal biopsy
- Indirect immunofluorescence is always negative, by contrast with bullous pemphigoid and pemphigus vulgaris.

Differential diagnosis

Scabies, urticaria, bites, other immunobullous diseases.

Treatment

Sulphone drugs (dapsone usually) result in a prompt clinical response. A gluten-free diet should be commenced: response to this is slow, but should allow sulphone drugs to be withdrawn in the long term.

Prognosis

The prognosis is good if the diet is strict. Long-term dapsone may be required if a gluten-free diet is not strictly adhered to. There is a long-term risk of small bowel lymphoma.

Disease associations

Gluten-sensitive enteropathy (90%) and other autoimmune diseases.

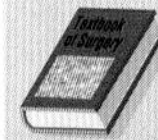

Fitzpatrick TB, Johnson RA, Wolff K *et al. Color Atlas and Synopsis of Clinical Dermatology. Common and Serious Diseases* (3rd edn). New York: McGraw-Hill, 1997.

2.6 Drug eruptions

Aetiology/pathophysiology/pathology

Drug eruptions can mimic a wide variety of idiopathic dermatoses and many drugs can trigger each clinical pattern. They are mediated by both non-immune and immune mechanisms (types I–IV hypersensitivity), and a genetic predisposition is probably important.

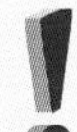

When you are assessing skin diseases, always suspect a drug trigger! In acute presentations, document the start and finish dates of all drugs taken in the preceding month. There is no test to identify the offending drug, but the most likely is chosen on the basis of timing and the track-record of the drugs consumed, some are more likely than others.

Epidemiology

Very common, occurring in around 3% of hospitalized patients. There is an increased incidence in HIV-positive individuals.

Clinical presentation

Common

- Maculopapular eruption (see Fig. 10, p. 171). Onset up to 3 weeks after starting drug. Usually 7–10 days. Within 48 h if previous exposure. Antibiotics (esp. penicillins, sulphonamides), gold, NSAIDs, phenytoin.
- Urticaria ± angioedema ± anaphlaxis (see Fig. 14, p. 172). Onset up to 2 weeks in unexposed, minutes/hours if sensitized. Antibiotics (esp. penicillins), contrast media, aspirin (NSAIDs), ACE-inhibitors, Ca-channel blockers, codeine, opiates.
- Fixed drug eruption. Red macules/patches/plaques. May blister. Often solitary. Resolve with hyperpigmentation (see Fig. 37, p. 187). Upon rechallenge, recurs at identical site (i.e. fixed). Antibiotics (esp. tetracyclines, sulphonamides), NSAIDs, barbiturates.

Uncommon

- Erythroderma (see Fig. 19, p. 175)—May evolve from a maculopapular eruption if the drug is continued. Sulphonamides, penicillins, phenytoin, antimalarials
- EM/SJS/TEN (see Figs 6, 11 and 13, pp. 167, 171 and 172)—Anticonvulsants, allopurinol, antibiotics (esp. sulphonamides, penicillins), NSAIDs. See Section 2.9 (p. 198).
- Drug hypersensitivity syndrome—Maculopapular or erythrodermic rash with fever, eosinophilia, lymphadenopathy ± hepatitis, pneumonitis, myocarditis. Onset 2–6 weeks after drug started. Anti-convulsants, sulphonamides, allopurinol, gold.
- Pigmentation—Usually a delayed onset (months). Amiodarone, minocycline, antimalarials, phenytoin, cytotoxics, phenothiazines, OCP, heavy metals.
- Necrosis—3–5 days after starting warfarin.
- Toxic pustuloderma (sheets of pustules on diffuse erythema) (see Fig. 15, p. 172)—Anticonvulsants, antibiotics (esp. penicillins).
- Acne (see Fig. 25, p. 179)—Phenytoin, lithium, cortico/anabolic steroids, androgens.
- Erythema nodosum (see Section 2.10, p. 200)—Sulphonamides, OCP.
- Lichen planus-like—Antimalarials, β-blockers, ACE-inhibitors, gold.
- Photosensitivity (Fig. 23, p. 178)—May not manifest until spring/summer. Antibiotics (esp. tetracyclines), NSAIDs, amiodarone, phenothiazines, thiazides.
- Hair loss—Cytotoxics, retinoids, anticoagulants, cimetidine.
- Vasculitis (see Fig. 12, p. 171)—Allopurinol, penicillin, sulphonamides.
- Pseudoporphyria—Furosemide (frusemide), NSAIDs, tetracyclines, sulphonylureas.
- Lupus-like—Procainamide, hydralazine, isoniazid, phenytoin, minocycline.
- Nail pigmentation—Anti-malarials, tetracyclines, lithium, heavy metals, cytotoxics
- Onycholysis—Tetracyclines, cytotoxics, captopril, phenothiazines.

Investigation/staging

- FBC may show eosinophilia
- Skin biopsy—Variable changes dependant on the type of reaction but the presence of eosinophils suggests a drug cause.

Treatment

- Emergency—Anaphylactic reactions: epinephrine (adrenaline), hydrocortisone, piriton. See *Clinical immunology and immunosuppression*, Sections 1.7 and 2.2.1.
- Short term—Stop the suspected drug and treat symptomatically. Systemic corticosteroids are used in drug hypersensitivity when there is visceral involvement and sometimes to hasten recovery in erythroderma and SJS/TEN (see Section 2.9, p. 198).

Prognosis

Generally good once the drug is stopped but SJS, TEN, anaphylaxis, erythrodermic drug reactions and drug hypersensitivity syndromes can be life-threatening.

Prevention

Avoid the drug. Document in medical records. Medical alert bracelet.

Breathnach SM, Hintner H. *Adverse Drug Reactions and the Skin.* Oxford: Blackwell Science, 1992.

Fitzpatrick TB, Johnson RA, Wolff K *et al. Color Atlas and Synopsis of Clinical Dermatology. Common and Serious Diseases* (3rd edn). New York: McGraw-Hill, 1997.

Habif TP. *Clinical Dermatology: A Colour Guide to Diagnosis and Therapy* (2nd edn). St Louis: CV Mosby, 1990.

2.7 Atopic eczema

Aetiology/pathophysiology/pathology

An itchy, chronically relapsing, inflammatory skin disease that often occurs in association with the other atopic conditions (hayfever and asthma). Genetic and environmental factors are important (70% of cases have a family history) but inheritance is polygenic.

Antigen challenge preferentially activates Th2 T-helper cells, which produce interleukin-4 and 5. These cytokines stimulate B cell IgE synthesis and IgE levels are raised in 60–80% cases. It is not clear how this leads to eczema.

Biopsies show a non-specific dermatitis (epidermal thickening, dermal and epidermal oedema, inflammatory cells).

Epidemiology

Males and females equally affected. Common, affecting between 5 and 15% of children by 7 years, with a prevalence of 2–10% in adults. Onset usually 2–6 months of age.

Clinical presentation

Common

- Itchy, macular erythema, papules and/or vesicles
- Lichenification (skin thickening with increased markings secondary to scratching)
- Excoriations
- Dry skin (xerosis)
- Secondary bacterial infection (impetiginized eczema)
- Distribution varies with age—cheeks/exposed sites in infants, limb flexures in children and adults (see Figs 21, p. 177, and 46).

Uncommon

- Inverse distribution of eczema—affecting extensor surfaces
- Nail pitting.

Investigation

The diagnosis is usually clinical. Take skin swabs if secondary infection is suspected. A raised IgE, positive radio-allergosorbent tests (RAST) or prick tests supports atopy.

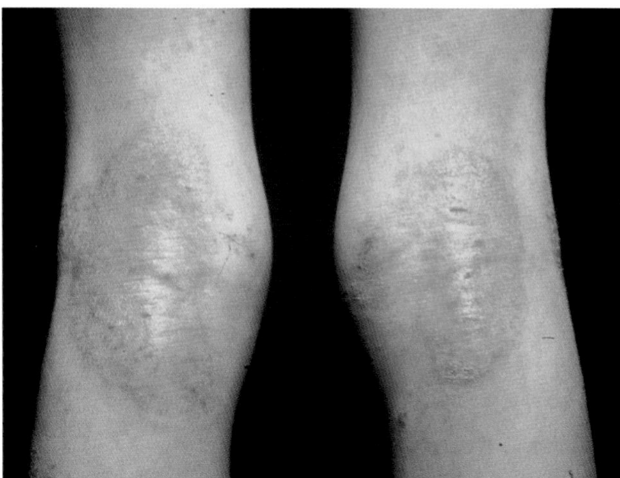

Fig. 46 Atopic eczema. There is erythema and lichenification of the skin in the popliteal fossae, a preferentially involved site. Excoriations due to scratching are also seen.

Differential diagnosis

Seborrhoeic dermatitis, allergic contact dermatitis, scabies.

Treatment

- Avoid soaps and detergents and avoid wearing wool. Reduce house dust mite exposure
- Emollients and topical steroids
- Treat secondary infections
- In more severe cases, phototherapy, oral steroids or second line immunosupression with azathioprine or cyclosporin may be required.

Complications

Secondary infection with bacteria, usually staphylococcus or streptococcus, or herpes simplex (eczema herpeticum) (see Fig. 2b, p. 166) (see Section 1.1, p. 165).

Prognosis

Gradual improvement through childhood. Fifty percent clear by 13 years.

Disease associations

Asthma, hayfever, food allergies, anaphylaxis.

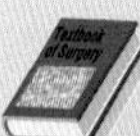

Holden CA and Parish WE. Atopic dermatitis. In: Champion R, Burton J, Burns A, Breathnach S (eds) *Textbook of Dermatology* (6th edn). Oxford: Blackwell Science, 1998.

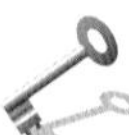

- The terms eczema and dermatitis are usually used synonymously.
- Eczema is the term commonly used in the atopic form.
- Dermatitis is the term used in contact and seborrhoeic forms.
- Seborrhoeic dermatitis is a very common form of eczema where the earliest sign is mild dandruff (see Fig. 20, p. 177) (see Section 1.4, p. 177). Pityrosporum yeasts are thought to play a causative role. Severe seborrhoeic dermatitis can occur with HIV.

2.8 Contact dermatitis

Aetiology/pathophysiology/pathology

Contact dermatitis (CD) is eczema of the skin induced by contact with exogenous substances. It is broadly divided into allergic and irritant reactions.

• Allergic CD is antigen specific and occurs only in some individuals. Memory T cells develop after the initial exposure and mediate type-IV (delayed) allergy upon subsequent exposure. Common allergens include rubber, nickel, perfumes, plants and cosmetics.
• Irritants directly damage the skin and irritant CD can develop in anyone after cumulative exposure, e.g. to detergents, or after a single exposure to a strong irritant, e.g. wet cement.

Epidemiology

Contact dermatitis is common. It accounts for approximately 50% of all reported cases of occupational disease.

Clinical presentation

Common

Allergic contact dermatitis

The physical signs are those of eczema (see Section 2.7, p. 196) and in very acute cases there may be severe blistering. Certain features suggest CD rather than atopic eczema. The onset later in life in a non-atopic individual or an atypical distribution, e.g. hand dermatitis with a cut off at the wrists if allergic to rubber in gloves, or dermatitis confined to the ear lobes and umbilicus if allergic to nickel in earrings and jeans studs (Fig. 47). CD may also occur at sites of topical medicament exposure, e.g. leg ulcers or pruritus ani. Think of CD in cases of eczema that are resistant to treatment.

Irritant contact dermatitis

Hand dermatitis is most common and particularly affects the finger webs. Often occurs in individuals whose occupation involves repeated hand washing or use of detergents.

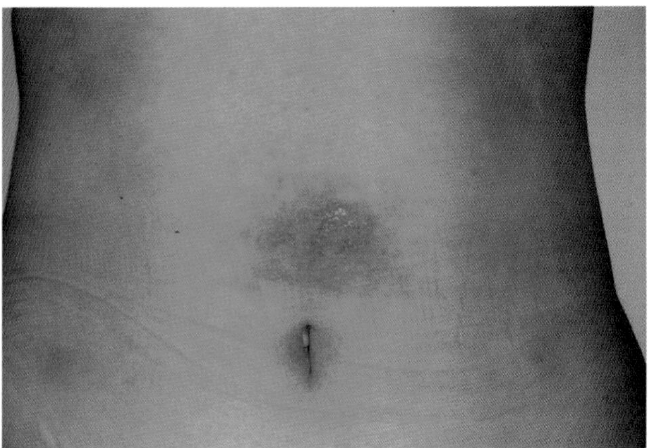

Fig. 47 Allergic contact dermatitis to nickel: a characteristic site (due to contact with the stud fastener of jeans).

Investigation

Patch testing to confirm or exclude allergic CD. See Section 3.3 (p. 213).

Differential diagnosis

Endogenous eczema, psoriasis, fungal infections.

Treatment

Avoidance of allergens and irritants. Topical use of emollients and corticosteroids. Systemic steroids are sometimes used in acute, severe CD.

Prognosis

Good if the patient is able to avoid specific allergens or avoid exposure to irritants. Rubber and nickel are ubiquitous and therefore difficult to avoid. Atopic patients have a worse prognosis.

Disease associations

Atopic patients are at increased risk of developing irritant CD.

Wilkinson JD, Willis CM, Shaw S. Contact Dermatitis. In: Champion R, Burton J, Burns A, Breathnach S (eds) *Textbook of Dermatology* (6th edn). Oxford: Blackwell Science, 1998.

2.9 Erythema multiforme, Stevens–Johnson syndrome, toxic epidermal necrolysis

Aetiology/pathophysiology/pathology

Erythema multiforme (EM), Stevens–Johnson syndrome (SJS) and toxic epidermal necrolysis (TEN) are thought to represent a spectrum of disease caused by an immunological reponse common to a number of stimuli. These include:
• infections, particularly herpes simplex and mycoplasma
• drugs (see Section 2.6, p. 195).

However, many cases (25–50%) are idiopathic. Biopsies show necrosis of keratinocytes which may be scanty in mild cases or full-thickness epidermal necrosis in TEN. Recent evidence implicates activation of the FAS death receptor on keratinocytes leading to apoptosis [1] (see Section 1.2, and *Cell Biology*, Section 3).

Clinical presentation

• Common—Skin rash (often tender) ± painful mucosal ulceration
• Uncommon—Mucosal ulceration alone; Recurrent EM (often herpes simplex virus (HSV) triggered).

Physical signs

Erythema multiforme

• Dusky red macules, papules and plaques (iris or target lesions typical but not always present) (see Fig. 11, p. 171)
• Typically distal limbs, including palms/soles, but may be more widespread
• Individual lesions may blister
• There may be mucosal ulceration
• ± Signs of mycoplasma pneumonia or HSV infection
• Patients often relatively well.

Stevens–Johnson syndrome

• Skin lesions as in EM, but tendency to be more widespread and bullous lesions are more common (see Fig. 6, p. 167).
• Painful mucosal inflammation/ulceration including (in order of frequency) mouth and lips, eyes, genitalia and respiratory epithelium (pneumonitis).
• Patient unwell ± fever.

Toxic epidermal necrolysis

• Diffuse erythema (>10% skin surface) with epidermal detachment (see Fig. 13, p. 172). Erythroderma occurs in 10% of cases.
• Nikolsky's sign positive
• Mucosal involvement as in SJS
• Patient very unwell with a fever.

Investigation/staging

• Skin biopsy
• Chest X-ray (looking for mycoplasma or pnemonitis)
• Mycoplasma and herpes simplex serology
• U+E, LFT, FBC.

Differential diagnosis

• EM—Hand, foot and mouth disease, cicatricial pemphigoid, PV
• TEN—Staphylococcal scalded skin syndrome.

Treatment

Treatment is largely supportive (see also Section 1.3, p. 175):
• Any suspected drug triggers should be stopped and triggering infections should be treated.
• If there is extensive skin involvement, nurse patients on an air-fluidized bed in an ITU.
• Skin handling should be minimal and aseptic and strong analgesia may be needed. Topical antiseptics are often used to minimize sepsis risk.
• Fluid replacement and nutritional supplementation will be needed. Monitor fluid balance carefully.
• Involve ophthalmology colleagues if there is ocular involvement.

No specific therapies are of proven benefit. Corticosteroids are controversial. The risks, especially if there are widespread erosions, may outweigh the short-term benefits. Recent experimental and clinical data supports the use of intravenous immunogobulin in TEN [1].

Complications

Common

• Fluid, electrolyte, protein loss and sepsis if extensive erosions
• Inability to eat/drink.

Uncommon

• Scarring of mucosal surfaces (may cause blindness)
• Pneumonitis.

Prognosis

The epidermis will regenerate after 3–4 weeks in TEN, but the mortality rate is 30%.

Prevention

Secondary

Avoid the precipitating drug. For HSV-triggered recurrent EM, prophylactic aciclovir is used. Azathioprine and other immunosuppressants are sometimes used in recurrent cases.

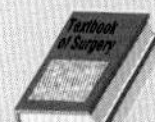

Fitzpatrick TB, Johnson RA, Wolff K *et al. Color Atlas and Synopsis of Clinical Dermatology. Common and Serious Diseases* (3rd edn). New York: McGraw-Hill, 1997.
1 Viard I, Wehrli P, Bullani R *et al.* Inhibition of toxic epidermal necrolysis by blockade of CD95 with human intravenous immunoglobulin. *Science* 1998; 282: 490–492.

2.10 Erythema nodosum

Aetiology/pathophysiology/pathology

Erythema nodosum (EN) is an idiopathic disorder but may be secondary to immune complex deposition following a number of different stimuli (Table 15). Histology shows a panniculitis (inflammation of fat).

Epidemiology

The annual UK incidence of EN is around 2.4 per 10 000, with a peak onset between 20 and 30 years. EN accounts for 0.5% of new dermatology outpatients and is commoner in females (F : M 3–6 : 1).

Clinical presentation

Common

Multiple, hot, tender, erythematous nodules on the anterior shins/lower legs (Fig. 48). These fade after 2–3 weeks to leave a bruised appearance. There may be a preceding upper respiratory infection and the eruption may be accompanied by fever, malaise and arthralgia.

Uncommon

Other sites may be involved such as arms, breasts, face.

Table 15 Causes of erythema nodosum.

Infections
Bacterial
- Streptococcus
- Mycobacterium
- Yersinia
- Chlamydia spp.

Viral
- Epstein–Barr virus

Fungal
- Trichophyton spp.
- Coccidioidomycosis

Drugs
Sulphonamides
Oral contraceptive

Others
Sarcoidosis
Crohn's disease
Ulcerative colitis
Behçet's disease
Malignancy, e.g. lymphoma

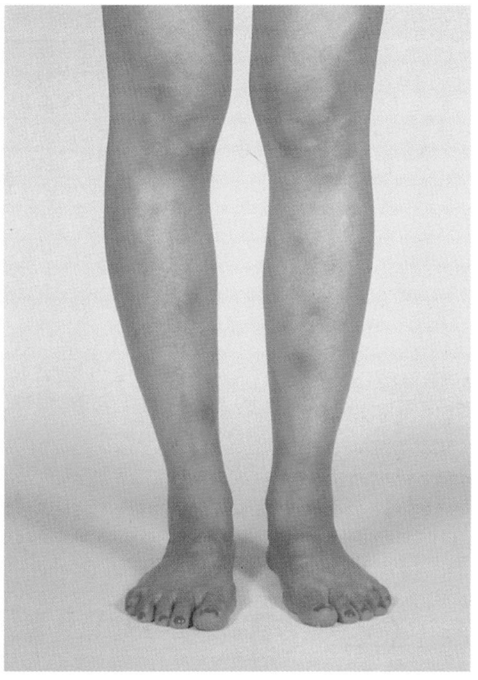

Fig. 48 Erythema nodosum. Painful, hot, red nodules which most commonly affect the lower legs. As they resolve, the colour changes simulate that of a bruise.

Investigation

- A skin biopsy can confirm the diagnosis, although this is usually made on clinical grounds.
- Throat swab, blood count, ESR, ASO titre, serum ACE, chest radiograph, virological and Yersinia titres. Consider a Mantoux test.

Differential diagnosis

- Consider cellulitis, abscess or superficial phlebitis.
- Nodular vasculitis, but lesions are smaller, harder and more persistent.

Treatments

- Leg elevation and support and removal of precipitating cause.
- Non-steroidal anti-inflammatory agents are most commonly used.
- Oral steroids are rarely used and are best avoided if an infectious aetiology has not been excluded.

Prognosis

Usually resolves in 3–6 weeks.

Disease associations

Erythema nodosum is associated with a number of other diseases (Table 15), but in many cases no definite cause is found.

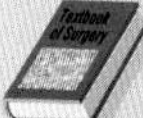

Ryan TJ. Erythema nodosum. In: Champion R, Burton J, Burns A, Breathnach S (eds) *Textbook of Dermatology* (6th edn). Oxford: Blackwell Science, 1998.
Du Vivier A. *Atlas of Clinical Dermatology* (2nd edn). London: Gower Medical Publishing, 1993.

2.11 Lichen planus

Aetiology/pathophysiology/pathology

Lichen planus (LP) is an inflammatory disease in which there is 'band-like', dense infiltrate of T cells in the upper dermis with damage to the overlying basal layer of the epidermis. The aetiology is unknown, but is likely to be immunologically based. LP-like rashes can be drug induced.

Epidemiology

LP accounts for approximately 1% of new dermatology outpatients. Females are more commonly affected. The peak onset is between 30 and 60 years.

Clinical presentation

Common

Violaceous (pink/purple), itchy, flat-topped papules distributed on the extremities, particularly the flexor surface of the wrists (Fig. 49a). White streaks (Wickham's striae) are usually visible on the papule surface. Fifty percent have white linear streaks in the oral cavity, particularly on the buccal mucosae (Fig. 49c). LP exhibits the Koebner phenomenon (Fig. 49b) and post-inflammatory hyperpigmentation is common.

Uncommon

The nails may be affected, for example by longitudinal grooves. LP can be generalized or may present with scarring alopecia or thick, hypertrophic plaques on the shins. Genital involvement can occur and mucosal LP can be erosive.

Investigation

Skin biopsy.

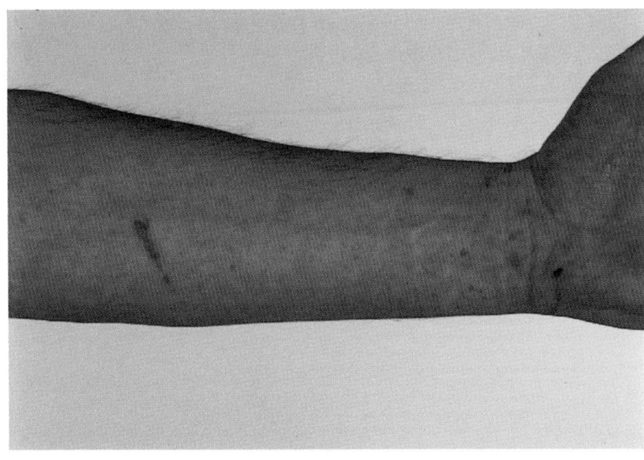

(a)

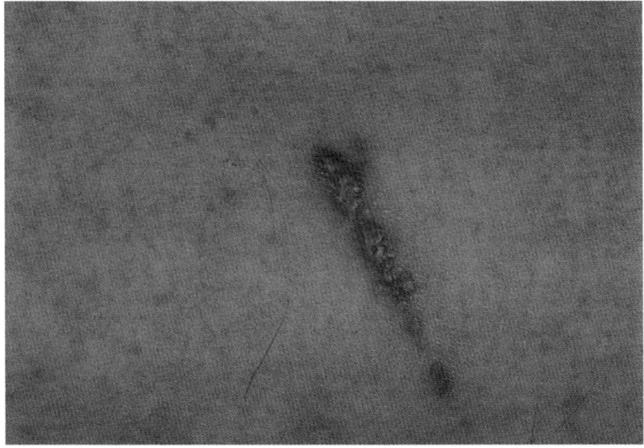

(b)

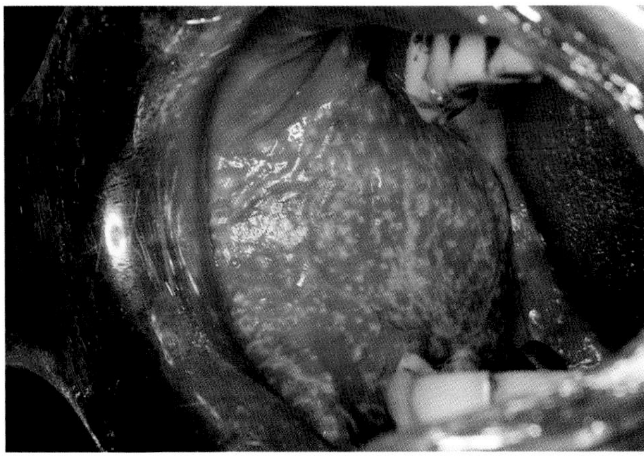

(c)

Fig. 49 Lichen planus. (a) An itchy eruption over the flexor surface of the forearm and wrist. (b) On close inspection, shiny purple/red, flat-topped papules with Wickham's striae on the surface (fine, white lines). The linear configuration is due to the Koebner phenomenon—the lesions have arisen at a site of trauma, in this case a scratch. (c) Always check the mucosal surfaces—Wickham's striae are seen here on the buccal mucosa

Differential diagnosis

- Drug-induced LP, psoriasis, lichen simplex
- Pemphigus vulgaris and cicatricial pemphigoid mimic erosive LP of the mucosal surfaces.

Treatments

- Potent topical steroids are most commonly prescribed.
- For severe or non-responsive cases, oral steroids (usually short courses) or PUVA are used.
- Occasionally, other immunosuppressive drugs are given, e.g. azathioprine.

Complications

Rarely, erosive mucosal LP has been complicated by the development of squamous cell carcinoma.

Prognosis

Most cases resolve within 6–9 months. Hypertrophic or mucosal, especially erosive, LP can persist for many years.

Disease associations

Rarely, ulcerative colitis, primary biliary cirrhosis, hypogammaglobulinaemia or chronic active hepatitis. In Mediterranean countries, hepatitis C is linked with LP.

Black MM. Lichen planus and lichenoid disorders. In: Champion R, Burton J, Burns A, Breathnach S (eds) *Textbook of Dermatology* (6th edn). Oxford: Blackwell Science, 1998.

2.12 Pemphigus vulgaris

Aetiology/pathophysiology/pathology

Pemphigus vulgaris (PV) is an autoimmune disease in which IgG binds to a desmosomal component, desmoglein 3, present on the cell surface of keratinocytes. This results in dyscohesion of the keratinocytes to produce the characteristic intra-epidermal blisters seen in skin biopsies. There is an association with HLA DR4 and 14; rare cases are drug induced.

Epidemiology

Onset at any age, including childhood, but most commonly the 3rd–6th decades. There is an increased incidence in Ashkenazi Jews and Indians.

Clinical presentation

Common

- Painful oral erosions—the first feature in around 70% of cases and may be the only sign (see Fig. 7b, p. 168).
- Cutaneous erosions that may be painful but do not itch, unlike BP (see Fig. 7a, p. 168). In fact blisters are less commonly seen because they are fragile, but these are usually round/oval with minimal surrounding erythema (cf. BP) and often on the upper trunk, scalp and sites of friction e.g. axillae. In the scalp, crusted plaques are commoner than erosions. Nikolsky's sign is positive in uncontrolled disease.
- Genital or nasal erosions.

Uncommon

- Ocular, laryngeal, oesophageal, anal erosions
- Childhood PV
- Neonatal PV (due to transplacental passage of pathogenic antibodies)
- Extensive areas of eroded skin (treatment usually prevents reaching this stage).

Investigation/staging

- Skin biopsy for histology and direct immunofluorescence—IgG on keratinocyte surface in lesional and 'normal' skin (see Section 3.2, p. 212).
- Serum for indirect immunofluorescence—Serum IgG binds to the keratinocyte surfaces of normal skin.

Differential diagnosis

- Pemphigus foliaceus (a rarer subtype that affects the skin only)
- Mucous membrane pemphigoid (cicatricial pemphigoid).

Treatment

- Short-term—Corticosteroids ± a steroid-sparing drug (usually azathioprine or cyclophosphamide). In rapidly progressing, extensive PV, consider pulsed corticosteroids, plasmapheresis or intravenous immunoglobulin.
- Long-term—Steroids with a steroid-sparing drug (doses are slowly reduced to the minimum required).

Complications

Common

- Treatment side effects.
- Secondary infection of erosions ± septicaemia.
- Difficulty eating and brushing teeth due to painful gums.

Uncommon

• Fluid, electrolyte and protein loss and septicaemia if there are extensive skin erosions.

Prognosis

PV is almost universally fatal without treatment. With treatment, there is a 6% mortality. Morbidity nowadays is mainly treatment related.

Disease associations

PV may be associated with other autoimmune diseases and is rarely paraneoplastic (lymphomas, CLL, thymomas, Castleman's tumours).

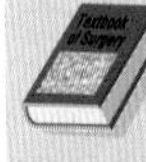

Fitzpatrick TB, Johnson RA, Wolff K *et al. Color Atlas and Synopsis of Clinical Dermatology. Common and Serious Diseases* (3rd edn). New York: McGraw-Hill, 1997.
Nousari HC, Anhalt GJ. Pemphigus and bullous pemphigoid. *Lancet* 1999; 354(9179): 667–672.

2.13 Superficial fungal infections

Aetiology/pathophysiology/pathology

Skin, hair and nails can all be affected by fungi, i.e. yeasts or moulds, which adhere to and invade keratin, causing thickening of the keratin layer and varying degrees of inflammation.

• Pityriasis versicolor is caused by Malassezia yeasts.
• 'Ringworm' is caused by a group of moulds termed dermatophytes, of which there are three types, *Microsporum*, *Trichophyton* and *Epidermophyton*.

Clinical presentation

Common

• Tinea corporis (ringworm affecting the body)—circular, well-defined lesions with a raised scaly edge that enlarge peripherancy with central clearing.
• Tinea capitis (ringworm of the scalp)—very variable. Erythema and scaling of the scalp with partial alopecia, often in localized patches but sometimes widespread (see Section 1.6, p. 183 and Figs 33 and 34, p. 184).
• Tinea pedis (ringworm of the feet, i.e. athlete's foot) —maceration and fissuring in toe web spaces. Toe nails often additionally affected.
• Tinea unguium (ringworm of the nails)—discoloration and thickening of the nail plate with subungual hyperkeratosis.

Uncommon

• Tinea corporis—pustules and blisters if inflammation severe.
• Tinea capitis—sometimes the host reaction is so great that an oozing, inflammatory mass occurs (a kerion) (see Fig. 34, p. 184).

Investigation

Direct microscopy and culture of skin scrapings, plucked hairs or nail clippings is required to confirm the diagnosis.

1 Scrape the active scaly edge of a suspected cutaneous lesion with a clean scalpel blade. Pluck hairs from affected hair-bearing areas and scrape keratin from beneath affected nails.
2 Transport specimen in folded pieces of paper to the microbiology lab for microscopy and culture.
3 Scrapings can be directly mounted in 30% potassium hydroxide on slides in clinic, and examined under a light microscope for signs of fungal spores and hyphae.

Differential diagnosis

Tinea corporis—eczema, psoriasis, Bowen's disease.

Treatment

Dermatophytes can be treated with the antifungals, itraconazole, terbinafine or griseofulvin. Localized cutaneous infections respond well to topical terbinafine. Widespread infections, tinea capitis and tinea unguium require oral therapy.

Disease associations

• Widespread dermatophyte infection can be associated with immunosupressive drug therapy.
• Oral candidiasis is particularly associated with HIV.

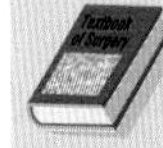

Hay RJ and Moore M. Mycology. In: Champion R, Burton J, Burns A, Breathnach S (eds) *Textbook of Dermatology* (6th edn). Oxford: Blackwell Science, 1998.

2.14 Psoriasis

Aetiology/pathophysiology/pathology

Psoriasis is an inflammatory disease in which epidermal turnover is greatly increased. It is believed to be T-cell mediated with both genetic and environmental factors playing a role. Inheritance is polygenic.

Biopsies show epidermal thickening, dilation of the

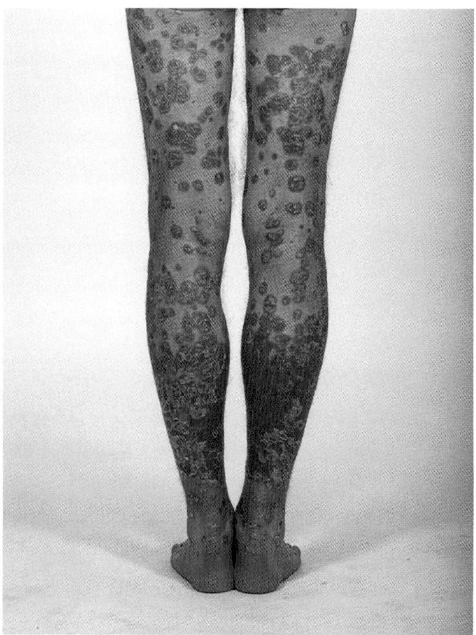

Fig. 50 Chronic plaque psoriasis: well-defined, round/oval, deep red, scaly erythematous plaques which are confluent on the lower legs. Note the homogeneity of lesions compared to mycosis fungoides, seen in Fig. 44.

dermal capillaries and a mixed inflammatory cell infiltrate, but CD4 lymphocytes predominate in early lesions.

Epidemiology

Psoriasis is common—prevalence 1.5–3%. Equal sex ratio. The onset can be at any age, but there are two peaks at 16–22 years and 57–60 years.

Clinical presentation

Common

• Well-defined, deep red, scaly plaques (Fig. 50). Removal of scale reveals pinpoint bleeding (Auspitz sign). Usually multiple, symmetrical plaques preferentially affecting the extensor surface of the elbows and knees, scalp, sacrum and umbilicus.

• Nails show pitting, thickening, onycholysis (separation of nail plate from the nail bed) and subungual hyperkeratosis (Figs 17b, p. 174, and 51).

Uncommon

• Guttate psoriasis—an acute shower of small (<1 cm) plaques ('rain drops') over the trunk and limbs. Particularly in children following a streptococcal throat infection.

• Palmoplantar pustular psoriasis—chronic, erythematous, scaly, plaques, studded with sterile pustules on the palms and soles (Fig. 52).

• Erythrodermic psoriasis—generalized erythema and scaling with loss of discrete plaques (Fig. 17a, p. 174).

• Generalized pustular psoriasis—widespread sheets of fiery red skin, studded with sterile pustules (see Figs 15, p. 172 and 18, p. 175).

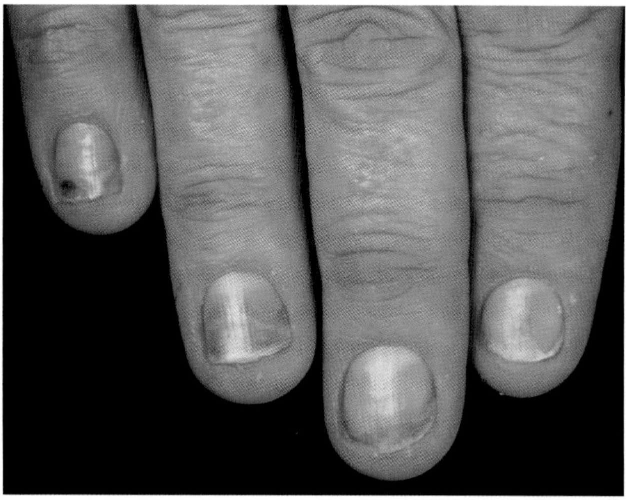

(a)

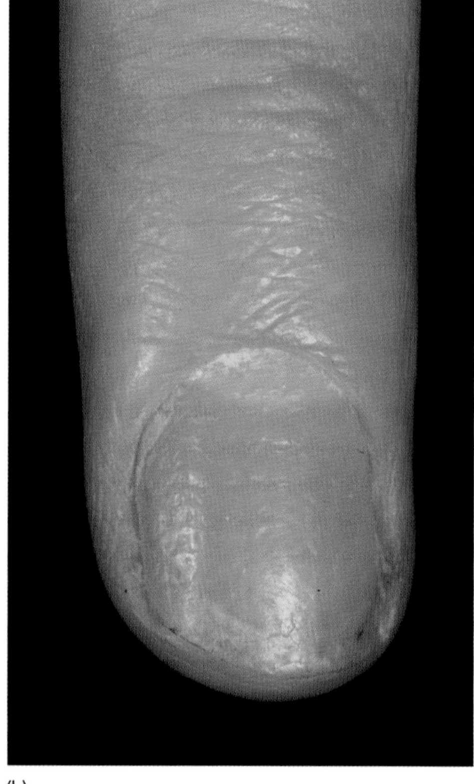

(b)

Fig. 51 Psoriatic nail changes: (a) Onycholysis is seen which is separation of the distal nail from the nail bed. (b) Pitting of the nail surface.

Investigation

• Skin biopsy if diagnosis in doubt.

• Throat swab and ASO titre in guttate psoriasis.

Differential diagnosis

• If atypical, may resemble eczema, discoid lupus or seborrheic dermatitis.

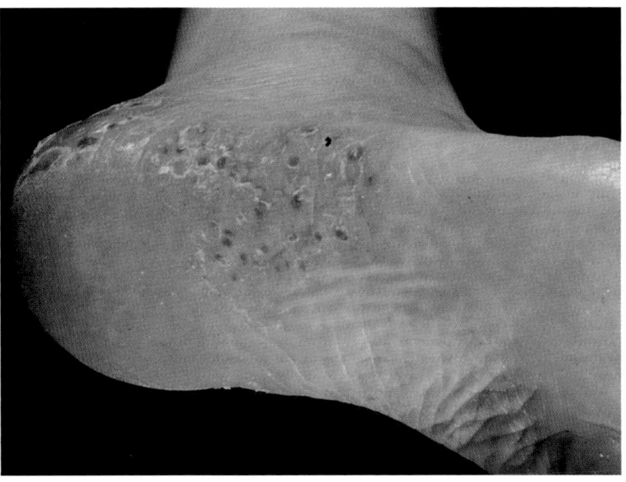

Fig. 52 Palmar-plantar pustular psoriasis: Pustules on an erythematous, scaly base which evolve to leave brown macules. This variety affects the palms and soles. The pustules are sterile if swabbed.

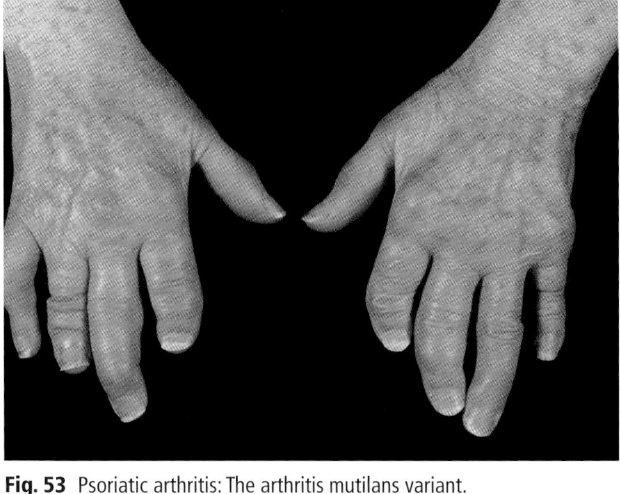

Fig. 53 Psoriatic arthritis: The arthritis mutilans variant.

- Single plaques may resemble Bowen's disease or lichen simplex.
- Guttate psoriasis may resemble pityriasis rosea or secondary syphilis.

Treatment

- Topical therapies—Emollients, vitamin D analogues (e.g. calcipotriol), steroids (particularly palms, soles, scalp, flexures), dithranol, tar.
- Phototherapy—UVB or PUVA
- Systemic therapies—Oral retinoids, methotrexate, cyclosporin, mycophenolate mofetil, hydroxycarbamide (hydroxyurea).

Complications

- Psoriatic arthritis (Fig. 53) (see *Rheumatology and clinical immunology*, Section 2.3)
- Patients with erythrodermic, especially pustular, psoriasis are at risk of hypoalbuminaemia, hypothermia, dehydration, renal failure, liver failure, septicaemia.

Prognosis

Very variable. Usually relapsing and remitting. Guttate psoriasis has a better prognosis.

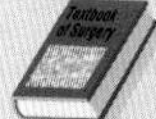

Camp RDR. Psoriasis. In: Champion R, Burton J, Burns A, Breathnach S (eds) *Textbook of Dermatology* (6th edn). Oxford: Blackwell Science, 1998.

Du Vivier A. *Atlas of Clinical Dermatology* (2nd edn). London: Gower Medical Publishing, 1993.

2.15 Scabies

Aetiology/pathophysiology/pathology

Scabies is due to an infestation by the mite *Sarcoptes scabiei* which is transmitted by skin-to-skin contact. Sensitization to *S. scabiei* takes several weeks to develop and results in the symptoms and majority of physical signs.

Scabies is a common but easily missed diagnosis that should be suspected in anyone complaining of pruritus. Search for the diagnostic burrows and scabetic nodules.

Epidemiology

Any age but particularly young adults (from intimate contact), institutionalized patients and healthcare workers.

Clinical presentation

Common

- Pruritus—Especially at night ± rash.
- Scabetic burrows—Tan/skin coloured linear ridges, several millimetres in length. Found especially in the finger webs, flexor surface of the wrists, lateral borders of hands/feet, axillae, penile shaft, palms/soles of infants (Fig. 31a, p. 182).
- Scabetic nodules—red/brown, 5–20 mm, particularly on penis, scrotum, buttocks, upper thighs, waist, axillae (Fig. 31b, p. 182).
- As a result of sensitization—Urticaria, eczema, maculopapular eruption, vesicles, excoriations.

Uncommon

• Norwegian scabies—Heavily crusted, localized or generalized eruption due to heavy mite infestation which occurs in the immunocompromised and those with neurological disorders.

Investigation/staging

Demonstrate a mite, egg or faeces. Scrape a burrow with a scalpel blade and view material with a light microsope.

Differential diagnosis

Urticaria, eczema, DH.

Treatment

• Permethrin, malathion or benzyl benzoate are applied topically from the neck down. In babies, the head must also be treated.
• All household members and any intimate contacts should be treated simultaneously, even if asymptomatic.
• Clothes/bedding should be washed (mites can survive up to 72 h off the host).

Complications

Treatment failure or re-infection is common. Secondary infection can occur and very occasionally results in septicaemia.

Prognosis

Itching may persist for several weeks following successful treatment (warn the patient) and scabetic nodules may persist for several months.

Occupational aspects

Healthcare workers are at risk.

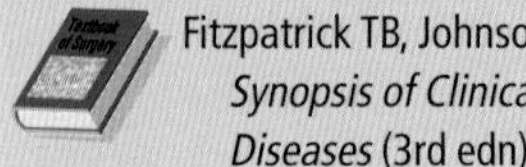

Fitzpatrick TB, Johnson RA, Wolff K *et al. Color Atlas and Synopsis of Clinical Dermatology. Common and Serious Diseases* (3rd edn). New York: McGraw-Hill, 1997.

2.16 Urticaria and angio-oedema

Aetiology/pathophysiology/pathology

Urticarial weals or hives are secondary to vasodilatation and leakage of capillary fluid into the dermis. Angio-oedema is produced when this process involves the deeper tissues. Urticaria can be classified according to aetiology and duration (Table 16). In most cases the final common pathway is mast cell degranulation, releasing inflammatory mediators including histamine.

Table 16 The classification of urticaria.

Subtype	Triggers/disease associations
Acute urticaria	Drugs, e.g. penicillins Foods, e.g. fish, nuts Infections, e.g. streptococcus Bee/wasp stings Idiopathic
Chronic urticaria (if occurs daily for more than 6 weeks duration)	Idiopathic (most cases) Drugs Infections SLE Autoimmune thyroid disease
Immune complex urticaria	Serum sickness Urticarial vasculitis
Physical	Dermographism Pressure Vibration Solar Cold Water
Cholinergic	Exercise, heat, emotion
Contact urticaria	Foods, e.g. fish
Angio-oedema alone	C1 esterase inhibitor deficiency
Others	Familial Mediterranean fever

Epidemiology

Urticaria is common, with a lifetime risk of 15–25%, and occurs at any age.

Clinical presentation

Common

Itchy, erythematous macules develop into weals (Fig. 14, p. 172). Can occur anywhere. In up to 50% there is associated angio-oedema with facial and mucosal swelling.

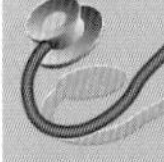

Weals are flesh coloured to pale pink, oedematous, itchy papules and plaques which may change in size and shape but always last less than 24 h and leave no mark. They are characteristic of urticaria and may be very large.

Uncommon

Consider urticarial vasculitis if individual weals last longer than 24 h or are associated with purpura.

Investigation

- The diagnosis is clinical.
- No investigations are required for most acute cases, but look for symptoms/signs of a triggering infection and investigate accordingly. Consider RAST to specific allergens.
- In chronic cases, screen for associated diseases including blood count, liver and thyroid function, ESR and an autoantibody profile. Challenge tests if a physical urticaria is suspected.
- C4 complement levels to exclude C1-esterase-inhibitor deficiency in angio-oedema.
- Skin biopsy and vasculitis screen (e.g. antinuclear antibody, complement) if urticarial vasculitis suspected.
- Stool should be sent for microscopy for parasites.

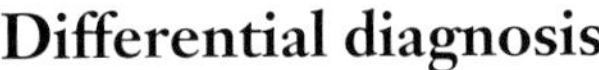

Differential diagnosis

Erythema multiforme, early bullous pemphigoid or insect bites, but in all of these lesions last >24 h.

Treatments

- Avoid any precipitating factors and direct histamine releasers, e.g. aspirin and opiates.
- Nonsedating or sedating H_1 antihistamines are the cornerstone of treatment.
- Oral steroids are rarely needed.
- Adrenaline for life-threatening anaphylaxis or angio-oedema (see *Immunology and immunosuppression*, Sections 1.7 and 2.2.1).
- Hereditary angio-oedema is treated with danazol and whole plasma or C1 esterase inhibitor concentrate is given in acute, severe attacks.

Complications

Severe angio-oedema with respiratory compromise ± anaphylaxis.

Prognosis

Fifty percent of individuals with urticaria clear within 6 months. Approximately 25% will persist for many years.

Disease associations

Hereditary or acquired C1-esterase-inhibitor deficiency. Systemic vasculitis.

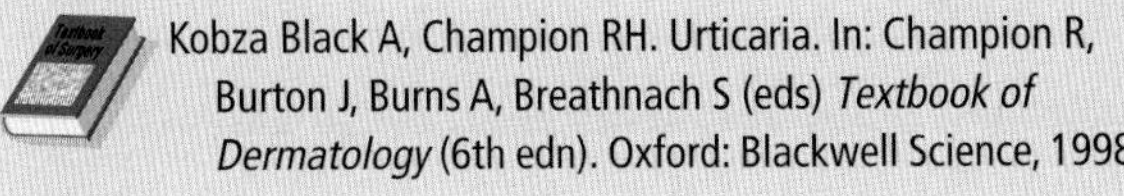

Kobza Black A, Champion RH. Urticaria. In: Champion R, Burton J, Burns A, Breathnach S (eds) *Textbook of Dermatology* (6th edn). Oxford: Blackwell Science, 1998.

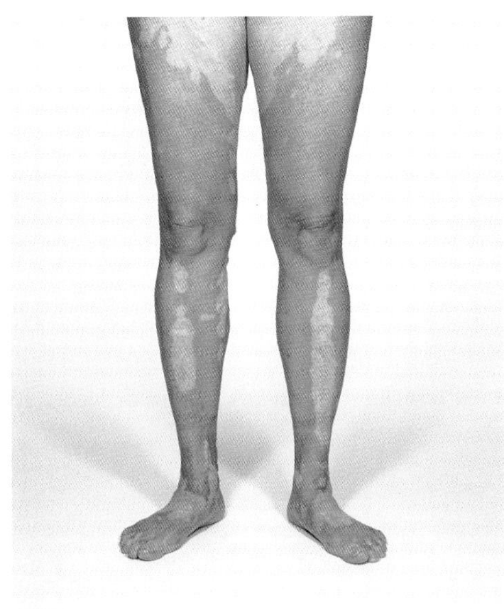

Fig. 54 Vitiligo—note the remarkable symmetry that is often a feature of this condition.

2.17 Vitiligo

Aetiology/pathophysiology/pathology

Vitiligo is believed to be an organ-specific autoimmune disease. There is selective loss of melanocytes within lesions and an infiltrate of T cells at the margins.

Epidemiology

Vitiligo is common and affects all races (0.5–1% worldwide prevalence). Thirty to forty percent of cases have a positive family history. In 50%, the onset is before 20 years of age.

Clinical presentation

Common

Depigmented macules, i.e. complete pigment loss, but the skin is otherwise normal. Often symmetrical, with a predilection for sun-exposed sites and sites of trauma (Koebner phenomenon). (Figs 38, p. 187, and 54).

Uncommon

Rapidly progressive and inflammatory in 1% of cases. There is a rare, restricted, segmental form that is not associated with autoimmune disease.

Investigation

Usually none. Some exclude associated autoimmune diseases.

Differential diagnosis

Post-inflammatory hypopigmentation and pityriasis versicolor, but pigment loss is usually only partial in these.

Treatments

Unsatisfactory.
- Camouflage can be used on visible areas.
- Sun-exposed patches should be protected with sunscreen.
- If severe, consider ultraviolet light or potent topical steroids.

Complications

Cutaneous malignancy in sun-exposed sites that have lost protective melanocytes.

Prognosis

Slowly progressive in most cases. Ten to twenty percent of cases show spontaneous repigmentation.

Disease associations

Autoimmune diseases, particularly thyroid disease, pernicious anaemia, diabetes mellitus and alopecia areata.

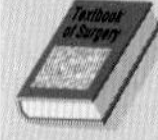

Bleehen SS. Vitiligo. In: Champion R, Burton J, Burns A, Breathnach S (eds) *Textbook of Dermatology* (6th edn). Oxford: Blackwell Science, 1998.

2.18 Pyoderma gangrenosum

Aetiology/pathophysiology/pathology

The aetiology is unknown, but there are numerous disease associations (Table 17). Histology shows a neutrophil-rich dermal infiltrate with necrosis, thrombosis and abscess formation.

Table 17 Diseases associated with pyoderma gangrenosum.

System	Disease
Gastrointestinal	Ulcerative colitis Crohn's disease
Liver	Chronic active hepatitis Primary biliary cirrhosis Sclerosing cholangitis
Joints	Rheumatoid arthritis Seronegative arthropathies
Blood	Leukaemias Lymphomas Monoclonal gammopathies
Others, malignant	Carcinoma of colon, prostate, breast
Others, non-malignant	Behçet's disease At sites of trauma (Koebner phenomenon) Thyroid disease Diabetes mellitus Systemic vasculitis Immunological defects

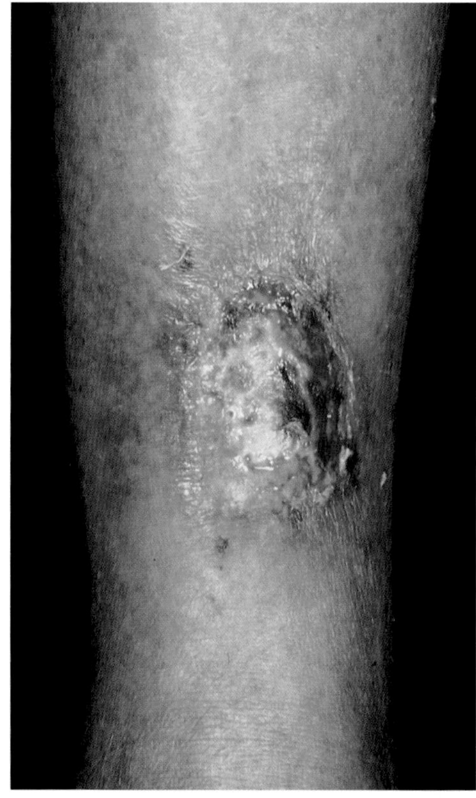

Fig. 55 Pyoderma gangrenosum. This ulcer on the shin was very painful, evolved rapidly and the medial border was overhanging. A swab was sterile. The patient had an underlying uterine carcinoma.

Epidemiology

Pyoderma gangrenosum (PG) is uncommon, but around 50% of cases are disease associated (Table 17).

Clinical presentation

Common

A very painful, erythematous nodule, commonly on the lower leg, which enlarges and ulcerates rapidly. The edge is typically irregular, blue/purple, raised and undermined with surrounding erythema (Fig. 55). Ulcers may be single or multiple and may be accompanied by high fever and malaise during the active phase.

Uncommon

Haemorrhagic, bullous, superficial and pustular forms. Peristomal PG.

PG should be considered whenever atypical ulcers are encountered, including surgical wounds that have broken down. Repeated surgical debridement can be avoided if the diagnosis is considered early.

Investigation

• Skin biopsy.
• Ulcer swab for microscopy and culture.
• Investigations to screen for associated diseases: Blood count and film, ESR, immunoglobulins and electrophoresis. Liver and thyroid function. Blood glucose. Rheumatoid factor. Further tests will depend on clinical suspicion.

Differential diagnosis

Infection, e.g. streptococcal, Clostridium, Behçet's disease, vasculitis, e.g. Wegener's granulomatosis, factitial.

Treatments

• High dose oral or intravenous steroids.
• Other systemic treatments may include sulphones, cytotoxics, cyclosporin. Minocycline is useful for subacute cases.
• Treat any underlying disease or secondary infection.

Complications

Usually related to any underlying disease. Also septicaemia and atrophic scars.

Prognosis

Variable but usually related to underlying disease.

Disease associations

See Table 17.

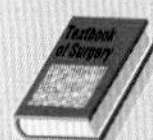
Ryan TJ. Pyoderma gangrenosum. In: Champion R, Burton J, Burns A, Breathnach S (eds) *Textbook of Dermatology* (6th edn). Oxford: Blackwell Science, 1998.

2.19 Cutaneous vasculitis

Aetiology/pathophysiology/pathology

Cutaneous vasculitis has numerous triggers, including:
• infections
• drugs
• malignancy
• some autoimmune conditions.

The underlying pathogenesis is thought to be vessel-wall damage triggered by immune complex deposition. Other contributing factors include stasis due to gravity or pressure, previous damage to vessel walls, blood viscosity and cold.

Biopsies show destruction and fibrinoid change of the vessel walls. The inflammatory infiltrate is predominantly neutrophils, which fragment to form 'nuclear dust'.

Epidemiology

Very common. Any age affected, men and women equally.

Clinical presentation

Common

• Palpable, purpuric (does not blanch on pressure) papules and plaques (Fig. 12, p. 171). Commonly on the lower legs and arms.
• Fever, arthralgia, malaise.

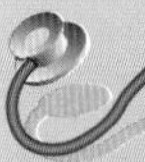
Extravasation of red cells into the dermis results in purpura. When due to platelet or coagulation abnormalities, this is non-palpable. However, purpura due to a vasculitis is usually palpable because of the associated perivascular inflammation.

Uncommon

• Nodules, haemorrhagic blisters and skin necrosis.
• Renal, pulmonary, gastrointestinal and central nervous system involvement.

Investigation

Skin biopsy to confirm vasculitis. Direct immunofluorescence will show perivascular IgA in the Henoch–Schoenlein purpura subtype.

Screening for visceral involvement

Renal function, liver function, blood pressure, urine dipstick for blood and microscopy for casts, chest X-ray.

Investigating the cause

• FBC (white count high if infection).
• ASO titre
• Blood cultures
• Throat swab
• Hepatitis serology
• ANA, ds DNA (to investigate possible lupus)

- ANCA
- VDRL
- Complement (Usually high. C4 low in cryoglobulinaemia.)
- Cryoglobulins
- Protein strip.

Differential diagnosis

Meningococcaemia, subacute bacterial endocarditis, DIC, viral haemorrhagic fevers, other vasculitides, e.g. PAN, Wegener's granulomatosis. In the context of thrombocytopaenia, many rashes may be purpuric.

Treatment

- Rest and elevation of the lower legs if affected.
- Treatment of any triggering infection or associated disease.
- Oral prednisolone if severe, acute vasculitis or systemic involvement. Adjuvant drugs, e.g. immunosuppressants, dapsone, may be required for chronic or recurrent disease.

Disease associations

Viral and bacterial infections, e.g. group A streptococcus, hepatitis B and C, drugs (see Section 2.6, p. 195), connective tissue diseases, e.g. lupus erythematosus, rheumatoid arthritis, Sjögren's syndrome, malignancies, cryoglobulinaemia, cryofibrinogenaemia, paraproteinaemia.

Prognosis

Cutaneous disease alone is largely benign, but multisystem disease may be life-threatening.

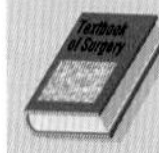

Ryan TJ. Cutaneous vasculitis. In: Champion R, Burton J, Burns A, Breathnach S (eds) *Textbook of Dermatology* (6th edn). Oxford: Blackwell Science, 1998.

2.20 Acanthosis nigricans

Aetiology/pathophysiology/pathology

In acanthosis nigricans (AN) epidermal proliferation is thought to occur due to stimulation of the keratinocyte insulin-like growth factor 1 receptor.

- Benign AN can be inherited, drug induced (e.g. nicotinic acid, oral contraceptive pill) or associated with various insulin resistance syndromes.
- Pseudoacanthosis nigricans is associated with obesity and is more common in racially pigmented skin.
- Malignant AN is usually associated with adenocarcinomas.

Clinical presentation

Common

Pigmented, thickened, papillomatous skin with a velvety texture commonly affecting the axillae, back of neck and groin (Fig. 41, p. 188).

Uncommon

- Other flexural sites and the umbilicus can be affected.
- Generalized forms exist (more common in malignant AN).
- Mucous membrane involvement (50% cases of malignant AN).
- Palmar involvement: 'tripe palms' (usually malignant AN).

Investigation

- Skin biopsy if there is any diagnostic uncertainty.
- Blood tests to investigate possible diabetes and insulin resistance syndromes.
- Look for underlying malignancy if suspected.

Treatment

None specific.

Prognosis

- Pseudo AN may improve with weight reduction and drug-induced AN will improve when the drug is stopped.
- Malignant AN may improve with removal of the underlying tumour.

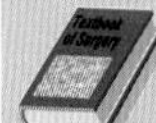

Griffiths WAD, Judge MR, Leigh IM. Disorders of Keratinization. In: Champion R, Burton J, Burns A, Breathnach S (eds) *Textbook of Dermatology* (6th edn). Oxford: Blackwell Science, 1998.

3 Investigations and practical procedures

3.1 Skin biopsy

Principle

To obtain a sample of skin for histological, immunohistochemical or microbiological analysis.

Indications

- Aid to diagnosis
- Tumour grading and staging
- Excision of cutaneous neoplasm.

Contra-indications

Relative contra-indications include:
- local anaesthetic hypersensitivity
- coagulation abnormalies
- sites of poor healing, e.g. lower leg
- high risk of keloid formation, e.g. upper trunk, black skin.

Practical details

Before procedure

Prepare your equipment

The basic equipment includes a sterile biopsy pack, suture material, local anaesthetic and dressing.

- An elliptical scalpel biopsy provides more information than a 3–4 mm punch biopsy and is the preferred method when possible.
- The choice of suture material depends on the site and size of the biopsy. In general, for a diagnostic biopsy of 0.5–1 cm a non-absorbable suture can be used: 5/0 for face and 4/0 elsewhere.
- Prepare a specimen tube for receipt of the sample. The choice of transport medium depends on the analysis; 10% formalin is most commonly used for routine histology, but must be avoided for immunofluorescence and microbiological analysis. Contact your local lab for their preferred transportation conditions.

Choice of anaesthetic

0.5–2% lignocaine ± epinephrine (adrenaline) is the most commonly used local anaesthetic. Epinephrine vasoconstricts, thus aids haemostasis and prolongs anaesthesia but must be avoided for the digits and penis where intense vasoconstriction can result in tissue necrosis.

Plan the procedure

- If possible, choose a covered site with a low risk of keloid formation and away from vital structures, e.g. the temporal artery (know your anatomy!).
- It can be helpful to include both normal and abnormal skin within the biopsy (ask a senior colleague because the optimum placement of the biopsy is disease dependant).
- Mark the site before anaesthetizing using a surgical marker.
- The wound should run parallel with natural skin tension lines.

Ask the patient whether they have a history of local anaesthetic allergy, latex allergy, bleeding tendency, poor healing or keloid scars and whether they take aspirin or warfarin.

Consent must be obtained from all patients with advice on the risk of scar formation (including keloids), infection and bleeding.

The procedure

1 Protective glasses and sterile gloves should be worn.
2 After preparing a sterile field, local anaesthetic is infiltrated into the subcutis.
3 The incision can be made with a scalpel or punch biopsy.
4 The sample should be carefully separated from underlying tissue (avoid crushing with forceps) and placed in an appropriately labelled container.
5 Sutures are usually needed to achieve haemostasis and good wound-margin apposition.
6 A sterile dressing is applied and sharps disposed of in an appropriate receptacle.

After procedure

- Give the patient wound-care instructions (leaflets are handy).
- The sutures are routinely removed in 5 days from the face; 7 days from the trunk and arms; and 10 days from the back and legs.

• The specimen should be transported and stored according to the recommendations of the local pathology or microbiology departments.

Clinical–pathological correlation is crucial when interpreting skin biopsies so give as much information as possible on your request form.

Complications

• Local anaesthetic or latex allergy can rarely result in anaphylaxis.
• Damage to underlying structures is possible.
• Less serious complications include bleeding, local infection or keloid scar formation.

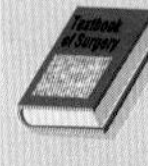

Cerio R. Histopathology of the skin: general principles. In: Champion R, Burton J, Burns A, Breathnach S (eds) *Textbook of Dermatology* (6th edn). Oxford: Blackwell Science, 1998.

3.2 Direct and indirect immunofluorescence

Principle

Most commonly used to detect antibodies and complement deposited in the skin *in vivo* (direct immunofluorescence, DIF) or serum antibodies that react with normal skin *in vitro* (indirect immunofluorescence, IIF).

Indications

• DIF—Diagnosis of diseases associated with immunoreactant deposition (Table 18).
• IIF—A less sensitive alternative to DIF in some diseases but allows measurement of antibody titre which can be helpful for disease monitoring.

Practical details

Before investigation

• DIF—take a skin biopsy (see Section 3.1, p. 211). Transport according to local guidelines (usually in Michel's medium or snap frozen in liquid nitrogen). A small punch biopsy will usually be sufficient. Lesional (affected) skin should be sampled in most diseases but normal, unaffected skin is better in immunobullous diseases because false negatives can be obtained if blistered (lesional) skin is sampled.
• IIF—Take serum.

Table 18 Diseases in which direct or indirect immunofluorescence may be helpful.

Disease	DIF findings	IIF findings
Pemphigus	Intercellular IgG + C3	± Intercellular IgG
Pemphigoid (all forms)	IgG + C3 along DEJ	± IgG along DEJ
Dermatitis herpetiformis	IgA + C3 in dermal papillae	Negative
SLE	IgG, M, A + C3 along DEJ	± ANA
DLE	IgG, M, A + C3 along DEJ	Negative
LP	Fibrinogen along DEJ	Negative
Porphyria cutanea tarda	± Perivascular IgG.	Negative
Vasculitis	Perivascular C3 and fibrin ± IgG, IgM (IgA in HSP)	Negative
Amyloid	Clumps of Ig in papillary dermis	Negative

ANA, antinuclear antibodies; DEJ, Dermo-epidermal junction; DIF, direct immunofluorescence; DLE, discoid lupus erythematosus; HSP, Henoch–Schönlein purpura; IIF, indirect immunofluorescence; LP, lichen planus; SLE, systemic lupus erythematosus.

The investigation

• DIF—Five sections of the patient's skin are incubated with fluorescein-labelled antibodies (Ab) to IgG, IgA, IgM, C3 and fibrinogen. After washing, Ab bound to sections is viewed with a fluorescence microscope.
• IIF—Patient's serum at several dilutions is incubated with sections of normal skin. After washing, steps are identical to DIF (anti-IgG or IgA only, according to the suspected disease). The result is expressed as the highest serum dilution at which Ab is detected, e.g. 1 in 100.

After investigation

The results are interpreted along with the clinical and pathological findings (Table 18). However, DIF is the gold standard investigation in immunobullous disorders (Fig. 56).

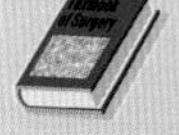

Bhogal BS, Black MM. Diagnosis, diagnostic and research techniques. In: *Management of Blistering Diseases* (Wojnorowska F, Briggaman RA, eds), London: Chapman and Hall Ltd, 1990: 15–34.

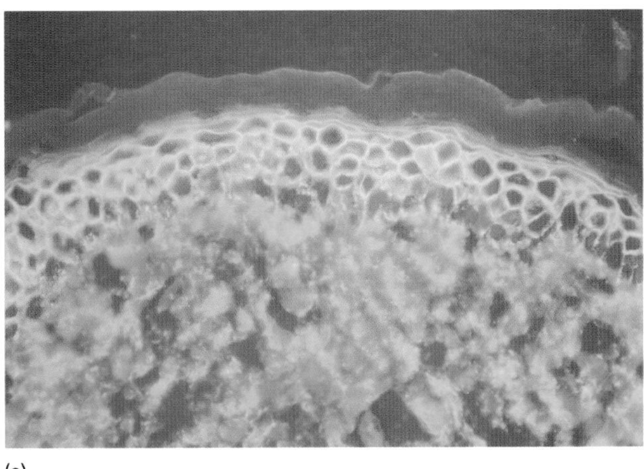

(a)

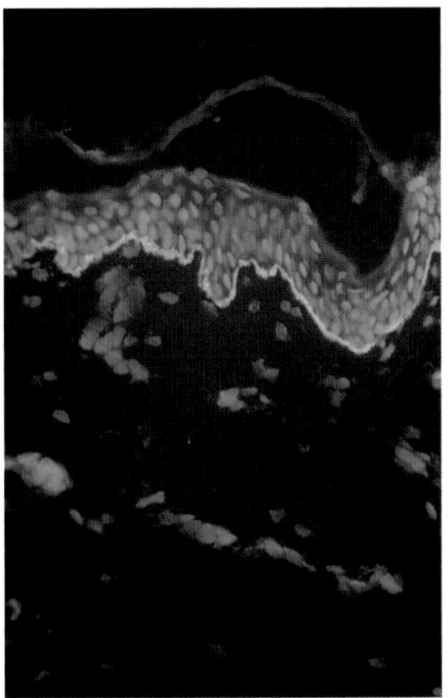

(b)

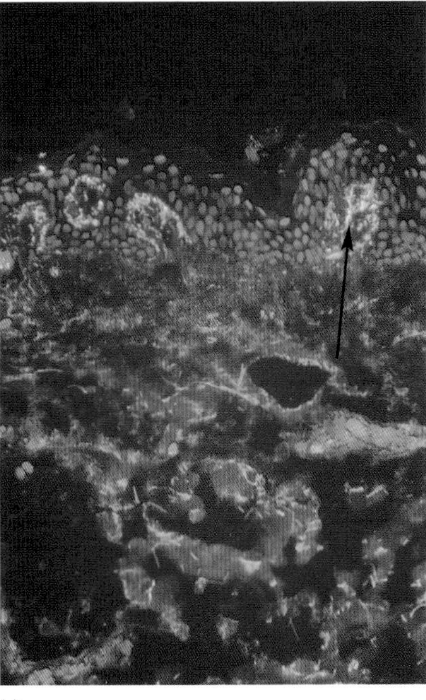

(c)

Fig. 56 Direct immunofluorescence. Antibodies in the skin fluoresce green. Cell nuclei have been counterstained red, allowing easy identification of the epidermis. D, dermis; E, epidermis. (a) Pemphigus vulgaris: IgG antibodies bind to the cell surface of keratinocytes and show up as fine green lines around cells in the epidermis. The overall appearance resembles a chicken wire fence. (b) Bullous pemphigoid: a green line runs beneath the epidermis due to binding of IgG at the dermo-epidermal junction. (c) Dermatitis herpetiformis: Granular deposits of IgA are present within the dermal papillae (arrow). (Courtesy of Professor M. Black, St. Thomas' Hospital.)

3.3 Patch testing

Principle

To identify substances that provoke a type 4 (delayed) allergy and may be the cause of an allergic contact dermatitis. Patients are tested against a standard battery of the most frequently encountered allergens. Additional series are available if relevant to the individual patient, e.g. hairdressing chemicals, plants, plastics.

Indications

Any patient suspected of having an allergic contact dermatitis (see Section 2.8, p. 197).

Contra-indications

Testing is unreliable if the patch test site (usually upper back) is not clear of eczema, or if the patient is taking oral steroids or other immunosuppressants.

Practical details

Before procedure

- Take a full history and examine the patient to elicit possible allergens. Ask specifically about allergens encountered at work and via hobbies.
- Minor complications are explained (see below) and the patient is asked to avoid disturbing the patches.

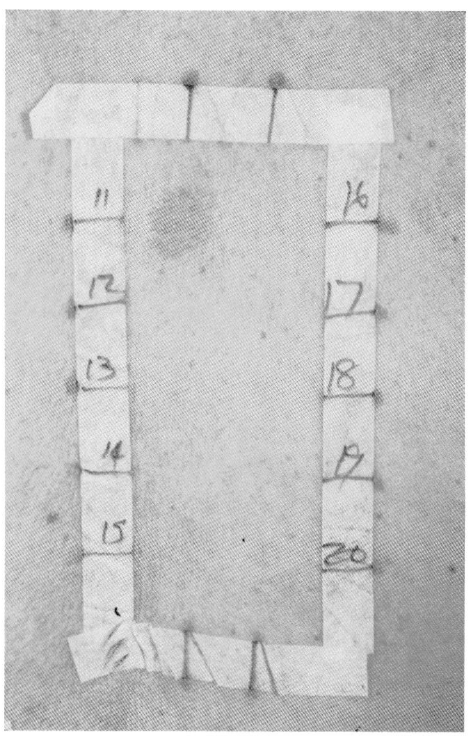

Fig. 57 Patch tests: a car mechanic presented with hand eczema. There is a positive reaction to patch 11 which is a preservative used in black rubber such as car tyres.

The procedure

• Allergens are usually purchased from manufacturers at specific concentrations in a petrolatum base. Small quantities are placed in chambers, usually small, aluminium 'finn' chambers, and secured to the upper back with hypoallergenic tape. The application sites are marked on the back and recorded in the notes.
• Patch tests are commonly 'read' after 2 days, when the patches are removed, and again after 4 days. Allergic reactions, which are erythematous, palpable and sometimes vesicular, are graded and recorded (Fig. 57).

After the procedure

The patch test results are interpreted with respect to the history and examination. Advice and leaflets on which substances to avoid are given to the patient.

Complications

• Major—Small risk of sensitizing the patient to a new allergen.
• Minor—Itching or postinflammatory hyper/hypopigmentation at the site of a positive reaction. Aggravation of eczema at distant sites due to percutaneous absorption of an antigen.

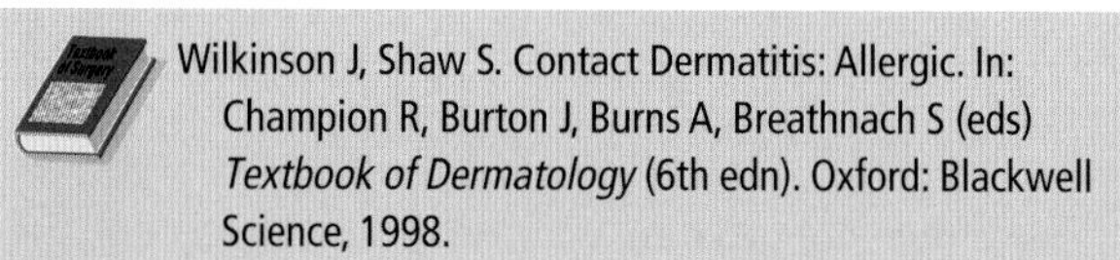

Wilkinson J, Shaw S. Contact Dermatitis: Allergic. In: Champion R, Burton J, Burns A, Breathnach S (eds) *Textbook of Dermatology* (6th edn). Oxford: Blackwell Science, 1998.

3.4 Topical therapy: corticosteroids

Principle

The skin lends itself to local delivery of therapy, which allows maximal concentration at the site of disease whilst minimizing systemic toxicity. Many medicaments are available in topical forms, e.g. corticosteroids, antibiotics, antihistamines, antifungals, retinoids. However, not all drugs can be applied topically because of poor epidermal penetration. The following notes will deal with corticosteroids (used very commonly in dermatological practice).

Indications

Eczema (all types), lichen planus, discoid lupus erythematosus, alopecia areata, lichen sclerosis, lichen simplex, keloid scars, vitiligo, psoriasis (particularly palmar–plantar and flexural varieties).

Contraindications

• Caution treating widespread plaque psoriasis.
• Infections, acne, rosacea.

Practical details

• Many topical steroids are available mainly in cream and ointment formulations.
• They are divided according to potency: Very potent, potent, moderate and mild (see the BNF).
• Initiate treatment with a steroid of adequate strength (disease dependant) for initial control then reduce the strength/frequency to the minimum for satisfactory disease control.
• Mild steroids only on face (very susceptible to side effects).
• Palms/soles need potent steroids as the skin is thick.
• Milder steroids used in children compared to adults.
• Ointments are greasy. Good if skin very dry.
• Creams are water based. They achieve better penetration than ointments if the skin is weepy. More cosmetically acceptable. Contain preservatives—risk of contact dermatitis.

Complications

• Local—Facial acne and steroid-rosacea, atrophy and fragility, easy bruising, telangiectasiae, striae, infections

(e.g. tinea incognito), contact dermatitis (especially creams), hypopigmentation.
• Systemic—Inhibition of pituitary/adrenal axis and other systemic effects due to absorption (if potent and used over large areas). Withdrawal of systemic or extensive topical steroids may precipitate erythrodermic or pustular psoriasis.

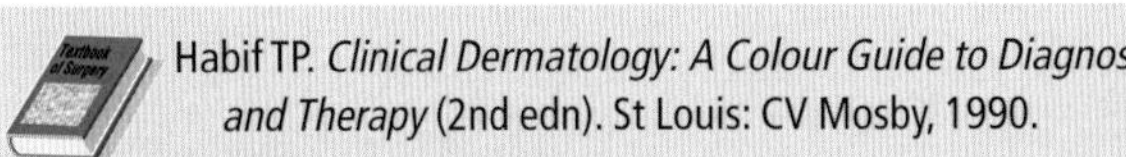

Habif TP. *Clinical Dermatology: A Colour Guide to Diagnosis and Therapy* (2nd edn). St Louis: CV Mosby, 1990.

3.5 Phototherapy

Principle

Phototherapy is the use of artificial ultraviolet (UV) radiation to treat skin diseases. UVB or psoralens with UVA (PUVA) are used for this purpose. Psoralens are photosensitizing drugs that enhance the effect of UVA. They are most commonly given orally but can be applied topically. Narrow-band UVB (TL01) covers a tighter wavelength range than conventional UVB and is more effective.

Indications

Clearance of dermatoses responsive to UV therapy, e.g. psoriasis, mycosis fungoides, atopic eczema or, less commonly, prevention of some photodermatoses, e.g. polymorphic light eruption.

Contra-indications

• Patients with a past history of excessive phototherapy and/or cutaneous malignancies.
• Light aggravated disease, e.g. systemic lupus erythematosus, porphyria.
• Use of PUVA in patients with renal or liver disease.

Practical details

Before procedure

• Choose the most appropriate phototherapy (narrow or broad-band UVB, topical or oral PUVA). This will depend on the patient, the disease and local facilities.
• Discuss possible complications/side effects.
• For oral PUVA, weigh the patient to calculate the psoralen dose.
• Assess the patient's sensitivity to phototherapy by phototesting to establish the starting UV dose.

The procedure

• For oral PUVA, patients must wear UVA protective glasses as soon as psoralens are swallowed and for the remaining daylight hours.
• Patients stand/lie inside the cabinets in which bulbs emit UV of specific wavelengths.
• The eyes, face and male genitalia are shielded.
• UVB is typically given three times a week and PUVA twice a week. Treatment times and UV doses are usually increased at each visit. The length of courses varies depending upon the response to treatment.

Complications

• Major—Increased risk of cutaneous malignancies with long-term use (particularly with PUVA).
• Minor—Burning, nausea with oral psoralens, photo-aging and PUVA freckling and PUVA itch/cutaneous pain.

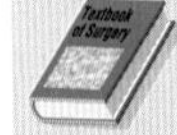

Camp RDR. Psoriasis. In: Champion R, Burton J, Burns A, Breathnach S (eds) *Textbook of Dermatology* (6th edn). Oxford: Blackwell Science, 1998.

3.6 Systemic retinoids

Principle

This term covers both synthetic and natural forms of vitamin A. The mode of action is unknown but there are effects on cell proliferation and differentiation. Specific receptors belong to the family of steroid-thyroid-vitamin D receptors.

Indications

• Severe recalcitrant acne
• Psoriasis
• Other disorders of keratinization, e.g. keratoderma, Darier's disease.

Contra-indications

• Absolute—pregnancy, renal disease, liver disease, breast feeding, dry eyes syndrome.
• Relative—concurrent tetracyclines or vitamin A supplements, hyperlipidaemia, diabetes, children, depression.

Practical details

Before treatment

- Fasting lipids, liver function tests.
- Exclude pregnancy (by laboratory test) and ensure effective contraception for at least 1 month prior to starting treatment.
- Some also check full blood count and urinalysis prior to starting treatment.

The treatment

- Isotretinoin is used for at least 16 weeks for acne. Dose schedules are debated but some use 0.5 mg/kg/day for first few weeks and then increase to 1 mg/kg/day depending on response.
- Acitretin is used for psoriasis and disorders of keratinization. Treatment tends to be prolonged with a dose in the range 10–50 mg/day.

For both isotretinoin and acitretin, fasting lipids and liver function tests are performed 1 month after starting treatment and then at intervals of 3 months. Investigate any atypical musculoskeletal symptoms and perform regular radiographic assessment in those on long-term therapy.

After treatment

- Avoid pregnancy for 2 years (acitretin) or 1 month (isotretinoin) after stopping treatment.
- Avoid giving blood for 1 year (acitretin) or 1 month (isotretinoin) after stopping treatment.

Outcome

- Sixteen weeks of isotretinoin produces dramatic sustained improvement in acne for the majority of patients.
- In those with psoriasis or chronic disorders of keratinization the effects are usually to offer suppression of symptoms rather than cure.

Complications

There are several potential complications but the most important are: teratogenicity; depression; derangement of plasma lipids and liver function tests; initial worsening of acne.

Important information for patients

Side effects should be explained. Common side effects are: rough, dry mucous membranes; dry eyes; myalgia; arthralgia. Less common but important side effects include: teratogenicity; worsening of acne; benign intracranial hypertension; diffuse thinning of hair; photosensitivity; diffuse interstitial skeletal hyperostosis; depression; disturbances of lipids and liver function tests.

Strong emphasis should be placed on the risk of teratogenicity and females should sign a consent form indicating that they understand the risks and the importance of effective contraception for 1 month prior to treatment, during treatment and for 2 years (acitretin) or 1 month (isotretinoin) after stopping treatment.

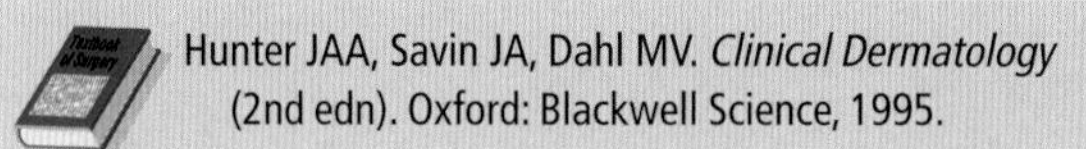

Hunter JAA, Savin JA, Dahl MV. *Clinical Dermatology* (2nd edn). Oxford: Blackwell Science, 1995.

Acknowledgements

The senior editor would like to thank Dr A Du Vivier, Dr E Higgins, Dr C Fuller and Dr JD Creamer for helpful advice in the selection of photographs for this section which are reproduced with kind permission of King's College Hospital, London.

4 Self-assessment

Answers are on pp. 227–229.

Question 1

Figure 58 shows a 24-year-old woman who developed an acute papular rash on her trunk and proximal limbs. She was not unwell or feverish, but had suffered from a sore throat one week previously. On close inspection, the surface of the red papules was scaly. What is the likely diagnosis?

A chickenpox
B eczema herpeticum
C psoriasis
D pemphigoid
E pemphigus

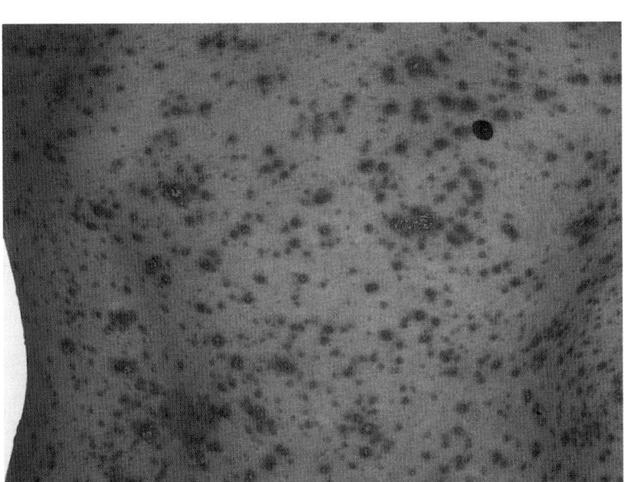

Fig. 58 Question 1.

Question 2

Figure 59 shows a 19-year-old woman who developed a rash on her abdomen. What is the likely diagnosis?

A erythema multiforme
B psoriasis
C irritant contact dermatitis
D allergic contact dermatitis
E atopic eczema

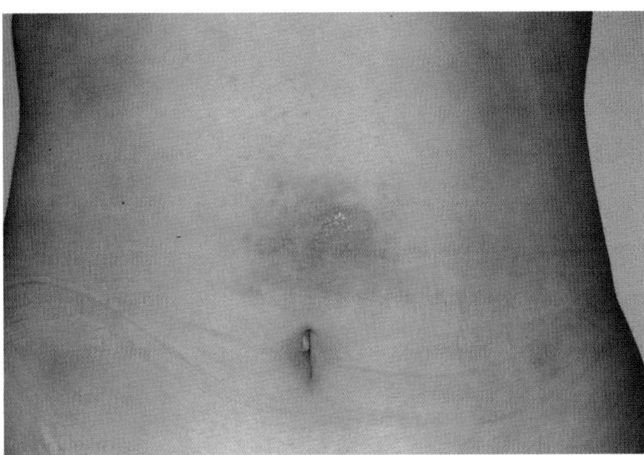

Fig. 59 Question 2.

Question 3

A 64-year-old man developed a scaly, itchy rash on his face and hands (see Figure 60). What is the likely diagnosis?

A psoriasis
B systemic lupus erythematosus
C irritant contact dermatitis
D allergic contact dermatitis
E photosensitive eczema

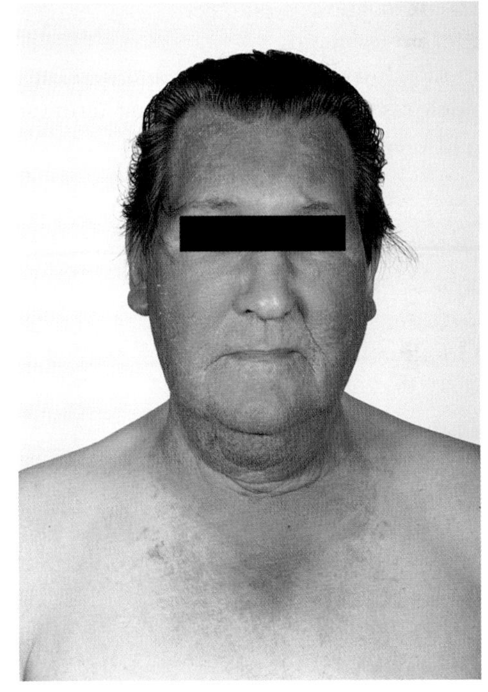

Fig. 60 Question 3.

Question 4

A 48-year-old man developed a chronic rash on his forehead, nose, cheeks and chin (see Figure 61). What is the likely diagnosis?

A rosacea
B acne
C atopic eczema

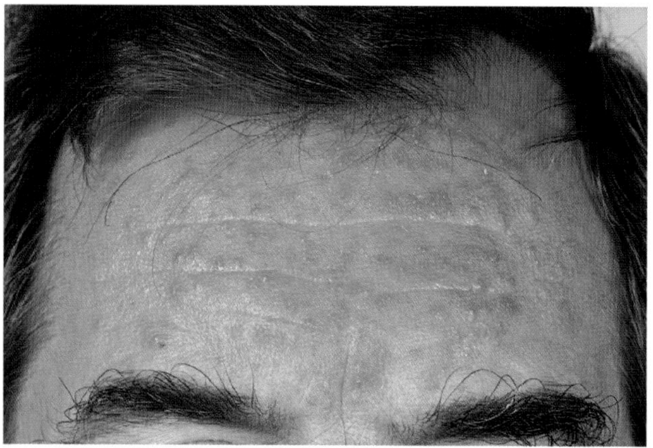

Fig. 61 Question 4.

D dermatomyositis
E photosensitive eczema

Question 5

A 20-year-old trainee hairdresser develops an intensely itchy, erythematous scaly rash on her hands. The two most common diagnoses would be:

A irritant hand dermatitis
B contact allergic dermatitis
C psoriasis
D lichen planus
E urticaria
F porphyria
G mycosis fungoides
H erythema multiforme
I bullous pemphigoid
J hand, foot and mouth disease

Question 6

A 28-year-old woman presents with painful lumps on her legs (see Figure 62). What are the two most likely diagnoses?

A Sezary syndrome
B erythema nodosum
C nodular vasculitis
D necrobiosis lipoidica
E mycosis fungoides
F discoid lupus erythematosus
G contact dermatitis
H pre-tibial myxoedema
I insect bites
J psoriasis

Question 7

A 40-year-old Indian man presents with mouth ulcers, a sore penis and ulcers on the skin. Which would be the two most helpful investigations in reaching a diagnosis?

A patch tests
B direct immunofluorescence

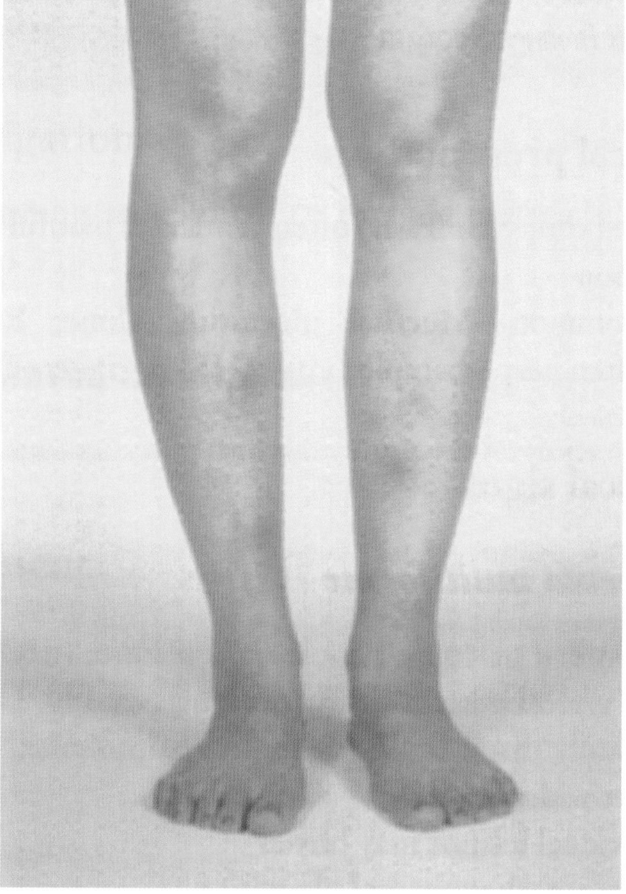

Fig. 62 Question 6.

C pathergy test
D autoantibody screen
E skin prick tests
F skin biopsy
G skin scrapings
H skin swab
I Tzanck smear
J IgE level

Question 8

A 28-year-old man presents with a 3-month history of the daily development of itchy erythematous weals each of which lasts several hours and then resolve without scaling. Which two of the following statements are true of chronic urticaria?

A with a careful history, it is possible to identify the trigger in virtually all cases
B it is thought to be predominantly IgE-mediated
C it is associated with internal malignancy
D it can be associated with systemic lupus erythematous (SLE)
E vasculitic changes are often seen on biopsy
F H1-antagonists provide an important therapeutic option
G H2-antagonists have no significant role in therapy
H most patients have disease lasting longer than 10 years

I essential investigations would include a chest radiograph
J non-steroidal anti-inflammatory drugs are often useful therapeutically

Question 9

A 60-year-old woman with rheumatoid arthritis presents with a rapidly enlarging, painful, sloughy leg ulcer on the anterior shin. Doppler examination is normal. There has been no improvement with dressings and bandages. What would be the most appropriate next step in management?
A referral to surgeons for debridement
B referral to surgeons for grafting
C maggot therapy
D compression
E immunosupression

Question 10

A 50-year-old man presents with hair loss. Examination reveals patches of scarring alopecia with surrounding inflammation. Which is the most likely diagnosis?
A lichen planopilaris
B androgenetic alopecia
C alopecia areata
D traction alopecia
E trichotillomania

Question 11

A 16-year-old girl presents with an itchy rash 3 days after arriving on holiday in the Mediterranean. Examination reveals an erythematous papular rash over the arms and trunk, sparing sites under her swimming costume and sparing her face and hands. What is the most likely diagnosis?
A systemic lupus erythematosus
B polymorphic light eruption
C photoallergic contact dermatitis
D scabies
E xeroderma pigmentosum

Question 12

A 30-year-old woman presents with a 5-year history of flushing of her facial skin and a spotty rash. Examination reveals a pustular rash on the cheeks with no comedones. What is the most likely diagnosis?
A rosacea
B acne vulgaris
C carcinoid syndrome
D systemic lupus erythematosus (SLE)
E allergic contact dermatitis

Question 13

A 17-year-old girl has developed an eczematous patch just below her umbilicus, thought to be due to allergy to a stud fastener in her jeans. Which one of the following statements is true regarding allergic contact dermatitis to nickel?
A it is diagnosed by prick testing
B it is a type 3 allergic reaction
C it affects males and females equally
D it occurs more commonly in atopic patients
E it can be caused by wearing gold jewellery

Question 14

A 60-year-old cleaner presents with a rash on both hands. An irritant hand dermatitis is suspected. Which one of the following statements is true regarding this condition?
A it classically causes a finger tip dermatitis
B it is diagnosed by patch testing
C it is more common in atopic patients
D it can be differentiated from allergic contact dermatitis histologically
E it should not be treated with topical steroids

Question 15

A 58-year-old man presents with a scaly rash. You consider the diagnosis of psoriasis. Which one of the following statements is true of this condition?
A psoriasis shows the Koebner phenomenon
B nail involvement in psoriasis is rare
C guttate psoriasis is the commonest form
D sterile pustules are frequently seen within lesions
E intense pruritus is a typical symptom

Answers to Self-assessment

Infectious diseases

Answer to Question 1

A

Figure 101 shows suppurative lymphadenitis caused by atypical mycobacterial infection.

The appearance of this problem 4 weeks after starting anti-retroviral treatment is an immune reconstitution phenomenon, when previously subclinical opportunistic infection—commonly TB or CMV—becomes apparent as a result of improvement in immune function.

Anti-retroviral treatment can usually be continued, but sometimes steroids are given to damp down the inflammatory response.

Answer to Question 2

B

The patient has extensive warts caused by papilloma virus. Disease of the extent shown would be most unusual in an immunocompetent host and suggests cell-mediated immunodeficiency.

Papilloma viruses are oncogenic and associated with genital and cutaneous squamous cell carcinomas. There is no specific antiviral therapy: treatment in this case will be by prolonged topical therapy, e.g. podophyllin preparations or cryotherapy, also probably by reduction in immunosuppression dosage.

Answer to Question 3

C

The most likely cause is an amoebic liver abscess, with a pyogenic abscess next on the list of differential diagnoses.

A specific serological test, e.g. immunofluorescent antibody test (IFAT), would be positive in 90% of cases, and cysts may be visible in the stool of 20–30%, but diagnostic/therapeutic aspiration may be needed to exclude pyogenic disease.

Metronidazole is used for acute treatment and diloxanide furoate to eradicate cysts in the bowel lumen.

Answer to Question 4

D

The blood film shows Howell-Jolly bodies, indicating hyposplenism. Patients without a functioning spleen are at particular risk from encapsulated bacteria and pneumococcal sepsis is the most likely diagnosis in this case. His illness could have been prevented by prophylactic penicillin.

Answer to Question 5

E

Figure 105 shows a precipitate of cryoglobulins revealed after blood is taken and kept warm until clotted, centrifuged and the serum removed and stored at 4°C. The cryoprecipitate has settled at the bottom of the tube.

Cryoglobulins are found in some lymphoproliferative disorders, autoimmune diseases and infections, the latter including EBV, hepatitis B and C, and mycoplasma. Hepatitis C causes mixed essential cryoglobulinaemia and can present with the nephrotic syndrome, making this the most likely diagnosis in this case.

Answer to Question 6

E

Figure 106 shows conjunctivitis, most likely due to adenoviral infection in this clinical context.

Herpes simplex can also cause conjunctivitis, and fluorescein instillation is essential to look for ulceration if this is suspected. Possible bacterial causes include *Haemophilus* spp, staphylococci and rarely *Neisseria* spp, but these do not fit well with the clinical scenario in this case.

Answer to Question 7

D

Figure 107 shows Gram-positive rods due to *Clostridium perfringens* causing gas gangrene.

Extensive surgical debridement of all necrotic tissue is essential, along with treatment with high-dose intravenous benzylpenicillin.

Answer to Question 8

C

The patient has had a thoracoplasty where the upper ribs on the left side have been removed to compress the chest cavity to treat pulmonary tuberculosis in the pre-antibiotic era. This was successful in many cases, but often produced a severe kyphoscoliosis, as seen here.

Answer to Question 9

A, B

The differential diagnosis is wide in this context. In this early stage, before a precise diagnosis has been made, he needs good broad-spectrum antibiotics aimed at covering immediate life-threatening infections such as meningococcal, pneumococcal or gram-negative sepsis. Drug, mode of delivery and dosing should allow adequate CSF penetration in the event that he has meningitis. Given his age and predisposing haematological condition listeria must be considered, hence ampicillin should be given in addition to a broad-spectrum agent such as ceftriaxone. The addition of aciclovir whilst awaiting PCR on CSF is not inappropriate but this should be administered intravenously.

Answer to Question 10

C, D

This would be a typical picture of a Gram negative or *Staphylococcus aureus* bacteraemia complicating surgical instrumentation. Often there is no immediate febrile response. The antibiotic regimen selected should have good Gram-negative cover and also activity against MRSA given his screening result. Other causes of acute post-operative deterioration, e.g. myocardial infarction, must be excluded and standard resuscitation performed.

Answer to Question 11

C, I

This woman has several pointers to potentially severe malarial disease – she is drowsy, jaundiced and pregnant.

Even when patients have severe cerebral malaria, CT seldom adds anything to diagnosis, and jaundice is common in malaria due to red-cell breakdown. Low platelets are almost invariable in this condition and require no treatment unless a patient is bleeding. Prophylactic antibiotics and phenobarbitone are seldom helpful, even in severe cases. Steroids are actively unhelpful. Exchange transfusion should only be contemplated in those with very high peripheral parasite loads (10% would be a minimum, usually more – always ask for specialist advice).

The key to managing malaria is an appropriate antimalarial given early, and this takes priority over all else. In potentially severe cases this should always be parenteral and as she has low platelets, intravenous is preferable to intramuscular. Hypoglycaemia is a common complication in severe malaria, especially in pregnant women, and those who are drowsy should have their glucose measured repeatedly.

Answer to Question 12

C, J

British Thoracic Society guidelines for the treatment of severe community-acquired pneumonia suggest parenteral treatment with a second- or third-generation cephalosporin, with high dose parenteral erythromycin in suspected Legionnaire's disease, which proved to be the diagnosis in this case.

Answer to Question 13

G, H

The most likely diagnosis is gas gangrene with clostridial infection. Bacteraemia complicates about 15% of patients with gas gangrene. Treatment includes emergency surgical exploration and debridement. The combination of intravenous penicillin and clindamycin is a widely used treatment once the diagnosis has been confirmed.

Further information should be obtained about the nature of this man's job. Though less likely, anthrax is also a possibility. Cases have been reported in postal workers in the USA and those who work with contaminated hides and leather. Intravenous ciprofloxacin is the recommended antibiotic, though mortality at this stage of infection is high.

Answer to Question 14

E, G

The fluid levels within cavities are due to lung abscesses. In an intravenous drug user, *Staphylococcus aureus* would be the most likely aetiological agent and was grown from this patient. *Klebsiella pneumoniae* is another common cause of lung abscess. Other bacteria are less likely causes of lung abscesses.

Answer to Question 15

C, H

The clinical picture can be explained by a diagnosis of right-sided endocarditis with secondary septic pulmonary emboli. The Gram stain shows a candidal species. Candidal endocarditis is seen in the intravenous drug using population where the organism is inadvertently introduced as a contaminant of the intravenous cocktail.

Answer to Question 16

E, I

This presentation is typical of depression. HIV encephalopathy may present with neuropsychiatric manifestations, focal neurology or dementia. Cerebral atrophy is usually present but is also common in patients with advanced HIV disease without clinical evidence of neurological involvement. MRI scans may show areas of increased signal but can also be normal. There is a substantial increase in psychiatric morbidity in patients with HIV/AIDS and acute psychiatric illness may be precipitated by a new HIV diagnosis.

Answer to Question 17

D, E

The clinical picture suggests an acute glandular fever-like viral illness. Epstein-Barr virus (EBV) and cytomegalovirus (CMV) would both need to be considered and a likely diagnosis of EBV can be quickly established by the Paul–Bunnell test. Acute CMV infection is confirmed by detection of anti-CMV IgM (not IgG). HIV seroconversion is also likely: HIV antibody is often negative early during seroconversion and the diagnosis can be established by measuring p24 antigen or detection of high level viraemia with PCR. Acute hepatitis B would need to be considered but acute hepatitis C is subclinical. Syphilis and disseminated gonorrhoea should be considered in any sexually active person presenting with fever and rash, but in this patient an acute viral infection is suggested by the reactive lymphocytosis.

Answer to Question 18

A

Primary HBV infection in susceptible hosts can either be symptomatic or asymptomatic, the latter being commoner. Most primary infections in adults are self-limiting, but 5% do not resolve and develop into persistent infection. Asymptomatic chronic HBV carriers have normal aminotransferase levels and normal or near normal liver biopsies. Patients with chronic hepatitis B have abnormal liver function tests and histological abnormalities on liver biopsy. Cirrhosis will develop in about 20% of patients with chronic hepatitis B.

Answer to Question 19

B

There are two forms of necrotising fasciitis. Type 1 is a mixed infection of anaerobes plus facultative species such as streptococci or enterobacteriacae. It is characterised by an acute, rapidly developing infection of deep fascia, marked pain, tenderness, swelling and often crepitus with bullae and necrosis of underlying skin. Type 2 is infection with group A streptococci and is characterised by acute infection often accompanied by toxic shock, rapid progression of oedema to bullae, and necrosis of subcutaneous tissue. There is no crepitus in this form of the condition.

MRI is useful in distinguishing cellulitis from necrotising fasciitis with a 100% sensitivity and 88% specificity, but wait for this test should not delay surgical exploration for a definitive diagnosis and treatment, although the prognosis is bleak.

Answer to Question 20

A

Other than rickettsial infection, which usually presents with a localised lymphadenopathy +/– eschar and rash and normal white blood count, all the other conditions listed can be associated with peripheral neutrophilia. Malaria is rarely associated with raised neutrophils but should always be excluded in travellers returning from endemic areas. Amoebic liver abscess is associated with neutrophilia and not eosinophilia. Always remember that many travellers with fever will have cosmopolitan rather than exotic causes for their illness, but a careful history and examination should be undertaken to exclude the exotic causes.

Answer to Question 21

C

Schistosomiasis is not endemic in the Indian subcontinent, although it would be a cause of this presentation elsewhere in the tropics. Heavy worm loads with *Trichuris* can cause bloody diarrhoea. Cosmopolitan causes of bloody diarrhoea should always be considered as a cause despite the travel history and *C. difficile* disease excluded when antibiotics have been taken.

Answer to Question 22

E

Important organisms to consider in this context are resistant gram negative rods, including pseudomonas. The only drug with such cover in this list is tazocin, but other anti-pseudomonal regimens may be suitable. Benzylpenicillin and cefuroxime cover community-acquired pneumonias but have weaker gram negative cover.

Answer to Question 23

B

VREs are an emerging problem in hospitals, where extensive glycopeptide use may select for resistant strains. Some are teicoplanin sensitive. The new agents linezolid and quinupristin with dalfopristin (Synercid) may be active. Co-trimoxazole (Septrin) is active against some highly resistant gram negative bacteria such as *Stenotrophomonas maltophilia*.

Answer to Question 24

C

MRSA is resistant to beta-lactam antibiotics. Glycopeptides such as vancomycin are commonly used. An alternative is teicoplanin. Other drugs such as gentamicin, rifampicin and doxycycline may be active.

Answer to Question 25

A

Polyoma virus BK is associated with interstitial nephritis, can cause fever and haematuria, but more commonly presents with impairment of transplant function (rising creatinine). Reduction of immunosuppression can reduce viral replication. The other viruses listed can reactivate during immunosuppression but do not cause haematuria. Cytomegalovirus (CMV) primary infection or reactivation is the most common and most feared infective complication in the early post transplant period.

Answer to Question 26

C

Aciclovir is safe in pregnancy and chickenpox is dangerous. Steroids exacerbate chickenpox. The immunosuppression of pregnancy puts the mother as well as the fetus at risk. In early pregnancy there is a risk of fetal abnormalities (about 2%). At this late stage the main danger is that a new born child would become infected with no transfer of antibody from the mother. In that case varicella-zoster immune globulin should be given to the child, but it has no role in therapy of the mother.

Answer to Question 27

D

Pseudomonas species are very common causes of nosocomial pneumonia on the ICU. *Strep pneumoniae* is a very common cause of community-acquired pneumonia. Staphylococcal disease due to methicillin-resistant *S. aureus* (MRSA) or methicillin-susceptible *S. aureus* (MSSA) is also reasonably common. *Legionella* is usually community-acquired and can lead to ICU admission, but is now an uncommon nosocomial infection.

Answer to Question 28

B

Erythema multiforme is a common complication of genital herpes infection. The target-like lesions appear either as the genital lesion is evolving or soon after. Attacks can be controlled with continuous oral aciclovir to prevent HSV reactivation, but aciclovir has no effect on the erythema multiforme during an acute attack.

Answer to Question 29

D

Sexually transmitted infections (STI) are unlikely with this history. Toxic shock syndrome is associated with retained tampons and can present with fevers, hypotension and rash. Unless diagnosed early patients may deteriorate rapidly and fatalities have been reported. Removal of the foreign body should be accompanied by antibiotic therapy regardless of the risk for STI.

Answer to Question 30

D

Patients often report as allergies side effects of a drug that are not related to allergic phenomenon. These commonly include nausea, diarrhoea and headache. If a patient reports a drug allergy you should always determine what the allergy was, how severe it was, and who diagnosed and/or documented it. Erythromycin is well known to cause nausea and gastrointestinal symptoms as a side effect.

Clinical manifestations of drug reactions	Onset
Anaphylaxis, urticaria	0–24 hours
Haemolytic anaemia, neutropenia, thrombocytopenia	>72 hours
Drug fever, serum sickness	7–14 days
Contact dermatitis	Variable
Rash, fixed drug reactions	>7–14 days

Answer to Question 31

D

The combination of long history, focal signs, very high protein, low glucose and a lymphocytic CSF make a diagnosis of tuberculous meningitis the most likely. The diagnosis of neurosyphilis cannot be made without a positive serum specific treponemal antibody (TPHA); the positive VDRL is a biological false positive.

Answer to Question 32

D

Penicillin allergy is reported after 0.7–4% of courses of the drug, with anaphylaxis reported following 1/32 000 to 1/100 000 courses.

Standard treatment of severe community-acquired pneumonia would involve parenteral administration of a second or third-generation cephalosporin (e.g. cefotaxime) and a macrolide (e.g. erythromycin). Patients with penicillin allergy often tolerate cephalosporins, but there is a 5–10% chance of cross-reactivity. If the previous reaction to penicillin were simply a rash you should not be dissuaded from giving a cephalosporin if there is good indication, and option A would be appropriate in this case. However, with a history of anaphylactic reaction this would clearly NOT be the correct treatment in this case and high dose intravenous erythromycin would be the treatment to use.

Answer to Question 33

C

Infective endocarditis is the only diagnosis that would explain all of the symptoms and investigative findings. Vertebral osteomyelitis/discitis and stroke are both recognised complications of infective endocarditis and either can be the presenting feature of the disease.

Answer to Question 34

C

The British Thoracic Society has published guidelines for assessment and management of adult community-acquired pneumonia. Adverse prognostic features include:

- Pre-existing factors: age > 50 years; co-existing disease
- Core clinical adverse prognostic features (CURB criteria): confusional state; urea > 7 mmol/l; respiratory rate > 30/min; systolic BP < 90 mmHg and/or diastolic BP < 60 mmHg.
- Additional features: hypoxaemia, SaO_2 < 92% or PaO_2 < 8 kPa; bilateral/multi-lobe disease.

Patients with two or more core features are at high risk of death and should be managed as severe pneumonia in hospital.

Answer to Question 35

A

The persistence of fever, timing and description of the lesions fits best with disseminated yeast infection, most likely *Candida* species. The diagnosis can usually be made on blood cultures, but the organisms can also be seen in the lesions on biopsy. Do not forget to look in the fundi in such cases. The presentation is too early for graft versus host disease.

Answer to Question 36

E

The presentation with fever, diarrhoea, shock and a macular rash are characteristic of staphylococcal toxic shock syndrome due to focal infection with a toxin-producing strain of *S. aureus*. Confusion, breathlessness (due to metabolic acidosis) and oliguria are commonly present. The toxin acts as a superantigen bypassing the normal antigen-restricted pathway of T-cell activation and leading to widespread cytokine release shock and organ failure. Approximately 50% of cases occur in young women due to vaginal infection with *S. aureus* at the time of menstruation. A retained vaginal tampon increases the risk and should be looked for in this type of presentation. A similar syndrome may also be seen with toxin producing streptococci.

Answer to Question 37

C

Tetanus and strychnine poisoning both produce muscle spasm that may lead to respiratory failure, but they do not cause muscle weakness. Rabies produces a uniformly fatal encephalitis characterised by pharyngeal spasm triggered by water. Diphtheria presents with a pharyngitis and a membrane over the tonsils: the toxin may cause myocarditis and neurotoxicity with palatal paralysis and cranial nerve palsies. Botulism typically produces a descending paralysis which starts with diplopia or blurred vision (due to difficulty with accommodation) and progresses to weakness of the neck, arms and respiratory muscles.

Answer to Question 38

C

Pneumococcus remains the commonest cause of community-acquired pneumonia. In giving empirical treatment you would want to cover for the possibility of Legionella and other atypicals (by giving clarithromycin or erythromycin), but these would be a less likely cause of this man's illness.

Answer to Question 39

D

The undetectable HIV viral load implies that the patient is receiving therapy. The blood tests point to a partially compensated metabolic acidosis with abnormal liver function tests. This syndrome is seen with nucleoside reverse transcriptase inhibitors (AZT group of drugs) and is thought to result from inhibition of mitochondrial DNA. In addition to lactic acidosis, most patients have fatty infiltration of the liver with a cholestatic pattern of liver enzymes. The initial clinical presentation is often non-specific with vague abdominal pain and bloating. Alternative diagnostic possibilities include bacterial sepsis and poisoning from salicylate or methanol, but there is nothing else to suggest these in this case.

Lactic acidosis is one of the most feared adverse effects of anti-HIV therapy and may be fatal if not recognised promptly. Most patients gradually improve after withdrawal of anti-retroviral therapy, in severe cases haemofiltration may be required to control acidosis.

Answer to Question 40

D

This is the typical presentation of someone with dengue fever, which has an incubation period of 5 to 8 days. Both malaria (usually falciparum in Thailand) and typhoid would have to be excluded. The diagnosis of dengue is confirmed serologically.

Dermatology

Answer to Question 1

C

The appearances are those of guttate psoriasis. This is often triggered by a streptococcal throat infection and presents as an acute shower of small (<1 cm) plaques ('rain drops') over the trunk and limbs.

Guttate psoriasis can be confused with pityriasis rosea or secondary syphilis, but the clinical context in this case is typical of guttate psoriasis.

Answer to Question 2

D

This is allergic contact dermatitis to nickel, caused in this typical case by contact with the stud fastener of a pair of jeans.

Answer to Question 3

E

The V-shaped cut off at the neck is absolutely typical of a photo-induced rash. The patient had been prescribed a thiazide diuretic in the autumn, but the rash did not appear until the following spring when he began spending time outdoors gardening.

Answer to Question 4

A

Rosacea causes erythematous papules and scattered pustules on the convex surfaces of the face, including the forehead as shown here. Telangiectasiae are a common feature. By contrast with acne, comedones are absent. There is no rash on the body.

Answer to Question 5

A, B

Although many of the diagnoses listed above can affect the hands, the commonest diagnoses in this setting would be an irritant hand dermatitis or a contact allergic dermatitis. Possible precipitants for the latter could include rubber (including latex), hair-dye and nickel. It would be important to undertake patch testing to a wide range of potential contact allergens in order to identify the precipitant and advise on her future career.

Answer to Question 6

B, I

This is a typical case of erythema nodosum, but insect bites can give a similar picture, as can nodular vasculitis, which is much rarer. Erythema nodosum can be caused by a variety of infections (streptococci, tuberculosis, yersinia, chlamydia, Epstein-Barr virus, *Trichophyton*, coccidiomycosis), drugs (sulphonamides, oral contraceptives), as well as other conditions such as sarcoidosis, Crohn's disease, ulcerative colitis, Behçet's disease and malignancy.

Answer to Question 7

B, F

Oral and genital ulceration may be part of Behçet's disease, for which a pathergy test is helpful, but cutaneous ulcers makes this diagnosis unlikely. Skin scrapings, which are generally sent for mycology and thus for diagnosis of fungal infections, would not be helpful. The history is not suggestive of an allergic contact dermatitis or atopic dermatitis so investigations such as patch tests, skin prick tests and IgE levels would not be helpful.

Ulceration of the skin, genitalia and mouth can occur in autoimmune blistering diseases such as pemphigus vulgaris (PV). The patient is the right age and ethnic group for PV that tends to present more commonly in the 3rd–6th decades and in Jewish and Indian patients. A skin biopsy for routine histology is a useful investigation, but the gold standard is direct immunofluorescence (performed on a skin biopsy), which demonstrates the intercellular IgG in the epidermis, which characterises PV.

Answer to Question 8

D, F

A precipitant is identified in about 50% of patients with chronic urticaria, but IgE-mediated chronic urticaria is a relatively minor cause. It is not associated with internal malignancy, but can rarely be associated with systemic vasculitides although in the vast majority of cases there are no vasculitic changes on biopsy. H1-antagonists can be very helpful and H2-antagonists can help some patients. Most patients with chronic urticaria will have improved within a year, but relapses are not infrequent. For uncomplicated chronic urticaria with no clear clues from the history or examination of systemic disease or an exogenous precipitant, the current UK guidelines (2003) recommend full blood count, ESR and antinuclear antibodies as reasonable screening investigations for those with moderate-severe disease. Non-steroidals are a common cause of exacerbation of urticaria.

Answer to Question 9

E

Rheumatoid arthritis is a risk factor for pyoderma gangrenosum (PG). The anterior shin is an unusual site for venous ulceration and Dopplers are normal, making arterial disease unlikely. PG ulcers are often painful and do not respond to conventional treatment.

PG is associated with pathergy, such that trauma to the ulcer via debridement, or removal of skin at a distant site for grafting, would be contraindicated. PG is diagnosed by exclusion of other causes of ulceration and by its improvement with immunosuppression.

Answer to Question 10

A

The two most common causes of scarring alopecia are lichen planopilaris (lichen planus affecting the scalp hair follicles) and discoid lupus erythematosus. Both conditions cause inflammation and can be difficult to differentiate clinically.

Androgenetic alopecia and alopecia areata are both non-scarring causes of alopecia. Traction alopecia can cause scarring but is not usually associated with inflammation: it occurs at sites of traction and is usually caused by hair styling practices, such as braiding.

Answer to Question 11

B

Polymorphic light eruption is a common photosensitivity disorder that particularly affects young women. The skin shows 'hardening', whereby areas frequently exposed to the sun, such as the face and hands, may not be affected whilst newly exposed sites are most severely affected. The rash often develops after a few days of sun exposure and is most severe at the beginning of the summer.

Systemic lupus erythematosus is a photoaggravated disorder in which the face is usually affected. Photoallergic contact dermatitis can occur due to sunscreen allergy, but a rash would appear at all sites where sunscreen had been applied and subsequently exposed to the sun. Scabies is not photoaggavated. Patients with xeroderma pigmentosum describe easy burning after minimal sun exposure and subsequently develop freckling, chronic solar damage and skin tumours.

Answer to Question 12

A

Rosacea often presents with easy facial flushing before the onset of a pustular rash. Rosacea is often mistaken for acne, but comedones are the clinical hallmark of acne and are absent in rosacea.

Carcinoid syndrome often presents with flushing but is not associated with a pustular rash. SLE can cause erythema of the cheeks but pustules are not seen. Allergic contact dermatitis would most commonly present with a scaly, eczematous rash.

Answer to Question 13

E

Allergic contact dermatitis is a type 4 (delayed) hypersensitivity reaction and is diagnosed by patch testing. Nickel is one of the commonest causes, with an increased frequency in women, probably due to increased exposure to nickel-containing jewellery, particularly through earrings for pierced ears. Men with nickel allergy are more likely to have an occupational cause. Atopic patients are thought to be less prone to developing allergic contact dermatitis (other than to medicaments). Low carat gold often contains significant amounts of nickel. This can be detected by the nickel spot test: dimethylglyoxime rubbed against a metal will turn pink in the presence of nickel.

Answer to Question 14

C

Irritant hand dermatitis classically causes dermatitis in the finger webs, beneath rings and over the dorsum of the hands. It can be caused acutely by contact with strong alkalis or acids, but is usually a chronic problem caused by repeated exposure to detergents and wet work. Atopic patients are more prone to develop irritant dermatitis.

Patch tests demonstrate type IV allergic reactions and are used to diagnose allergic contact dermatitis: they are negative in an irritant dermatitis. Histology is similar in allergic and irritant dermatitis hence the diagnosis of an irritant contact dermatitis is based on the history, clinical signs and negative patch tests. The treatment of irritant and allergic dermatitis is similar and involves avoidance of irritants/allergens, use of soap substitutes, regular emollients and topical steroids.

Answer to Question 15

A

The Koebner phenomenon is the localization of cutaneous disease to sites of trauma and is shown by several disorders including psoriasis, lichen planus, viral warts and vitiligo.

Nail involvement in psoriasis is common and characterized by the presence of 'thimble pitting', onycholysis (separation of the nail from the nail bed) and subungual hyperkeratosis. Chronic plaque psoriasis localising to the extensor surfaces is by far the commonest form. Widespread pustules within lesions or on erythematous skin should raise the possibility of generalized pustular psoriasis, which is a rare but serious complication with a significant mortality. Although pruritus can be feature of psoriasis, it is rarely intense.

The Medical Masterclass series

Scientific Background to Medicine 1

Genetics and Molecular Medicine

1 Nucleic acids and chromosomes
2 Techniques in molecular biology
3 Molecular basis of simple genetic traits
4 More complex issues

Biochemistry and Metabolism

1 Requirement for energy
2 Carbohydrates
3 Fatty acids and lipids
4 Cholesterol and steroid hormones
5 Amino acids and proteins
6 Haem
7 Nucleotides

Cell Biology

1 Ion transport
2 Receptors and intracellular signalling
3 Cell cycle and apoptosis
4 Haematopoiesis

Immunology and Immunosuppression

1 Overview of the immune system
2 The major histocompatibility complex, antigen presentation and transplantation
3 T cells
4 B cells
5 Tolerance and autoimmunity
6 Complement
7 Inflammation
8 Immunosuppressive therapy

Anatomy

1 Heart and major vessels
2 Lungs
3 Liver and biliary tract
4 Spleen
5 Kidney
6 Endocrine glands
7 Gastrointestinal tract
8 Eye
9 Nervous system

Physiology

1 Cardiovascular system
  1.1 The heart as a pump
  1.2 The systemic and pulmonary circulations
  1.3 Blood vessels
  1.4 Endocrine function of the heart
2 Respiratory system
  2.1 The lungs
3 Gastrointestinal system
  3.1 The gut
  3.2 The liver
  3.3 The exocrine pancreas
4 Brain and nerves
  4.1 The action potential
  4.2 Synaptic transmission
  4.3 Neuromuscular transmission
5 Endocrine physiology
6 Renal physiology
  6.1 Blood flow and glomerular filtration
  6.2 Function of the renal tubules
  6.3 Endocrine function of the kidney

Scientific Background to Medicine 2

Statistics, Epidemiology, Clinical Trials, Meta-analyses and Evidence-based Medicine

1 Statistics
2 Epidemiology
  2.1 Observational studies
3 Clinical trials and meta-analyses
4 Evidence-based medicine

Clinical Pharmacology

1 Introducing clinical pharmacology
  1.1 Preconceived notions versus evidence
  1.2 Drug interactions and safe prescribing
2 Pharmacokinetics
  2.1 Introduction
  2.2 Drug absorption
  2.3 Drug distribution
  2.4 Drug metabolism
  2.5 Drug elimination
  2.6 Plasma half-life and steady-state plasma concentrations
  2.7 Drug monitoring
3 Pharmacodynamics
  3.1 How drugs exert their effects
  3.2 Selectivity is the key to the therapeutic utility of an agent
  3.3 Basic aspects of a drug's interaction with its target
  3.4 Heterogeneity of drug responses, pharmacogenetics and pharmacogenomics
4 Adverse drug reactions
  4.1 Introduction
  4.2 Definition and classification of adverse drug reactions
  4.3 Dose-related adverse drug reactions

Clinical Skills

General Clinical Issues

Pain Relief and Palliative Care

Medicine for the Elderly

Emergency Medicine

Infectious Diseases and Dermatology

Infectious Diseases

Dermatology

Haematology and Oncology

Haematology

Oncology

Cardiology and Respiratory Medicine

Cardiology

Respiratory Medicine

Gastroenterology and Hepatology

Neurology, Ophthalmology and Psychiatry

Neurology

Ophthalmology

Psychiatry

Endocrinology

Nephrology

Rheumatology and Clinical Immunology

Index

Note: page numbers in *italics* refer to figures, those in **bold** refer to tables.